Kostoris

R026

D1757281

8

2r

IARC Handbooks of Cancer Prevention

Volume 9

Cruciferous Vegetables, Isothiocyanates and Indoles

THIS BOOK BELONGS TO:
Medical Library
Christie Hospital NHS Trust
Manchester
M20 4BX
Phone: 0161 446 3452

WORLD HEALTH ORGANIZATION

INTERNATIONAL AGENCY FOR RESEARCH ON CANCER

IARC Handbooks of Cancer Prevention

Volume 9

Cruciferous Vegetables, Isothiocyanates and Indoles

IARCPress

Lyon, 2004

Published by the International Agency for Research on Cancer,
150 cours Albert Thomas, F-69372 Lyon Cedex 08, France

© International Agency for Research on Cancer, 2004

Distributed by Oxford University Press, Walton Street, Oxford, OX2 6DP, UK (Fax: +44 1865 267782) and in the USA by Oxford
University Press, 2001 Evans Road, Carey, NC 27513, USA (Fax: +1 919 677 1303).
All IARC publications can also be ordered directly from IARC*Press*
(Fax: +33 4 72 73 83 02; E-mail: press@iarc.fr)
and in the USA from IARC*Press*, WHO Office, Suite 480, 1775 K Street, Washington DC, 20006

Publications of the World Health Organization enjoy copyright protection in
accordance with the provisions of Protocol 2 of the Universal Copyright Convention.
All rights reserved.

The designations used and the presentation of the material in this publication do not imply the
expression of any opinion whatsoever on the part of the Secretariat of the World Health Organization
concerning the legal status of any country, territory, city, or area or of its authorities,
or concerning the delimitation of its frontiers or boundaries.

The mention of specific companies or of certain manufacturers' products does not imply
that they are endorsed or recommended by the World Health Organization in preference to others
of a similar nature that are not mentioned. Errors and omissions excepted,
the names of proprietary products are distinguished by initial capital letters.

The authors alone are responsible for the views expressed in this publication.

The International Agency for Research on Cancer welcomes requests for permission to
reproduce or translate its publications, in part or in full. Applications and enquiries should be addressed
to the Communications Unit, International Agency for Research on Cancer,
which will be glad to provide the latest information on any changes made to the text, plans for new
editions, and reprints and translations already available.

IARC Library Cataloguing in Publication Data

Cruciferous vegetabes, isothiocyanates and indoles / IARC Working Group on the
  Evaluation of Cancer Preventive Strategies (2003 : Lyon, France)

(IARC Handbooks of Cancer Prevention ; 9)

1. Brassica. 2. Indoles 3. Isothiocyanates 4. Neoplasms - prevention & control
I. IARC Working Group on the Evaluation of Cancer Preventive Strategies.

ISBN   92 832 3009 4   (NLM Classification: QZ39)
ISSN   1027 - 5622

Printed in France

International Agency For Research On Cancer

The International Agency for Research on Cancer (IARC) was established in 1965 by the World Health Assembly, as an independently financed organization within the framework of the World Health Organization. The headquarters of the Agency are in Lyon, France.

The Agency conducts a programme of research concentrating particularly on the epidemiology of cancer and the study of potential carcinogens in the human environment. Its field studies are supplemented by biological and chemical research carried out in the Agency's laboratories in Lyon and, through collaborative research agreements, in national research institutions in many countries. The Agency also conducts a programme for the education and training of personnel for cancer research.

The publications of the Agency contribute to the dissemination of authoritative information on different aspects of cancer research. Information about IARC publications, and how to order them, is available via the Internet at: http://www.iarc.fr/

This publication represents the views and opinions of an IARC Working Group on the Evaluation of Cancer Preventive Strategies which met in Lyon, France, 18–24 November 2003

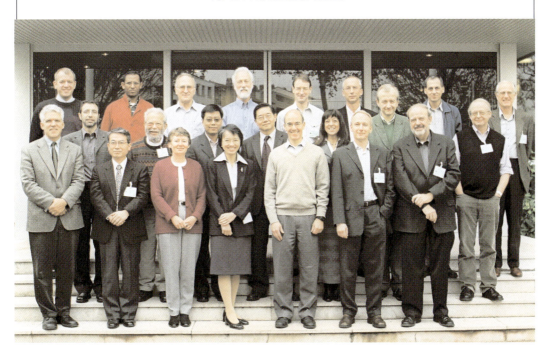

From left to right:
Front: T. Byers; A. Nishikawa; M. Manson; A. Seow; S. Hecht, L. Dragsted; G. Stoner
Middle: A. Agudo, L. Bradlow; Y. Zhang; F.L. Chung; E. Taioli; J. Thornalley, I. Johnson
Back: O. Vang, F. Kassie; H. Schut, G. Bailey; J. Hayes, S. Loft, R. Mithen, A. Miller

Note to the Reader

Anyone who is aware of published data that may influence any consideration in these *Handbooks* is encouraged to make the information available to the Unit of Chemoprevention, International Agency for Research on Cancer, 150 Cours Albert Thomas, 69372 Lyon Cedex 08, France

Although all efforts are made to prepare the *Handbooks* as accurately as possible, mistakes may occur. Readers are requested to communicate any errors to the Unit of Chemoprevention, so that corrections can be reported in future volumes.

Acknowledgements

We would like to acknowledge generous support from the Foundation for Promotion of Cancer Research, Japan (the 2nd Term Comprehensive 10-Year Strategy for Cancer Control), and from the World Cancer Research Fund, London, United Kingdom (WCRF Grant 2001/45).

Contents

List of participants

A. Agudo
Department of Epidemiology
Catalan Institute of Oncology
Av. Gran Via s/n km 2.7
08907 L'Hospitalet de Llobregat
Spain

G.S. Bailey
MFBS Center
Department of Environment and
Molecular Toxicology
Oregon State University
435 Weniger Hall
Corvallis, OR 97331
USA

H.L. Bradlow
David and Alice Jurist Institute for
Research
Hackensack University Medical
Center
30 Prospect Avenue
Hackensack, NJ 07601
USA

T. Byers (Chairman)
Department of Preventive Medicine &
Biometrics
University of Colorado School of
Medicine
Box C245
4200 East Ninth Avenue
Denver CO 80262
USA

F.-L. Chung
Division of Carcinogenesis &
Molecular Epidemiology
Institute for Cancer Prevention
American Health Foundation
Valhalla, NY 10595
USA

L.O. Dragsted
Institute of Food Safety and Nutrition
Danish Veterinary & Food
Administration
19 Morkjoj Bygade
2860 Søborg
Denmark

J. Hayes
University of Dundee
Biomedical Research Centre Level 5
Ninewells Hospital & Medical School
Dundee DD1 9SY
Scotland
United Kingdom

S.S. Hecht
University of Minnesota Cancer
Center
Mayo Mail Code 806
420 Delaware St, SE
Minneapolis, MN 55455
USA

I.T. Johnson
Institute of Food Research
Norwich Research Park
Colney
Norwich NR4 7UA
England
United Kingdom

F. Kassie
Institute of Indoor & Environmental
Toxicology
University of Giessen
Aulweg 123
35385 Giessen
Germany

S. Loft
The Panum Institute of Public Health
University of Copenhagen
Blegdamsvej 3
2200 Copenhagen N
Denmark

M.M. Manson
Cancer Biomarkers and Prevention
Group
Biocentre
University of Leicester
University Road
Leicester LE1 7RH
England
United Kingdom

A.B. Miller
Department of Public Health
Sciences
University of Toronto
Box 992
Niagara on the Lake
Ontario LOS 1JO
Canada

R. Mithen
Institute of Food Research
Norwich Research Park
Colney
Norwich NR4 7UA
England
United Kingdom

A. Nishikawa
National Institute of Health Sciences
Division of Pathology
1-18-1 Kamiyoga
Setagaya-ku
Tokyo 158-8501
Japan

H.A.J. Schut
Department of Pathology
HEB 202
Medical College of Ohio
3055 Arlington Avenue
Toledo, OH 43614-5806
USA

A. Seow
Faculty of Medicine
National University of Singapore
16 Medical Drive MD3
Singapore 117597

G. Stoner
School of Public Health
Ohio State University
1148 CHRI
300 W. 10th Avenue
Columbus, OH 43210-1240
USA

E. Taioli
Unit of Molecular and Genetic
Epidemiology
Ospedale Policlinico IRCCS
Padiglione Marangoni
Via F. Sforza 35
20122 Milano
Italy

J.P. Thornalley
Department of Biological Sciences
University of Essex
Central Campus
Wivenhoe Park
Colchester
Essex C04 3SQ
England
United Kingdom

O. Vang
Roskilde University
Department of Life Sciences &
Chemistry
Bldg 18-1
PO Box 260 – Universitetsvej 1
4000 Roskilde
Denmark

Y. Zhang
Roswell Park Cancer Institute
Department of Cancer
Chemoprevention
Basic Science 711
Elm and Carlton Streets
Buffalo, NY 14263
USA

Observers

**World Cancer Research Fund
International**

E. Stone
International Research Manager
World Cancer Research Fund
International
First Floor
19 Harley Street
London W1G 9QU
England
United Kingdom

WHO

I. Keller
Noncommunicable Diseases and
Mental Health
Nutrition and NCD Prevention
World Health Organization
CH-1211 Geneva 27
Switzerland

Secretariat

W. Al-Delaimy
F. Bianchini (co-responsible officer)
P. Brennan
V. Cogliano
M. Friesen
Y. Grosse
J. Hall
E. Heseltine (Editor)
C. Malaveille
H. Ohshima
T. Sawa
B. Secretan
N. Slimani
K. Straif
H. Vainio (Head of programme, co-responsible officer)

Post-meeting scientific assistance

F. Bianchini
H. Vainio

Technical assistance

J. Mitchell
A. Rivoire
J. Thévenoux

Preface

Why a Handbook on cruciferous vegetables, isothiocyanates and indoles

Nutritional epidemiology provides the only direct approach to the assessment of the health effects of the human diet. During the past 10 years, various study designs and sophisticated methods have been used to establish relationships between dietary habits and risks for noncommunicable diseases, including cancer. In the light of reports that fruit and vegetables are important dietary components for reducing the risks for various cancers, IARC considered it important to evaluate the current evidence on the health effects of a diet rich in fruit and vegetables.

Volume 8 of the *IARC Handbooks of Cancer Prevention* confirmed that a high consumption of fruit and vegetables is associated with lower risks for cancer at several sites. More specifically, the final evaluation stated that consumption of fruit probably lowers

the risks for cancers of the oesophagus, stomach and lung, while consumption of vegetables probably lowers the risks for cancers of the oesophagus and colorectum. Various fruit and vegetables have been investigated separately, to identify the most effective cancer preventing groups and active ingredients. Cruciferous vegetables have been considered good candidates.

Consumption of cruciferous vegetables, such as broccoli, cabbage, cauliflower, watercress and Brussels sprouts, was shown to be associated with decreased risks for cancer in epidemiological studies In the 1980s. These vegetables contain substantial amounts of glucosinolates, which are hydrolysed to isothiocyanates and indoles when normal portions of these raw vegetables are chewed or otherwise macerated. Experimental studies

have shown that these compounds inhibit carcinogenesis, and plausible mechanisms of action have been investigated extensively.

This *Handbook* provides an up-to-date review of knowledge on the efficacy of cruciferous vegetables and naturally occurring isothiocyanates and indoles as chemopreventive agents. Data from human, experimental and mechanistic studies are reviewed. In the epidemiological studies, cancer risk was examined in relation to consumption of cruciferous vegetables, which was assessed either from food frequency questionnaires or by measuring markers of cruciferous vege-table intake. In some recent studies of intake, individuals were stratified on the basis of genetic polymorphisms.

The volume also provides recommendations for future research and public health action.

Chapter 1

Cruciferous vegetables

Botanical classification

From the botanical point of view, the term 'vegetable' broadly refers to any plant, whether edible or not (IARC, 2003). In common language, however, it applies to one of the main groups of edible plant foods apart from fruit and cereals. Specific types of vegetables, such as tubers, legumes and pulses, are often considered separately. In epidemiological studies, vegetables are further classified into subgroups, mainly on the basis of their content of nutrients or bioactive compounds. Cultural and culinary groupings are often used in household and nutritional surveys, for reporting food supply and food consumption, as well as in dietary assessments.

The botanical classification of vegetables is based on the structure, organization and physiological characteristics of plants. Cruciferous vegetables belong to the botanical family Brassicaceae, order Capparales (National Resources Conservation Services, 2003). Within this order, there are 16 families, all of which contain glucosinolates; some of these are minor vegetable crops (Mithen, 2001).

Brassicaceae is a large family, with about 3000 species in 350 genera, including several types of edible plants. It was formerly known as Cruciferae or Cruciferaceae, and is sometimes referred to as 'the cabbage family' or 'the mustard family', after the names of some of its components. The

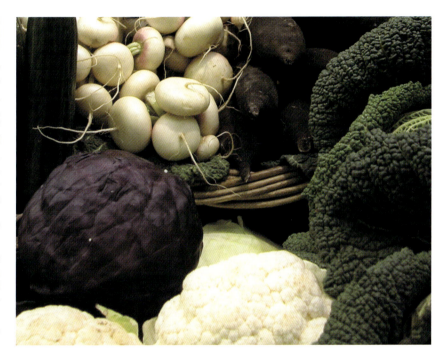

petals of plants of this family have a distinctive cruciform arrangement, which is the origin of the terms 'Cruciferae' and 'cruciferous'. These plants can be annuals, biennials or perennials. They are well adapted to average temperatures of 16–18 °C and are thus grown during the cool season in temperate areas. Crops of Brassicaceae are distributed mainly in temperate regions of the Northern Hemisphere: in areas of Southwest and Central Asia, China and Japan, Europe, the Mediterranean region and North America.

Despite the great diversity among the Brassicaceae, members of only a few genera are eaten. The most commonly eaten cruciferous vegetables belong to the genus *Brassica,* and many belong to several varieties of the species *B. oleracea,* including cabbage, cauliflower, broccoli and Brussels sprouts. Other edible species in the genus *Brassica* are *B. rapa* and *B. napus,* which include, respectively, Chinese cabbage and rape. Other cruciferous vegetables used in the human diet, such as radish and cress, belong to other genera of the Brassicaceae family. A list of the main cruciferous

Table 1. Main cruciferous vegetables in the human diet: Scientific and common names

Genus	Species and variety	Common name
Brassica	*B. oleracea* var. *botrytis*	Cauliflower
	B. oleracea var. *capitata*	Cabbage, white cabbage
	B. oleracea var. *costata*	Portuguese cabbage
	B. oleracea var. *gemmifera*	Brussels sprouts
	B. oleracea var. *gongyloides*	Kohlrabi, turnip cabbage, stem turnip
	B. oleracea var. *italica*	Broccoli
	B. oleracea var. *rubra*	Red cabbage
	B. oleracea var. *sabauda*	Savoy cabbage
	B. oleracea var. *sabellica*	Curly kale
	B. oleracea var. *viridis*	Kale, collards
	B. oleracea var. *alboglabra*	*Kai lan,* Chinese kale
Brassica	*B. rapa* var. *chinensis*	Chinese cabbage, *pak-choi, bok choi*
	B. rapa var. *oleifera*	Turnip rape
	B. rapa var. *pekinensis*	Chinese cabbage, *pe-tsai,* Napa cabbage, celery, cabbage
	B. rapa var. *rapa*	Turnip
	B. rapa var. *parachinensis*	*Choi sum*
Brassica	*B. napus* var. *napobrassica*	Swede, Swedish turnip, rutabaga
	B. napus var. *oleifera*	Rape, canola, colza
Brassica	*B. alba*	White mustard
	B. juncea	Indian mustard, brown mustard, spinach mustard
	B. juncea var. *rugosa*	*Kai choi*
	B. nigra	Black mustard
Raphanus	*R. sativus*	Radish
Armoracia	*A. rusticana*	Horseradish
Nasturtium	*N. officinalis*	Watercress
Lepidium	*L. sativum*	Cress, garden cress
Eruca	*E. vesicaria*	Arugula, rocket, Italian cress
Wasabia	*W. japonica*	Wasabi
Beta	*B. vulgaris flavescens*	Swiss chard
Crambe	*C. abyssinica*	Crambe

vegetables with their botanical classification is given in Table 1 (National Resources Conservation Services, 2003).

Estimated intake by region and country

Methods used

Consumption of cruciferous vegetables in several countries and world regions was assessed from published data. To ensure that the information was up-to-date and took into account any time trends in intake, only papers published in 1993 or later were included; when two or more papers reported data on the same population or study, the most recent one was used. A review based on data that were originally published before 1993 was therefore also used. The two main criteria for including a paper were that intake of cruciferous vegetables was explicitly reported or could be easily estimated from the data, and that the population to which the consumption applied was clearly identified. Furthermore, the search was restricted to adult populations. The results and the main features of the studies included are summarized in Table 2.

Various methods are used for estimating food intake, as reviewed in the *Handbooks of Cancer Prevention* on fruit and vegetables (IARC, 2003). Usually, data on dietary intake are derived from dietary surveys of representative populations. In most of these studies, however, data on energy and nutrient intake and on the consumption of main food groups are reported, while individual food consumption or the intake of specific subgroups is not.

Table 2. Estimated intakes of cruciferous vegetables by control subjects in epidemiological studies

Reference	Country	Sex	Age (years)	Type of study and no. of controls	Diet information method	Cruciferous vegetables included	Mean or median	Intake (g/day)	Proportion of all vegetable intake (%)
Asia									
Bosetti et al. (2002)	Japan	M, W	NR	CC, 365	FFQ	Broccoli, cabbage, radish, turnip, mustard greens	Mean	83.5	21.2
Memon et al. (2002)	Kuwait	M, W	≤ 70	CC, 311	FFQ, 13 items	Broccoli, Brussels sprouts, cabbage, cauliflower	Median	59.8	NR
National Institute of Health & Nutrition (2002)	Japan	M, W	30–70	Survey, no. not given	Household food intake	Cabbage, Chinese cabbage, Japanese radish	Mean	59.8	8.1
Seow et al. (2002a)	Singapore	M, W	45–74	CC, 1194	Semi-quantitative FFQ, 165 items	Chinese white cabbage, Chinese mustard, Chinese flowering cabbage, water-cress, Chinese kale, head cabbage, celery cabbage, broccoli, cauliflower	Mean	W: 43.4 M: 42.1	NR
Shannon et al. (2002)	Thailand	W	30–60	CC, 509	FFQ, 80 items	Cruciferous, unspecified	Median	46.3	NR
Chiu et al. (2003)	Shanghai, China	M, W	30–74	CC, 1552	FFQ, 86 items	Bok choi, cabbage, Chinese cabbage, cauliflower	Median	W: 102.4 M: 101.8	W: 24.4 M: 24.2
Rajkumar et al. (2003)	Southern India	M, W	18–80	CC, 582	FFQ, 21 items	Cruciferous, unspecified	Median	17.1	15
North America									
Lin et al. (1998)	Southern California, USA	M, W	50–74	CC, 507	Semi-quantitative FFQ, 126 items	Broccoli, Brussels sprouts, cabbage kale, coleslaw, cauliflower, mustard, chard greens	Mean	40	11.7
Yuan et al. (1998)	Los Angeles, USA	M, W	25–75	CC, 1204	FFQ, 90 items	Broccoli, cabbage, coleslaw, Brussels sprouts, collard, kale, mustard, turnip greens	Median	29.7	NR

Table 2 (contd)

Reference	Country	Sex	Age (years)	Type of study and no. of controls	Diet information method	Cruciferous vegetables included	Mean or median	Intake (g/day)	Proportion of all vegetable intake (%)
Cohen *et al.* (2000)	Seattle, USA	M	40–64	CC, 602	FFQ, 99 items	Broccoli, coleslaw, cabbage, sauerkraut, Brussels sprouts, cauliflower	Geometric mean	20.5	9.6
Feskanich *et al.* (2000)	Boston, USA	M, W	W: 30–55 M: 40–75	Prospective: W: 77 283 M: 47 778	Semi-quantitative FFQ, 116 items (W), 131 items (M)	Broccoli, cabbage coleslaw, sauerkraut, cauliflower, Brussels sprouts, kale, mustard, chard greens	Median	32.0	14.3
Johnston *et al.* (2000)	USA	M, W	25–75	Survey, 4806	Two non-consecutive 24-h recalls	Broccoli, cauliflower, kale Brussels sprouts	Mean	16	5.6
Kolonel *et al.* (2000)	Canada & USA	M	65–84	CC, 1618	Diet history	Broccoli, Brussels sprouts, green mustard cabbage, head cabbage, mustard greens, *pak-choi*, red cabbage, turnip greens, watercress, *won bok*	Median	29	15.4
Slattery *et al.* (2000)	USA, several areas	M, W	> 55	CC, 1989	Diet history	Broccoli, Brussels sprouts, cauliflower, cabbage, coleslaw, greens, turnip, rutabaga	Mean	30.8	
Smith-Warner *et al.* (2000)	Minnesota, USA	M, W	30–74	Randomized controlled trial, 101	Diet records	Cruciferous, unspecified	Mean	26.4	8.9
Spitz *et al.* (2000)	Texas, USA	M, W	60.9 (mean)	CC, 465	Semi-quantitative FFQ, 135 items	Broccoli, cauliflower, Brussels sprouts, coleslaw, cabbage, sauerkraut, mustard greens, turnip greens, collard greens, kale	Mean	29.1	NR
Lanza *et al.* (2001)	USA	M, W	35–89	Intervention, 1042	FFQ & 4-day food records	Cruciferous, unspecified	Mean	23.6	8.9

Table 2 (contd)

Reference	Country	Sex	Age (years)	Type of study and no. of controls	Diet information method	Cruciferous vegetables included	Mean or median	Intake (g/day)	Proportion of all vegetable intake (%)
Bosetti et al. (2002)	Hawaii, USA	M, W	NR	CC, 441	FFQ	Broccoli, cabbage, Chinese cabbage, cauliflower, Brussels sprouts, turnip, rutabaga, mustard cabbage, Swiss chard	Mean	33.2	14.8
	Connecticut, USA	M, W	NR	CC, 184	FFQ	Brussels sprouts, broccoli, cabbage	Mean	28.5	NR
Smith-Warner et al. (2002)	Minnesota, USA	M, W	30–74	CC, 1237	Semi-quantitative FFQ, 153 items	Broccoli, cabbage, cauliflower	Mean	W: 38.8 M: 27.5	W: 12.6 M: 10.3
Cerhan et al. (2003)	Iowa, USA	W	55–69	Prospective, 29 368	Semi-quantitative FFQ, 127 items	Cabbage, cauliflower, broccoli	Median	27.5	12.1
South America Pacin et al. (1999)	Argentina	M, W	18–50	Survey, 449 W, 378 M	24-h recall	Broccoli	Mean	W: 2.43	NR
Atalah et al. (2001)	Chile	M, W	> 20	CC, 1066 W, 547 M	FFQ, 58 items	Cabbage, cauliflower, broccoli, Brussels sprouts	Median	W: 11.1 M: 14.3	W: 5.0 M: 6.6
Australia Nagle et al. (2003)	Australia	W	18–79	CC, 609 cases	Semi-quantitative FFQ, 119 items	Broccoli, cauliflower, cabbage coleslaw, Brussels sprouts	Median	49.6	13.1
Europe Bosetti et al. (2002)	Sweden	M, W	NR	CC, 252	FFQ	Cabbage, broccoli, Brussels sprouts, cauliflower	Mean	11.5	14.7
	Norway	M, W	NR	CC, 173	FFQ	Cabbage, broccoli, Brussels sprouts, cauliflower	Mean	17.2	23.1
	Italy	M, W	NR	CC, 617	FFQ	Cruciferous, unspecified	Mean	11.5	6.9
	Switzerland	M, W	NR	CC, 412	FFQ	Cruciferous, unspecified	Mean	11.5	6.7
	Greece	M, W	NR	CC, 140	NR	Broccoli, cauliflower	Mean	5.7	7.8

Table 2 (contd)

Reference	Country	Sex	Age (years)	Type of study and no. of controls	Diet infor- mation method	Cruciferous vegetables included	Mean or median	Intake (g/day)	Proportion of all vegetable intake (%)
Terry et al. (2002)	Sweden	W	50–74	CC, 2887	FFQ	Cabbage, Chinese cabbage, broccoli, cauli- flower	Median	28.5	NR
Michaud et al. (2002)	Finland	M	50–69	Prospective, 27 111	FFQ, 276 items	Broccoli, cauli- flower, cabbage, Brussels sprouts, rutabaga	Median	9.7	9.8
Voorrips et al. (2000a)	Nether- lands	M, W	55–69	Prospective, 1497 W, 1456 M	Semi- quanti- tative FFQ, 150 items	Brussels sprouts, kale, cauliflower	Mean	W: 31.6 M: 32.7	W: 16.5 M: 17.5
Africa									
Steyn et al. (2003)	South Africa	M, W	≥ 10	National food survey, no. not given	FFQ, 24-h recall	Brassica	Mean	15.0	16.5

M, men; W, women; CC, case–control study; FFQ, food frequency questionnaire; NR, not reported

Most of the data in this Handbook come from analytical studies of the effects of intake of cruciferous vegetables on several disease outcomes; these are mainly case–control studies, with some intervention studies. From these studies, data for the controls or the reference group were used. In prospective or intervention studies, estimates are made from information collected at baseline. It should be borne in mind that the results are for specific populations and are not nec- essarily representative of the country in which the study was conducted.

In this Handbook, intake of cruciferous vegetables is always expressed in grams per day, as the mean or the median of consumption, depending on how it was reported in the original work or on the data avail- able. Intake of cruciferous vegetables was estimated directly in grams in a few cases, but usually it was reported in servings per day or per week. Except when the authors explicitly stated the portion size assigned to a serving, it was assumed that a stan- dard serving of vegetables corre- sponds to 80 g (Williams, 1995; Department of Health and Human Services, 2000). Usually, consumption of cruciferous vegetables was report- ed for both sexes together; when the data were available, separate estimates are given for men and women. In addition to the absolute amount, the consumption of crucifer- ous vegetables is given as the propor- tion of total vegetable intake, when the information was available for such a calculation.

In order to improve the inter- pretability of the results, the following data were reported: place, sex and age of the population studied, type and size of study, method used to assess intake of cruciferous vegeta- bles and the individual foods consid- ered within the group 'cruciferous vegetables'.

Various countries and regions

In the studies that were reviewed (Table 2), the highest intake of crucifer- ous vegetables was reported to be that of people in Shanghai, China, who consumed more than 100 g/day, repre- senting about one-fourth of their total vegetable intake (Chiu et al., 2003). Other Asian and some Middle Eastern populations (in Japan, Singapore and Thailand and Kuwait) had relatively high intakes of cruciferous vegetables, ranging from 40 to 80 g per day (Bosetti et al., 2002; Memon et al., 2002; National Institute of Health and Nutrition, 2002; Seow et al., 2002a; Shannon et al., 2002); the only study carried out in India (Rajkumar et al., 2003) showed a lower daily intake, of about 17 g. Studies in China (Chiu et al., 2003) and Singapore (Seow et al., 2002a) that gave separate estimates for men and women, showed similar intake by sex.

Studies of cruciferous vegetable intake in North America covered a variety of populations (Table 2). Overall, the daily estimated consumption was about 25–30 g, with a range of 16–40 g, representing 5–15% of total vegetable intake. Although most of the studies included both men and women, only one gave separate results, showing higher consumption by women (38.8 g per day) than by men (27.5 g per day). Two studies in South America showed low consumption of cruciferous vegetables, with 2.4 g per day for women in Argentina (Pacin et al., 1999) and 14 g per day for men and 11 g per day for women in Chile (Atalah et al., 2001).

The only study with data for Australia was a case–control study of women with ovarian cancer (Nagle et al., 2003), who were reported to have a consumption of 49.6 g per day, comparable to the intake observed in most Asian countries.

In Europe, the lowest intake of cruciferous vegetables was reported for Greece, at 5.7 g per day (Bosetti et al., 2002), whereas the estimates for Finland, Italy, Norway, Sweden and Switzerland were between 10 and 30 g per day (Bosetti et al., 2002; Terry et al., 2002). The results of two prospective studies in which information on diet was based on answers to extensive, detailed questionnaires showed an estimated intake of 9.7 g per day in Finland (Michaud et al., 2002) and a daily consumption of 32.7 g by men and 31.6 g by women in The Netherlands (Voorrips et al., 2000a).

In one study performed in South Africa, the combined results of several surveys among adults showed a mean consumption of Brassica vegetables of 15 g per day (Steyn et al., 2003).

European countries

The European Prospective Investigation into Cancer and Nutrition (the EPIC study) is a multicentre prospective study being carried out in 27 centres in 10 countries of Europe (Riboli et al., 2002). Information on intake of cruciferous vegetables, obtained from a 24-h dietary recall interview, is available for a subset of 35 644 persons, about one-third of whom were men (36%) and two-thirds women (64%) with mean ages of 57 and 55 years, respectively. The participants were interviewed during 1 year between 1995 and 2000, on any day of the week. The quality of the instrument and the logistics of the study resulted in valid, reliable and comparable data on dietary consumption across countries. Further details about the study and the participants have been given elsewhere (Slimani et al., 2002). The results presented below were derived from an extension of analyses previously reported for all vegetables (Agudo et al., 2002). Although most of the participants represented the general population, the estimates given below cannot be considered to reflect intake in a particular country.

Geographical pattern

The average daily consumption of cruciferous vegetables by the participants in each country is shown in Table 3. Overall, intake was about 21 g per day. Consumption by country varied markedly: intake in the United Kingdom was reported to be about three times that in Spain, which had the lowest intake. Three groups of countries can be distinguished: participants in Germany, Norway and the United Kingdom ate more than 30 g per day; those in France and The Netherlands ate between 20 and 30 g daily; and those in Denmark, Greece, Italy, Spain

and Sweden ate between 10 and 20 g per day. The pattern was consistent for individual centres and countries as a whole (results not shown).

This geographical pattern is quite different from that of consumption of all vegetables, which shows a clear south–north gradient (Agudo et al., 2002): consumption of cruciferous vegetables is high in countries of central Europe and Great Britain, while the lowest intake is seen in countries of southern Europe, with intermediate intake in France. The Scandinavian countries show differences in consumption, with a high intake in Norway and an intake in Sweden similar to that in southern countries. The discrepancy between intake of cruciferous and of all vegetables is even clearer when expressed as a proportion: about 13% of all vegetables eaten are of the cruciferous type, but cruciferous vegetables constitute more than 20% of total vegetable intake in countries with high consumption and account for only 5–10% in countries with low consumption.

Overall, about 80% of all cruciferous vegetables are eaten cooked by both men and women. Raw preparations represent 30–40% of cruciferous vegetable intake in Greece, Norway and Sweden and less than 10% in other countries (Figure 1). This pattern does not, however, appear to be related to the amount consumed but to the way all vegetables are eaten, and thus to the eating habits in each country.

Cruciferous vegetables eaten

Table 4 shows the contributions of individual cruciferous vegetables to total consumption. Of the 21 items reported, cauliflower was the most commonly consumed variety, accounting for 25% of the total; 'cabbage', comprising white cabbage, the commonest variety, plus unspecified cabbage, accounted for another 25%, and broccoli accounted for 18%. These three

Table 3. Consumption of cruciferous vegetables by participants in the EPIC study

Country	No. of participants	Intake (g/day)		
		Mean	Standard error	Proportion of total vegetable intake (%)
Denmark	3918	18.9	0.9	13
France[a]	4639	23.5	0.8	11
Germany	4418	30.2	0.9	18
Greece	2686	13.4	1.1	6
Italy	3956	18.4	0.9	9
Netherlands	3984	26.8	0.9	20
Norway[a]	1798	32.2	1.4	26
Spain	3220	12.0	1.0	6
Sweden	6050	15.8	0.8	13
United Kingdom	975	34.4	1.9	21

Means and standard errors adjusted by age, day of the week, season and sex when the two were combined
[a] Only women

Table 4. Consumption of cruciferous vegetables by participants in the EPIC study, as a proportion of total vegetable intake

Cruciferous vegetable	Proportion of all vegetables	
	%	Cumulative %
Cauliflower (including romanesco)	25	25
Broccoli	18	43
White cabbage	13	56
Cabbage, unspecified	12	68
Radish	6	74
Brussels sprouts	6	80
Red cabbage	5	84
Swede, Swedish turnip, rutabaga	4	88
Turnip	3	91
Other (12 items)	9	100

Only cruciferous vegetables accounting for at least 90% of total consumption are listed.

represented more than two-thirds of all cruciferous vegetables eaten.

Most of the cruciferous vegetables (90%) eaten by participants in the EPIC study belonged to the genus *Brassica*; cruciferous vegetables belonging to other genera accounted for more than 10% (22.3%) of intake only in France (Figure 2). Within the genus *Brassica*, several varieties and subspecies of the species *B. oleracea* (including cauliflower, cabbage and broccoli) predominated in most European countries.

Two or three commonly eaten cruciferous vegetables accounted for one-half of total intake, and six or fewer accounted for about 90%. In countries with the lowest absolute intake, there was also less variety in the vegetables eaten: only eight items were reported to be eaten in Greece and Spain, and only four accounted for more than 90% of total consumption. France was the only country where a frequently eaten cruciferous vegetable did not belong to the genus *Brassica*: radish (*Raphanus sativus*) accounted for 19% and ranked second. In Norway, the most commonly eaten cruciferous vegetable was rutabaga (*B. napus* var. *napobrassica*), which accounted for 27% of total intake, and this the only country where the most commonly consumed cruciferous vegetable was not a variety of *B. oleracea*.

Intake by sex, age and smoking habit
Table 5 shows the intake of cruciferous vegetables according to sex, age and smoking habits in the EPIC study. All the means were adjusted by day of the week, season and centre. No difference in cruciferous vegetable intake was found between men and women. Differences in consumption were seen by age but might reflect differences in recruitment among countries. Current smokers ate an average of 20 g per day of cruciferous vegetables, while former smokers and lifelong non-smokers ate 21 g per day. Nevertheless, the overall differences by smoking status did not reach statistical significance.

Production

Information on the production of cruciferous vegetables between 1961 and 2000 in selected regions of the world is shown in Figure 3. Total production (3a) and production per capita (3b) show similar trends. The highest

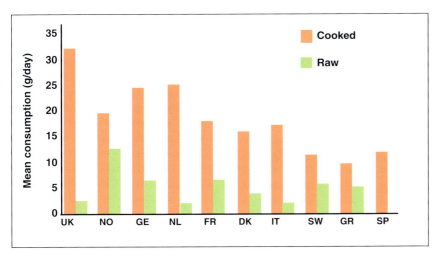

Figure 1 Mean consumption of cruciferous vegetables, cooked and raw, by participants in 10 countries in the EPIC study

UK, United Kingdom; NO, Norway; GE, Germany; NL, Netherlands; FR, France; DK, Denmark; IT, Italy; SW, Sweden; GR, Greece; SP, Spain

production volume was in eastern Europe, with little variation over time. A decreasing trend in production was seen in some regions over time, from 18% to 9% in western Europe and from 22% to 9% in Australia and New Zealand. The production volume in South and South-East Asia increased from about 10% in 1961 to 15% in 1980 and then fell to 10% in 2000. In Canada and the USA, cruciferous vegetables accounted for about 7% of all vegetable production. Per capita production changed little over time, except in western Europe, where it decreased from 20 to 13 kg per person per year, and in East and South-East Asia, where it increased from 7 to 19 kg per person per year.

Table 5. Consumption of cruciferous vegetables by participants in the EPIC study, by sex, age and smoking habit

	No. of participants	Mean consumption (g/day)
Sex		
Men	12 917	20.8
Women	22 727	21.4
Age (years)		
35–44	3 302	18.7
45–54	12 431	20.3
55–64	14 799	22.5
65–74	5 102	21.2
Smoking status		
Never	17 160	21.3
Former	10 138	21.5
Current	7 668	20.3

Intake adjusted by centre, day of the week and season and by age and sex for smoking status

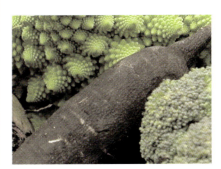

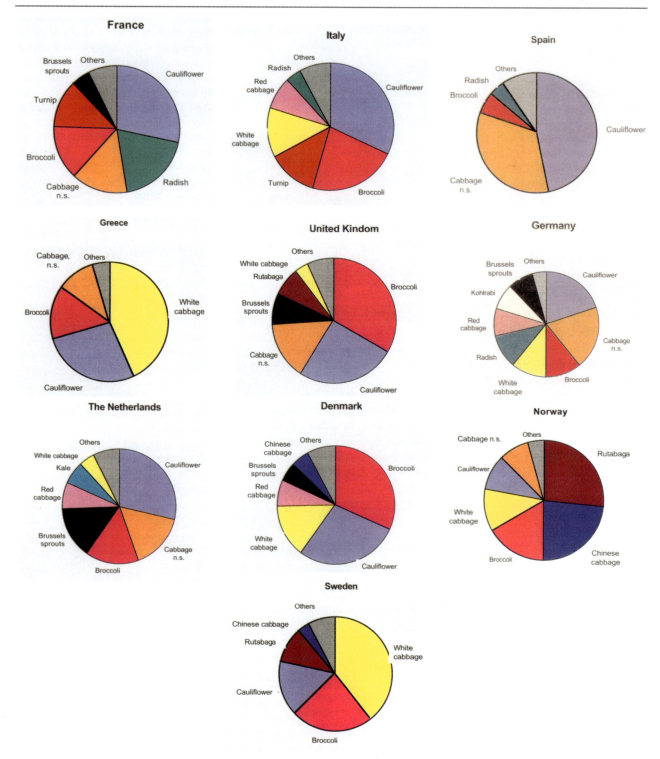

Figure 2 Consumption of cruciferous vegetables by participants in the EPIC study, as a proportion of consumption of all vegetables
Only women in France and Norway. Proportions for the United Kingdom exclude vegetarians. n.s., not specified

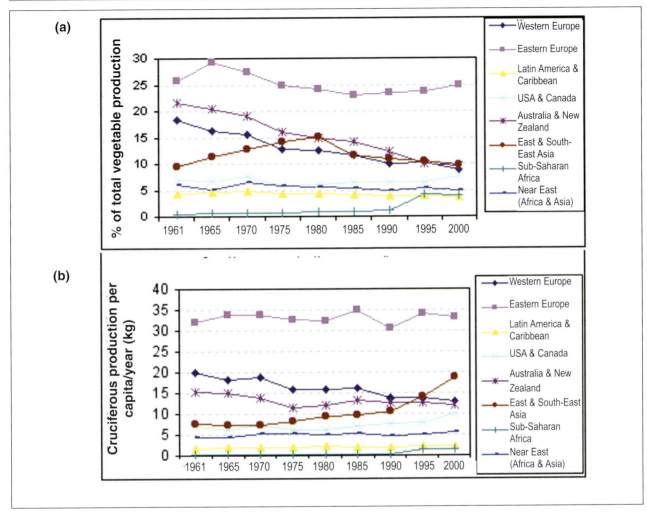

Figure 3 Production of cruciferous vegetables in selected regions worldwide: (a) relative to all vegetables and (b) per capita production

Sources: a) FAOSTAT (2000); b) FAOSTAT (2000), United Nations (2002)

The regions defined by FAO do not correspond exactly to those defined by the United Nations; furthermore, there are discrepancies in the countries included in western Europe, the near East and sub-Saharan Africa by the two bodies.

'Sub-Saharan Africa' comprises: all countries south of the Sahara Desert except South Africa, West Sahara and Sudan, which are included in the FAO data but not those from the United Nations.

East and South-East Asia comprise: Brunei Darussalam, Cambodia, China, Democratic People's Republic of Korea, Indonesia, Japan, Democratic Lao People's Republic, Malaysia, Mongolia, Myanmar, Philippines, Singapore, Thailand, Timor Leste and Viet Nam. Note that the data for China are not reliable.

'Near East' comprises: Algeria, Afghanistan, Azerbaijan, Bahrain, Cyprus, Egypt, Georgia, Palestine, Islamic Republic of Iran, Iraq, Israel, Jordan, Kuwait, Lebanon, Lybian Arab Jamahirya, Morocco, Oman, Qatar, Saudi Arabia, Syrian Arab Republic, Tunisia, Turkey, United Arab Emirates and Yemen. Azerbaijan, Georgia, Israel and Palestine are included in the United Nations data but not in those from FAO.

'Eastern Europe' comprises: Albania, Bosnia Herzegovina, Bulgaria, Croatia, Czech Republic, Hungary, Macedonia, Poland, Romania, Serbia-Montenegro, Slovakia and the former Yugoslavia.

Western Europe includes: Austria, Belgium, Denmark, Finland, France, Germany, Greece, Iceland, Ireland, Italy, Luxembourg, Malta, Netherlands, Norway, Portugal, Spain, Sweden, Switzerland and United Kingdom.

Chapter 2

Glucosinolates, isothiocyanates and indoles

Although isothiocyanate and indole compounds derived from cruciferous vegetables appear to be structurally unrelated, they are both derived from glucosinolates. These sulfur-containing glycosides are found in the order Capparales, which includes the large family Brassicaceae. The glucosinolate molecule comprises a common glucone moiety and a variable aglucone side-chain, derived from one of seven amino acids. Isothiocyanates are formed by the degradation of glucosinolates that have either aliphatic or aromatic side-chains (Figures 4 & 5), derived (mainly) from methionine and phenylalanine, respectively, whereas indoles are derived from glucosinolates with indolyl side-chains derived from tryptophan (Figures 6 & 7) (Rosa *et al.*, 1997). Cruciferous vegetables also contain other phytochemicals that have been associated with potential health benefits, including phenolics, vitamins and other sulfur-containing compounds.

Isothiocyanates are familiar to many of us as they are largely responsible for the characteristic hot, pungent flavours of salad vegetables such as radish, cress, mustard leaves and watercress, and contribute to the flavour of cooked cruciferous vegetables. Indoles do not contribute to the flavour of crucifers. Many of the biological and chemico-physical properties of these compounds (e.g. volatility and lipophilicity) are determined by the chemical structure of the isothiocyanate side-chain (Figure 5; Appendix 1), which, in turn, is determined by the structure of the parent glucosinolate molecule. The bioactivity of these compounds to humans is thus influenced by a combination of the chemical structure of the isothiocyanates and their concentration.

Major dietary sources of specific isothiocyanates and indoles

The concentrations and forms of glucosinolates in commonly eaten cruciferous vegetables are summarized in Table 6. Several surveys of variations in glucosinolate content between *Brassica* cultivars have been reported, for example for *B. rapa* (Carlson *et al.*, 1987a; Hill *et al.*, 1987) and *B. oleracea* (Carlson *et al.*, 1987b; Kushad *et al.*, 1999), and these are also summarized in Table 6. While over 90 different isothiocyanate (ITC) glucosinolates have been described, only about six occur frequently in the diet (Figure 5; Table 6). Sulforaphane (4-methylsulfinylbutyl-ITC) is obtained predominantly from broccoli but may also be obtained from rocket (*Eruca sativa*) and some cultivars of cabbage and Brussels sprouts. 2-Propenyl ('allyl')-,

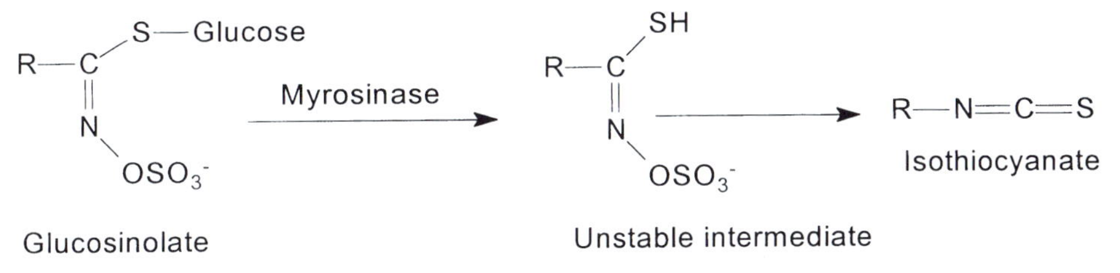

Figure 4 General scheme of the hydrolysis of glucosinolates to isothiocyanates

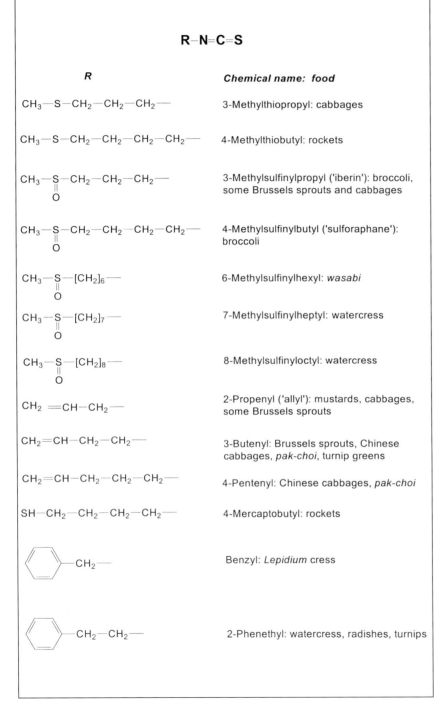

Figure 5 Structures of isothiocyanates and side-chain structures (R) found in commonly eaten cruciferous vegetables

3-butenyl- and 3-methylsulfinylpropyl-ITC ('iberin') are derived from consumption of certain cultivars of *B. oleracea*. Propenyl-ITC can also be obtained from leafy mustard vegetables. 3-Butenyl- and 4-pentenyl-ITC are obtained from leafy *B. rapa* crops and particularly Chinese cabbage. Phenyl-ethyl-ITC is obtained from watercress and to a lesser extent from root crops such as turnips and rutabaga. 6-Methylsulfinylhexyl-ITC is derived from the Japanese vegetable *wasabi* (*Wasabia japonica*). Benzyl-ITC is relatively rare in the diet, as it is obtained from *Lepidium* (cress) species. In addition to cruciferous vegetables, isothiocyanates may also be derived from mustard condiments, which are eaten mainly in western countries. Hydroxy-benzyl-ITC is found in 'English' mustard and is obtained from the seeds of white mustard, *Sinapis alba*. Allyl- (2-propenyl-) and 3-butenyl-ITCs are found in French and American mustards and are derived from the seeds of brown (or Indian) mustard, *B. juncea*. Allyl-ITC is also derived from the grated roots of horseradish (*Armoracia rusticana*), which is used as a condiment in western Europe and North America. Cruciferous vegetables may also be processed by pickling or fermenting, as in sauerkraut in western Europe and in some forms of *kimchi* in the Korean peninsula. Consumption of these products is an additional source of isothiocyanates in the diet.

Six different indolyl glucosinolates have been identified, but only four have been found in cruciferous crops (Figure 7), and, of these, only two, indolylmethyl ('glucobrassicin') and 1-methoxy-3-indolylmethyl ('neoglucobrassicin'), are found frequently. The types of indole glucosinolates vary from species to species (Table 6), and there is wide variation in the concentrations of specific indole glucosinolates. In broccoli, the concentration of

Table 6. Main glucosinolate side-chains of isothiocyanates occurring in cruciferous vegetables

Cruciferous vegetable	Glucosinolate side-chain	Content (µmol/100 g fresh weight)
Broccoli (*B. oleracea* var. *italica*)[a]	3-Methylsulfinylpropyl	0–330
	4-Methylsulfinylbutyl	29–190
	Indole-3-methyl	42–100
	1-Methoxyindole-3-methyl	2–18
Cabbage (*B. oleracea* var. *capitata*)[b]	2-Propenyl	4–160
	3-Methylsulfinylpropyl	5–280
	Indolylmethyl	9–200
Brussels sprouts (*B. oleracea* var. *gemmifera*)[c]	2-Propenyl	4–390
	3-Methylsulfinylpropyl	0–150
	3-Butenyl	0–220
	4-Methylsulfinylbutyl	0–23
	2-Hydroxy-3-butenyl	1–300
	Indole-3-methyl	45–470
	1-Methoxyindole-3-methyl	2–34
Cauliflower (*B. oleracea* var. *botrytis*)	2-Propenyl	1–160
	3-Methylsulfinylpropyl	0–330
	4-Methylsulfinylbutyl	2–190
	Indole-3-methyl	14–160
	1-Methoxyindole-3-methyl	1–32
Kale (*B. oleracea* var. *acephala*)	2-Propenyl	62–200
	3-Methylsulfinylpropyl	0–50
	3-Butenyl	6–38
	2-Hydroxy-3-butenyl	17–130
	Indole-3-methyl	67–160
Rape (*B. rapa,* including Chinese cabbage and turnip tops)[d]	3-Butenyl	38–290
	4-Pentenyl	20–150

All the crops can also contain low concentrations of other glucosinolates (Carlson *et al.*, 1987a,b; Hill *et al.*, 1987; Rosa *et al.*, 1997; Kushad *et al.*, 1999). The concentrations must be interpreted with care, as different methods of analyses were used in the different studies, and the concentrations are affected by a wide range of environmental factors. In addition, generalizations cannot be made about the glucosinolate content of cabbages and Brussels sprouts as there are large genetic differences between cultivars. The values quoted indicate the greatest range of values in the reviews referred to above.

[a] All broccoli cultivars produce predominantly 4-methylsulfinylbutyl glucosinolate, the precursor of sulforaphane.

[b] Some cabbage varieties produce the elongated glucosinolates, 3-butenyl and 4-methylsulfinylbutyl; some also produce their precursors, 3-methylthiopropyl and 4-methylthiobutyl.

[c] Surprisingly, the glucosinolate content of Brussels sprouts varies: some cultivars produce high concentrations of 2-propenyl, while others produce high concentrations of 3-butenyl and 2-hydroxy-3-butenyl. Recently developed cultivars either have low concentrations of these glucosinolates or moderate concentrations of 3-methylsulfinylpropyl or 4-methylsulfinylbutyl.

[d] Cultivars tend to have both 3-butenyl and 4-pentenyl (and hydroxylated forms) or just 3-butenyl

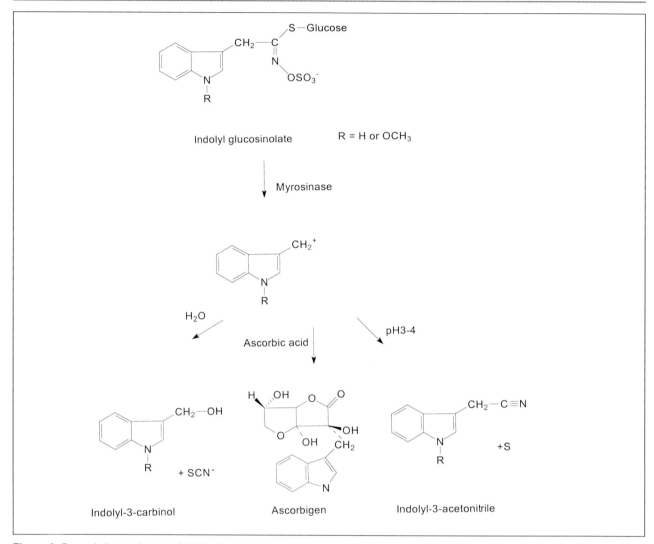

Figure 6 Degradation pathways of indole glucosinolates

neoglucobrassicin was found in some studies to be even higher than that of glucobrassicin (Vang *et al.*, 2001; Vallejo *et al.*, 2003a). In Brussels sprouts, neoglucobrassicin occurs at a much lower concentration than glucobrassicin (Kushad *et al.*, 1999; Ciska *et al.*, 2000), while 4-hydroxy-3-indolylmethyl glucosinolate and glucobrassicin are found at similar concentrations in cauliflower (Kushad *et al.*, 1999). In white cabbage, the main

indole glucosinolate is glucobrassicin, and 4-methoxy-3-indolylmethyl glucosinolate is present at half the concentration (Ciska *et al.*, 2000).

Four factors interact to determine the exposure of the gastrointestinal tract to isothiocyanates and indoles:

• the biochemical genetics of the biosynthesis of glucosinolates and isothiocyanates within the crop plant, which determines the chemical structure of the glucosinolate

side-chain and partially determines the overall amount;

• abiotic and biotic environmental factors, which can influence the overall amount of isothiocyanates produced by the plant;

• post-harvest storage, processing and cooking; and

• the thioglucosidase activity of the intestinal microbial flora.

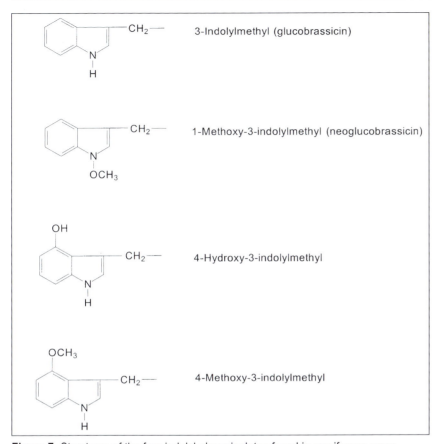

Figure 7 Structures of the four indolyl glucosinolates found in cruciferous crops

Biochemical genetics of glucosinolate biosynthesis

Side-chain structures

Glucosinolates with more than 115 side-chain structures derived from one of eight amino acids (alanine, valine, leucine, isoleucine, phenylalanine, methionine, tyrosine and tryptophan) have been described. These glucosinolates all form isothiocyanates upon hydrolysis, except for those derived from tryptophane, which release indoles. The glucosinolate contents of wild and cultivated plants have been surveyed by Daxenbichler *et al.* (1991) and Fahey *et al.* (2001).

Biosynthesis of these glucosinolates and their resultant isothiocyanates or indole derivatives can be separated into four parts: amino acid chain elongation, core glucosinolate synthesis, chain modification and production of isothiocyanates and indoles (Figure 8). The side-chain structure of glucosinolates in any one genotype is under strict genetic control, whereas the overall level is determined by interactions between genotype and environment. Only an overview is provided here; for further details, see Halkier and Du (1997) and Mithen (2001).

Amino acid elongation

While some glucosinolates are synthesized from chain-elongated forms of valine and phenylalanine, about 50% of all known glucosinolates, only from the Brassicaceae and the Capparaceae, are synthesized from elongated forms of methionine. Methionine can be elongated by the addition of one to nine methyl groups, but most taxa within the Brassicaceae have only a restricted chain length, which can be divided into three classes: 'short chains', from the addition of one, two, three or (rarely) four methyl groups to methionine, such as found in *Brassica* crops; 'long chains', from the addition of five or six methyl groups; and 'very long chains' from the addition of seven, eight or nine methyl groups.

Biochemical studies in which [^{14}C]acetate and ^{14}C-labelled amino acids were administered, with subsequent analysis of the labelled glucosinolates, suggest that the amino acid elongation is similar to that which occurs during synthesis of leucine from 2-keto-3-methylbutanoic acid and acetyl coenzyme A (Strassman & Ceci, 1963; Graser *et al.*, 2000). The amino acid is transaminated to produce an α-keto acid, followed by condensation with acetyl coenzyme A, isomerization involving a shift in the hydroxyl group, and oxidative decarboxylation to result in an elongated keto acid which is transaminated to form the elongated amino acid. It is likely that the elongated keto acid can undergo further condensation with acetyl coenzyme A to result in multiple chain elongations.

Molecular genetics studies in *Arabidopsis thaliana* resulted in identification of a small gene family, designated *MAM* (*methylthioalkylmalate*), which catalyse condensation of the keto acids with acetyl coenzyme A (Kroymann *et al.*, 2001). Differences in expression and allelic variants of the *MAM* genes appear to explain the variety of chain lengths observed, although the details remain to be clarified (Kroymann *et al.*, 2003). Thus, differences in the chain length of

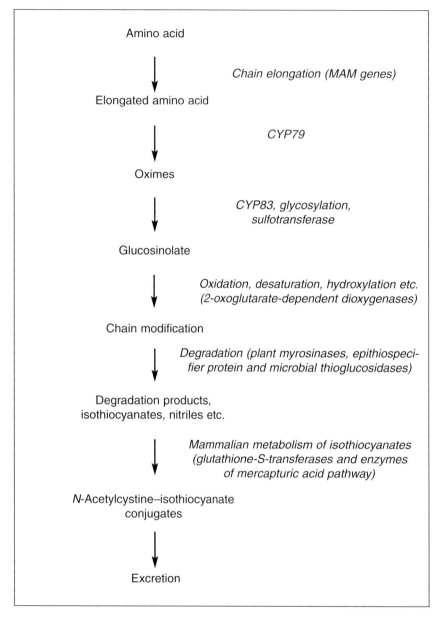

Figure 8 Biosynthesis and metabolism of glucosinolates and isothiocyanates
Indole glucosinolate degradation products are not metabolized via the mercapturic acid pathway

methionine-derived glucosinolates in cruciferous crops is probably due to allelic differences in *MAM* genes that result in different specificities of their enzymic products for elongated keto acids.

Core glucosinolate biosynthesis

The first step in glucosinolate biosynthesis is conversion of the amino acid to an oxime. Recent studies, largely with *A. thaliana*, suggest that all amino acid–oxime conversions are catalysed

by cytochrome P450 (CYP) monooxygenases of the CYP79 family. The best characterized system is conversion of tyrosine and phenylalanine to their corresponding oximes (Du *et al.*, 1995; Bak *et al.*, 1999) as precursors of benzyl and hydroxybenzyl glucosinolates. In *Arabidopsis*, oximes from chain-elongated methionine homologues are formed by the action of the *CYP79F1* and *CYP79F2* genes. The first of these can catalyse many homologues of chain-elongated forms of methionine, whereas the latter can catalyse only long-chain methionine homologues.

In *Arabidopsis*, conversion of the oxime to the thiohydroximate is probably catalysed by another cytochome P450, CYP83B1 (Hansen *et al.*, 2001). As thiohydroximates would be toxic to plant tissue, they are effectively detoxified by glycosylation by a soluble UDPG:thiohydroximate S-glucosyltransferase to produce a desulfoglucosinolate (Reed *et al.*, 1993; Grootwassink *et al.*, 1994; Guo & Poulton, 1994). This is sulfated by a soluble 3'-phosphoadenosine 5'-phosphosulfate: desulfoglucosinolate sulfotransferase (Jain *et al.*, 1990), to produce the glucosinolate.

Chain modification

The chain structure of glucosinolates derived from any amino acid can undergo modification. As for other aspects of glucosinolates, most attention has been paid to methionine-derived compounds.

After the biosynthesis of methylthioalkyl glucosinolates from methionine, the side-chain can undergo various modifications. Initial oxidation results in methylsulfinylalkyl, which accumulates in broccoli. Additional oxidation results in methylsulfonylalkyl glucosinolates, which accumulate in certain non-cultivated cruciferous vegetables. Removal of the methylsulfinyl group and desaturation result in alkenyl glucosinolates. Alternatively, hydroxylation results in 3-hydroxypropyl or 4-hydroxy-butyl glucosinolate (Mithen *et al.*, 1995; Giamoustaris & Mithen, 1996; Hall *et al.*, 2001). There is considerable scope for variation in this part of the pathway. For example, 4-methyl-sulfinylbutenyl glucosinolate, found exclusively in *Raphanus*, probably results from desaturation of the corresponding methylsulfinylbutyl glucosinolate but without associated methyl-sulfinyltransferase activity. The alkenyl glucosinolates 3-butenyl and 4-pentenyl can undergo β-hydroxylation, with important consequences for the nature of the hydrolytic products. While the details of the biochemical processes and the genes that determine these modifications are not fully understood, studies with *Arabidopsis* suggest that many of the processes are due to the activity of 2-oxogluturate-dependent dioxygenases (Hall *et al.*, 2001). As for side-chain elongation, genetic control of the side-chain structure is very strict. Thus, a specific genotype always produces the same chain structure, regardless of the environment in which it is grown.

Indole glucosinolates derived from tryptophan are also modified by addition of hydroxyl or methoxy groups (Figure 7), but the biochemical mechanisms and genetic basis of these modifications are unknown. Although modification of the side-chains of isothiocyanates, producing glucosinolates, is under strict genetic control, environmental factors can affect modification of indole side-chains.

Genetic basis of glucosinolate accumulation

While several genes that determine side-chain structure have now been cloned, the genetic control of total glucosinolate accumulation is still far from understood. Most studies have been conducted on spring or winter rape (*B. napus*), in which breeders have sought to reduce the content of 2-hydroxy-3-butenyl glucosinolate ('progoitrin') owing to the goitrogenic activity of its major hydrolysis product, 5-vinyloxazo-lidine-2-thione (goitrin), when incorporated into animal feed. Thus, glucosinolate concentrations have been reduced from greater than 80 µmol/g to less that 5 µmol/g in spring rape and to less than 15 µmol/g in winter rape. This was shown to be a complex genetic trait determined by alleles at four or five quantitative trait loci (Toroser *et al.*, 1995; Howell *et al.*, 2003). Studies in broccoli have focused on increasing the concentration of methylsulfinylalkyl glucosinolates. Surveys of glucosinolates in existing broccoli cultivars showed that the concentration of 4-methylsulfinyl-butyl glucosinolates varied from 0.8 mmol/g dry weight to 21.7 mmol/g (Kushad *et al.*, 1999). In an effort to obtain higher concentrations, Faulkner *et al.* (1998) used *B. villosa* and other wild members of the nine *B. oleracea* species complex. Hybrids between these accessions and broccoli contained concentrations in excess of 80 µmol/g dry weight. After several back-crosses, isothiocyanate-enriched broccoli was developed from these initial hybrids (Mithen *et al.*, 2003). Some of the quantitative trait loci important in enhancing the glucosinolate concentration of broccoli are in positions in the genome similar to those that determine reduction of glucosinolate levels in rape. Identification of the genes involved in these quantitative trait loci might facilitate a genetic approach to enhancing glucosinolates in horticultural crops.

Glucosinolate hydrolysis and formation of isothiocyanates

When tissue is disrupted, an endogenous plant thioglucosidase ('myrosinase', see below) causes cleavage of the thio–glucose bond to give rise to unstable thiohydroximate *O*-sulfonate (Figure 4). This aglycone sponta-neously rearranges to several products. Most frequently, it undergoes a Lossen rearrangement to produce an isothiocyanate. If the glucosinolate side-chain contains a double bond, and in the presence of an epithiospec-ifier protein (see below), the isothiocyanate may rearrange to produce an epithionitrile (Figure 9a). If the glucosinolate lacks a double bond, the sulfur may be lost and a nitrile formed. (Figure 9b). A few glucosinolates have been shown to produce thiocyanates, although the mechanism by which this occurs is unknown. Aglucones from glucosinolates which contain β-hydroxy-lated side-chains, such as progoitrin found in the seeds of oilseed rape and in the edible parts of Chinese cabbage and Brussels sprouts, spontaneously cyclize to form the corresponding oxazolidine-2-thiones (Figure 9c).

Glucosinolate hydrolysis and formation of indoles

The formation of indoles from indole glucosinolates has been reviewed by Vang and Dragsted (1996). After tissue disruption, myrosinase cleaves the thioglucose bond, like other glucosino-lates, but the resulting isothiocyanate is unstable and degrades to the corresponding alcohol (Figure 5). The alcohol can condense to 3,3′-diindoyl-methane. As with methionine-derived glucosinolates, indolyl-3-acetonitrile can be formed instead of an unstable isothiocyanate. The factors that determine the degradation pathway are largely unknown. Moreover, in the acidic conditions of the stomach, indole-3-carbinol (and related products from other indolyl glucosinolates) can undergo several condensation reactions, to produce at least 15 different oligomeric products (Anderton *et al.*, 2003). Indole-3-carbinol can also react with ascorbic acid to form ascorbigen (Piironen & Virtanen, 1962; Hrncirik *et al.*, 2001). As for isothiocyanate-producing glucosinolates, if cooking

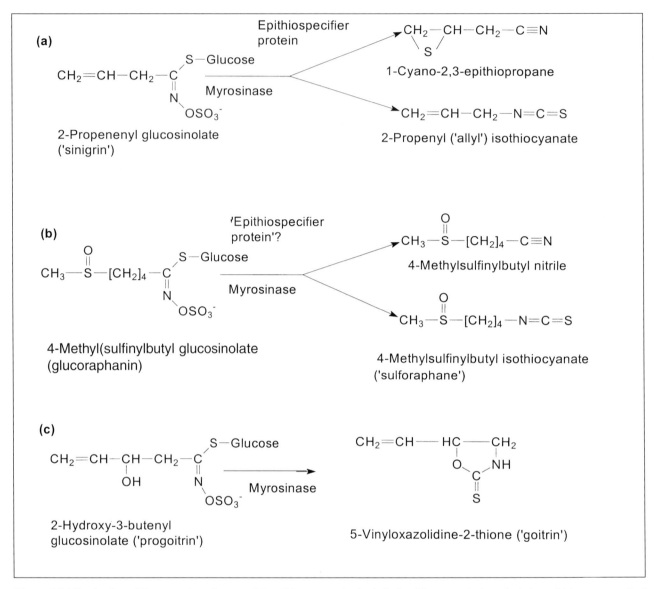

Figure 9 (a) Production of 2-propenyl- or 1-cyano-2,3-epithiopropane by hydrolysis of 2-propenyl glucosinolates, which are a result of expression of the epithiospecifier protein. **(b)** Production of 4-methylsulfinylbutyl isothiocyanate or nitrile by hydrolysis of the corresponding glucosinolate, as a result of expression of epithiospecifier-like protein. **(c)** Production of 5-vinyloxazolidine-2-thione (goitrin) from 2-hydroxy-3-butenyl glucosinolate

denatures myrosinase activitiy, the intact indole glucosinolate can be degraded in the colon, in which the contrasting pH may result in production of different degradation products and their absorption into the bloodstream.

Myrosinases
Bones and Rossiter (1996) and Rask et al. (2000) have reviewed the data on myrosinases, and only a brief summary is provided here. Many myrosinase isozymes have been detected in glucosinolate-containing plants, and myrosinase (i.e. thioglucosidase) activity has also been detected in insects, fungi and bacteria. In plants, the expression of isozymes varies both between species and within the organs

of the same individual (Lenman et al., 1993). In general, isozymes with activity towards the glucosinolate chain structure appear to have little substrate specificity, although a myrosinase highly specific to epiprogoitrin was described in Crambe (Bernardi et al., 2003). Molecular studies with A. thaliana, Brassica and Sinapis have shown that myrosinases comprise a gene family (Xue et al., 1992) with three subclasses, denoted MA, MB and MC. Members of each of these subfamilies occur in A. thaliana (Xue et al., 1995). As would be expected, many more copies occur in the B. napus genome, because of genome replication. All myrosinases are glyco-sylated, and the extent of glycosylation varies between subclasses. It is likely that the subdivision of myrosinases will be revised as new data on sequences become available. MB and MC myrosinases are linked with myrosinase-binding proteins and myrosinase-associated proteins, respectively (Lenman et al., 1990). The roles of these proteins are not understood, but they seem to have no significance for the generation of glucosinolate degradation products after consumption of cruciferous vegetables.

Epithiospecifier protein

The epithiospecifier protein was first described by Tookey (1973) and was purified from B. napus (Bernardi et al., 2000; Foo et al., 2000). This protein appears to have no inherent enzymatic activity; it does not interact with glucosinolates but only with the unstable thiohydroximate O-sulfonate after myrosinase activity. Foo et al. (2000) suggested that the mode of action of epithiospecifier protein is similar to that of a cytochrome P450, such as in iron-dependent epoxidation reactions. While this protein has been considered only in the context of the generation of epithionitriles, it might also be involved in the production of nitriles from glu-

cosinolates, such as those with methyl-sulfinylalkyl side-chains found in broccoli and watercress. In this case, the sulfur from the glucone is lost, as it cannot be re-incorporated into the degradation product since it lacks a terminal double bond.

The ratio of isothiocyanates:nitriles varies according to genotype (Matusheski et al., 2003; Mithen et al., 2003), and this may be related to expression of the epithiospecifier protein. Glucosinolates in ecotypes of A. thaliana vary with respect to the relative ratio of isothiocyanate to epithionitrile or to nitrile they form after tissue disruption, due partly to allelic variation at a quantitative trait locus associated with gene coding for epithiospecifier protein (Lambrix et al., 2001). Likewise, while in standard cultivars of broccoli hydrolysis results in about a 20:80% ratio of isothiocyanates:nitriles, isothiocyanate enriched broccoli produces about 95% isothiocyanates after hydrolysis (Mithen et al., 2003).

Factors that affect glucosinolate concentrations

Abiotic and biotic environmental factors

In general terms, while the ratio of individual glucosinolates within a particular class (e.g. those derived from methionine) is relatively constant and is unaffected by environmental factors, the total concentration is affected by several such factors. Our understanding of these is relatively poor, and it is likely that there are often significant genotype–environment interactions. Soil fertility is probably a major factor. Zhao et al. (1994) reported that the sulfur and nitrogen supply affected the glucosinolate content of rapeseed and described minor alterations in the ratios of individual methionine-derived

glucosinolates and larger alterations in the ratio of indolyl:methionine-derived glucosinolates. In contrast, sulfur fertilization alone had either a small effect or no effect at all on the glucosinolate content of broccoli (Vallejo et al., 2003a,b). It is likely that any effect of sulfur depends strongly on the nitrogen supply. Soil fertilization (combined N and S) was reported to have a significant effect on glucosinolates in broccoli (Mithen et al., 2003). This study also showed that certain genotypes have a greater response than others. Nitrogen fertilizer in a hydroponic system enhanced the concentration of glucosinolates in pak-choi (Shattuck & Wang, 1994). Water stress induced glucosinolates in rapeseed and rape (Bouchereau et al., 1996; Jensen et al., 1996) and is likely to have a similar effect in horticultural cruciferous vegetables. The effect of temperature has not been studied in detail, and, like other environmental factors, affects general plant growth parameters. Pereira et al. (2002) reported that temperature affected the glucosinolate concentrations in seedlings ('sprouts') of broccoli, those grown at higher temperatures having more glucosinolates than those grown at lower temperatures.

Not only abiotic factors but also insects and pathogens induce glucosinolate accumulation, although the effects are mainly on indolyl glucosinolates as opposed to methionine-derived (isothiocyanate-producing) glucosinolates (Birch et al., 1992; Shattuck & Wang, 1994). Jasmonic acid, a signalling molecule involved in several plant–insect or –pathogen interactions, also induced glucosinolates (Bodnaryk, 1994).

Post-harvest storage, processing and cooking

Few studies have been conducted on the effects of post-harvest events on the concentration of glucosinolates in horticultural cruciferous vegetables.

Vallejo et al. (2003c) reported a loss of 70–80% of the total glucosinolate content after a period of simulated cold storage during transport and storage before sale. Storage of cut cabbage reduced methionine-derived glucosinolates, as expected, but enhanced the concentration of indolyl glucosinolates (Verkerk et al., 2001). Storage of broccoli under various conditions also enhanced indole glucosinolates (Hansen et al., 1995).

As described above, myrosinase-mediated glucosinolate degradation results in initial formation of an unstable intermediate and then in the formation of an isothiocyanate or a nitrile (Figure 9a and b), the latter due to the presence of an epithionitrile specifier or an epithiospecifier nitrile-like protein. When raw Brassica vegetables are macerated, about 80% of the methionine-derived glucosinolates can be converted to nitriles, as opposed to isothiocyanates, the precise ratio of isothiocyanates:nitriles depending on genotype (Mithen et al., 2003). Both myrosinase and ethiospecific protein can be degraded by cooking. Mild cooking, for example steaming broccoli florets for less than 3 min, denatured the epithionitrile specifier protein while leaving at least some of the endogenous myrosinase intact, enhancing the isothiocyanate content. Further cooking, e.g. heating broccoli for 10 or 20 min at 50 °C, subsequently denatured myrosinase, preventing any immediate isothiocyanate production. Thus, the degree of cooking can have significant effects on the delivery of isothiocyanate to the gastrointestinal tract: consumption of raw vegetables may result in exposure to a significant amount of nitriles; mild cooking may result in consumption of large amounts of isothiocyanates, with topical exposure of the upper gastrointestinal tract to biologically significant concentrations; while more extensive cooking prevents isothiocyanate formation, and

intact glucosinolates will be consumed which may be degraded to isothiocyanates or other compounds by the intestinal microflora, as discussed below.

Glucobrassicin is chemically and thermally stable, as no degradation was observed after 2 h in aqueous media with pH values ranging from 2 to 11. Moreover, glucobrassicin was weakly degraded by heat treatment (10% after 1 h) (Chevolleau et al., 1997).

Intestinal microbial flora

Cooking glucosinolate-containing vegetables for more than 2 min inactivates myrosinase, as described above. Several studies have shown that isothiocyanate metabolites can be detected in blood and urine after cooked glucosinolate-containing foods are eaten, although to a lesser extent than when raw glucosinolate-containing foods are consumed (Getahun & Chung, 1999; Conaway et al., 2000). A likely source of isothiocyanates is microbial degradation of glucosinolates by the intestinal microflora. Thus, isothiocyanates can be generated by incubation of cooked (i.e. myrosinase denatured) watercress with human fæces under anerobic conditions (Getahun & Chung, 1999). Rouzaud et al. (2003) compared urinary isothiocyanate metabolites in gnotobiotic rats harbouring whole human faecal flora and in germ-free rats and found, as expected, that after feeding with glucosino-late-containing food the greatest excretion of isothiocyanates was observed when the plant myrosinase was intact. When the plant myrosinase was denatured by heat treatment, the amount of isothiocyanate produced was estimated to be reduced by > 85% in the gnotobiotic rats. Some isothiocyanates also appeared to be produced in the germ-free rats, and some evidence was obtained that the presence of human faecal flora actually reduced the amount of isothiocyanate available for absorption.

Indole glucosinolates are likely to be degraded in the gastrointestinal tract. When they were fed to rats, similar biological effects were seen as when degradation products were fed, suggesting microbial degradation of intact glucosinolates (Bonnesen et al., 1999).

Estimates of dietary intake of isothiocyanates and indoles

Estimates of dietary intake of isothiocyanates and indoles are clearly needed. The existing databases on consumption of crucifers (section 1) and glucosinolate content (Table 6) might be considered adequate to provide a basis for such estimates, but the wide variation in glucosinolate content due to the factors described above and the difficulty in estimating the conversion of glucosinolates to isothiocyanates and indoles during consumption reduce the confidence with which such estimates can be made.

Measurement of isothiocyanates in vegetables before consumption

Jiao et al. (1998) in Singapore and Shapiro et al. (1998) in the USA reported the isothiocyanate concentrations found in vegetables. In each case, the vegetables were analysed by condensation with 1,2-benzenedithiol (see section 3), which results in quantification of total isothiocyanates. Endogenous plant myrosinase was denatured by cooking before treatment with exogenous myrosinase (Table 7). Thus, the estimate of isothiocyanate production is probably higher than that which occurs within the gastrointestinal tract, on the assumption that myrosinase activity is a limiting factor.

Intake of indole glucosinolates

Estimates of the average daily intake of indole glucosinolates are based on

Table 7. Isothiocyanate (ITC) content of cruciferous vegetables in Singapore and the USA

Vegetable	Mean content (µmol/100 g fresh weight (range))	
	Singapore (Jiao *et al.*, 1998)	USA (Shapiro *et al.*, 1998)
Broccoli (*B. oleracea* var. *italica*)	38.6 (10.1–62.0)	6.7
Cabbage (*B. oleracea* var. *capitata*)	27.5 (11.9–62.7)	4.4
Cauliflower (*B. oleracea* var. *botrytis*)	11.6 (2.7–24.0)	
Kale (*B. oleracea* var. *acephala*)		18.2
Kai lan (*B. oleracea* var. *alboglabra*)	15.4 (3.1–35.9)	
Turnip (*B. rapa* var. *rapa*)		1.4
Bok choi (*B. rapa* var. *chinensis*)	4.9 (2.0–7.5)	
Choi sum (*B. rapa* var. *parachinensis*)	11.1 (3.5–23.4)	
Watercress (*Nasturtium officinale*)	81.3 (17.1–144.6)	
Kai choi (*B. juncea* var. *rugosa*)	71.2 (25.6–138.4)	

the intake of specific cruciferous vegetables and their content of the various indole glucosinolates. The estimates are only approximate, as the concentrations of indole glucosinolates vary considerably depending on growing conditions, the cultivar, storage and preparation conditions, as considerable amounts of glucosinolates can be lost during storage and processing.

Sones *et al.* (1984) estimated the per-capita intake of indole glucosinolates in the United Kingdom to be 19.4 mg/day for glucobrassicin and 3.1 mg/day for neoglucobrassicin. Vang and Dragsted (1996) estimated the per capita intake in Denmark to be 5 mg/day for glucobrassicin and 0.5 mg/day for neoglucobrassicin, and the respective values in Finland to be 2.5 mg/day and 0.3 mg/day. Broadbent and Broadbent (1998a) in the USA estimated the per capita intake of glucobrassicin to be 8.1 mg/day. The total intake of indole glucosinolates, including the two major ones and both fresh and cooked cruciferous vegetables, was about 22.5 mg/day per capita. The more recent estimates indicate wide variations between countries, which are due to the use of different methods for estimating intake of cruciferous vegetables and indole glucosinolates.

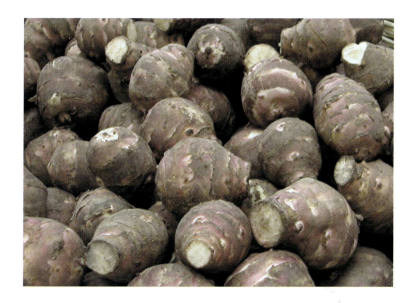

Chapter 3

Metabolism, kinetics and genetic variation

Observations in humans

Isothiocyanates
Metabolism and disposition
The $-N=C=S$ group of most isothiocyanates is electrophilic and can react readily with various nucleophiles, including thiols. Studies in both humans and experimental animals have established that isothiocyanates are metabolized in vivo to various dithiocarbamates principally by the mercapturic acid pathway. An initial conjugation with glutathione (GSH, the most abundant cellular thiol), which takes place spontaneously but is further promoted by glutathione S-transferase (GST), gives rise to the corresponding conjugates.

In the spontaneous reaction, isothiocyanates react reversibly with cysteinyl thiols, forming dithiocarbamates:

$$\text{cystine residue}-\text{SH} + \text{RN}=\text{C}=\text{S} \;\longleftrightarrow\; \text{cystine residue}-\text{S}-\underset{\underset{\text{S}}{\|}}{\text{C}}-\text{NHR}$$

The equilibrium position and the chemical relaxation time for equilibrium have been estimated for phenethylisothiocyanate (ITC) reacting with cysteinyl residues in blood plasma (cysteinyl thiol concentration, about 500 µmol/l) and cells (cysteinyl thiol concentration, 5 mmol/l). The equilibrium constant, K, was 730 per mol. At equilibrium, about 27% of phenethyl-ITC is bound to plasma thiols in blood, and about 88% is bound to thiols in cells. For a plasma concentration of 5 µmol/l of phenethyl-ITC, the equilibrium relaxation time for formation of adducts with protein thiols

is about 17 min in plasma and about 3 min in cells (Xu & Thornalley, 2000a).

The GSH conjugates undergo further enzymatic modification, in the GSH portion, to give rise sequentially to the cysteinylglycine, cysteine and N-acetylcysteine conjugates, which are excreted in urine (Brüsewitz et al., 1977), as shown in Figure 10. Urinary excretion of N-acetylcysteine conjugates is the principal route of disposition of ingested isothiocyanates. For example, when benzyl-ITC was administered orally to six men, 54% of a dose of 14.4 mg was recovered in the urine as N-acetyl-S-(N-benzylthiocarbamoyl)-L-cysteine (benzyl-ITC–N-acetylcysteine). This compound was excreted rapidly: maximum excretion occurred within 2–6 h, and the compound was essentially undetectable 10–12 h after dosing (Mennicke et al., 1988). Watercress is rich in gluconasturtiin (constituting more than 30% of total glucosinolates), the precursor of phenethyl-ITC. When four volunteers ate 30 g of watercress containing 21.6 mg of gluconasturtiin, an average of 47% of the amount was recovered as the N-acetylcysteine conjugate in 24-h urine (Chung et al., 1992). The amount of phenethyl-ITC–N-acetylcysteine in urine is probably greater when phenethyl-ITC is administered, because the myrosinase-catalysed conversion of gluconasturtiin to phenethyl-ITC may be incomplete after ingestion of watercress. In these studies, the

amount of urinary N-acetylcysteine –ITC might have been underestimated, because these conjugates are unstable and readily dissociate to isothiocyanates (Conaway et al., 2001). The metabolic disposition of other isothiocyanates, including allyl-ITC and sulforaphane, are similar in humans, as discussed below.

Measurement of isothiocyanates and isothiocyanate metabolites
The cyclocondensation assay is a highly sensitive quantitative method for measuring isothiocyanates and their metabolites (referred to collectively here as isothiocyanate equivalent) (Zhang et al., 1996) and is a valuable tool for studying dietary consumption of isothiocyanates and their metabolism. The assay is based on the almost universal ability of isothiocyanates to react quantitatively with 1,2-benzenedithiol, a vicinal dithiol, to give rise to a five-membered cyclic product and a free amine (Zhang et al., 1992a), as shown in Figure 11. Reactive isothiocyanates are converted to the same cyclic product, 1,3-benzodithiole-2-thione, and conversion is complete in the presence of excess 1,2-benzenedithiol. The resultant 1,3-benzodithiole-2-thione can be measured accurately in amounts as low as a few picomoles, with a simple high-performance liquid chromatography (HPLC) procedure. Conjugation products of isothiocyanates with thiols (dithiocarbamates), including N-acetyl-cysteine–isothiocyanate, also react quantitatively with 1,2-benzenedithiol, giving rise to the same cyclic product. Thus, this assay allows detection of the total amount of isothiocyanates and their

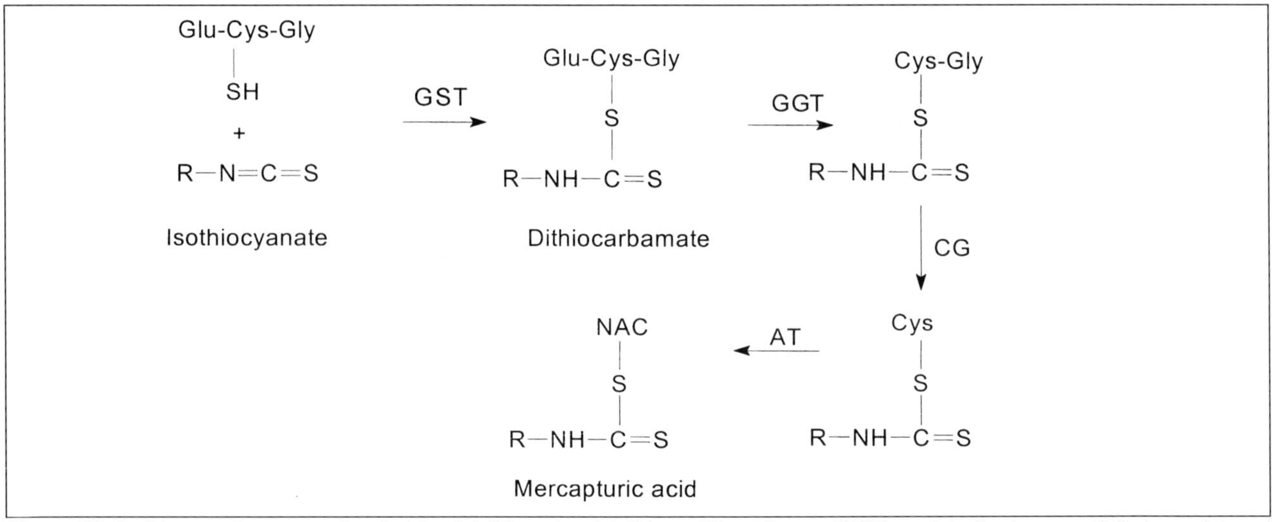

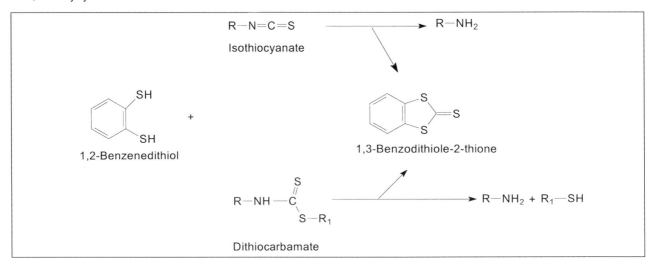

Figure 10 Isothiocyanates are conjugated to glutathione by glutathione S-transferase (GST), metabolized sequentially by γ-glutamyl transpeptidase (GGT), cysteinylglycinase (CG) and N-acetyltransferase (AT) to form, ultimately, mercapturic acid. NAC, N-acetylcysteine

Figure 11 Cyclocondensation reaction of isothiocyanate and dithiocarbamate with 1,2-benzenedithiol

thiol conjugates. The assay has allowed quantitative assessment of total isothiocyanates in cruciferous vegetables and isothiocyanate equivalents in human fluids, including blood and urine. Because it reveals both isothiocyanates and their thiol metabolites, the total urinary concentrations of these compounds are not affected by dissociation of thiol conjugates to

isothiocyanates. Even though individual isothiocyanates and isothiocyanate metabolites can be quantified sensitively by other methods, including HPLC–mass spectrometry (Ji & Morris, 2003; Vermeulen et al., 2003), such analyses might not provide accurate values, since the metabolites are unstable and can dissociate to isothiocyanates.

Use of the cyclocondensation assay is nevertheless subject to some caveats. Although there are no endogenous sources of urinary isothiocyanates or dithiocarbamates in humans (Shapiro et al., 1998), non-dietary sources may exist. The contributions of cigarette smoke (possibly due to the presence of carbon disulfide, which is also detected in the assay), agricultural chemicals, chemicals used in the rubber industry and medical compounds such as disulfiram and antiseptics, should be considered (Zhang et al., 1996; Shapiro et al., 1998; Ye et al., 2002). Shapiro et al. (1998) found that when urine samples were stored at –20 °C, the cyclocondensation reactivity remained stable, but 35% of the dithiocarbamate content was lost in samples stored for 18 months at the same temperature.

Measuring metabolic disposition of isothiocyanates

Studies on dietary intake of isothiocyanates are still extremely limited, and the information below was obtained from studies of a small number of volunteers. Ye et al. (2002) determined the metabolic disposition of isothiocyanates from broccoli sprouts by giving four volunteers a single serving of a myrosinase-treated extract of 3-day-old broccoli sprouts containing 200 μmol total isothiocyanate. The isothiocyanate composition of the preparation was 77.2% sulforaphane or iberin and 22.8% iberin (aliphatic isothiocyanates with closely related chemical structures). The isothiocyanates were absorbed rapidly and reached peak plasma concentrations of 0.94–2.27 μmol/l 1 h after ingestion, which declined according to first-order kinetics (half-life, 1.77 ± 0.13 h). The cumulative urinary excretion of isothiocyanate equivalent at 8 h was $58.3 \pm 2.8\%$ of the dose. In a similar experiment, the cumulative urinary excretion of isothiocyanate equivalent at 72 h was $88.9 \pm 5.5\%$ (Shapiro et al., 2001). Similar results were obtained in volunteers given horseradish isothiocyanates (Shapiro et al., 1998), most of which are allyl- or phenylethyl-ITC (Liebes et al., 2001; Ji & Morris, 2003). For example, after a single serving of 20 ml of horseradish juice containing 74 μmol of isothiocyanates to 10 volunteers, $42 \pm 5\%$ of isothiocyanate

equivalent was recovered in urine within 10 h (Shapiro et al., 1998). Thus, isothiocyanates are rapidly and efficiently absorbed, rapidly cleared from blood and eliminated almost exclusively in urine.

The molecular basis for the rapid metabolic disposition of isothiocyanates in humans was elucidated by studying cultured human cells with the cyclocondensation assay (Zhang & Talalay, 1998; Zhang, 2000, 2001; Zhang & Callaway, 2002). Exposure of cells to an isothiocyanate led to rapid accumulation of the compound through conjugation with cellular thiols. GSH, the most abundant intracellular thiol, is the major driving force for isothiocyanate accumulation, and cellular GST enhances isothiocyanate accumulation by promoting conjugation reactions. Peak intracellular isothiocyanate accumulation was achieved within 0.5–3 h after the beginning of exposure to isothiocyanate, reaching 100–200 times the extracellular isothiocyanate concentration. Intracellularly accumulated isothiocyanate and conjugates were also rapidly exported by membrane transporters, including the multidrug resistance-associated protein (MRP)-1 and P-glycoprotein-1: the half-life of the accumulated isothiocyanate and conjugates in human prostate cancer LNCaP cells was only about 1 h.

These studies have begun to reveal the pharmacokinetics of ingested isothiocyanates in humans; however, the question remains as to when urine should be collected for assessment of dietary isothiocyanate intake. As dithiocarbamates are excreted rapidly in urine after ingestion of isothiocyanates, continuous urine collection over a sufficient period (e.g. 8 or 24 h) after isothiocyanate ingestion might be important for comparing urinary total isothiocyanate equivalents among individuals. Analysis of random spot urine samples might lead to incor-

rect conclusions about long-term dietary intake of isothiocyanates.

Cellular uptake of isothiocyanates is enhanced by GST isozymes (Zhang, 2001); however, export of intracellular isothiocyanate–GSH conjugates is also highly efficient without GST involvement (Zhang & Calloway, 2002). While GSTs are likely to be important in isothiocyanate metabolism, current understanding does not allow a prediction of the consequences of GST polymorphism on exposure of tissues or the rates and extent of urinary excretion of isothiocyanates and isothiocyanate conjugates.

Bioavailability of isothiocyanates from cruciferous vegetables

In a study designed to compare the bioavailability of isothiocyanate in fresh and steamed broccoli, 12 men were asked to eat 200 g of fresh or steamed broccoli, and urine samples were collected during the subsequent 24 h. The total content of isothiocyanate in fresh and steamed broccoli after treatment with myrosinase was virtually identical (1.1 and 1.0 μmol/g wet weight); however, the average 24-h urinary excretion of isothiocyanate equivalent was $32.3 \pm 12.7\%$ and $10.2 \pm 5.9\%$ of the amount ingested in fresh and steamed broccoli, respectively. Thus, the bioavailability of isothiocyanates from fresh broccoli was approximately three times greater than that from steamed broccoli, in which myrosinase was inactivated by heat (Conaway et al., 2000). In another study (Getahun & Chung, 1999), 350 g of watercress (containing 475 μmol total glucosinolates) was cooked in boiling water for 3 min to inactivate myrosinase and then eaten by nine volunteers. The 24-h urine samples showed a total urinary excretion of isothiocyanate equivalent ranging from 5.6 to 34.8 μmol, corresponding to 1.2–7.3% of the total glucosinolates ingested. In contrast, ingestion of

150 g of uncooked watercress resulted in excretion of 17.2–77.7% of the total ingested glucosinolates in 24-h urine. Clearly, myrosinase in the original vegetable contributed to the release of isothiocyanates from glucosinolates. It can also be inferred from these results that human myrosinase, known to exist in the intestinal flora (Shapiro et al., 1998; Getahun & Chung, 1999; Krul et al., 2002), might hydrolyse only a fraction of the glucosinolates ingested and might also vary widely in activity among individuals. Nevertheless, when enteric flora were reduced by a combination of mechanical cleansing and oral antibiotics after ingestion of 100 µmol of a broccoli glucosinolate preparation in which myrosinase had been inactivated, a dramatic reduction was seen in 72-h urinary excretion of isothiocyanate metabolites, falling from 11.3 ± 3.1% of the dose before treatment to 1.3 ± 1.3% after treatment (Shapiro et al., 1998). Not surprisingly, the extent of glucosinolate conversion to isothiocyanates by the myrosinase in vegetables is also affected by the length of time the vegetable is chewed. In a study in which four volunteers were each given 12 g of fresh broccoli sprouts containing 109 µmol total glucosinolates and were asked to either swallow without chewing or chew thoroughly before swallowing, thorough chewing resulted in significantly greater excretion of isothiocyanate equivalent (42.4 ± 7.5 µmol and 28.8 ± 2.6 µmol, respectively) in 24-h urine (Shapiro et al., 2001).

Assessing consumption of cruciferous vegetables by measuring isothiocyanate equivalents in urine

Controlled metabolic studies have shown that urinary isothiocyanate equivalent assayed by the cyclocondensation reaction reflects the amount of cruciferous vegetables eaten. Shapiro and colleagues (1998) found that the disposition of ingested isothio-cyanates was consistent between volunteers in different studies and that the urinary concentration of dithiocarbamates was proportional to an escalating dose regimen ($r^2 = 0.976$). The urinary concentrations peaked within < 8 h of consumption, but complete excretion took 24–72 h. In studies in which volunteers were given glucosinolates and isothiocyanates from broccoli sprouts, measurements of urinary isothiocyanate equivalent with this assay were highly reproducible (coefficient of variation, ≤ 10%), and their concentrations accurately reflected the absorption, metabolism and excretion of the isothiocyanate consumed. A strict linear relationship was observed between isothiocyanate dose and isothiocyanate equivalent in 72-h urine over an eightfold range of isothiocyanate dose (25–200 µmol) (Shapiro et al., 2001), with no evidence of a threshold. Fowke and colleagues (2001) reported that an acceptable dose–response relationship between intake of cruciferous vegetables and urinary dithiocarbamate was found only at intake levels of 100–200 g/day. The intake levels were achieved in a planned dietary intervention and were much higher than the 0.2 serving per day (one serving = one cup of raw leafy or one-half cup of cooked or chopped raw) estimated to be the average intake of cruciferous vegetables by residents of the USA in 1994–96 (Johnston et al., 2000).

In an Asian population (n = 246) who frequently ate cruciferous vegetables (mean daily intake of cooked, 40.6 g; mean daily isothiocyanate intake, 9.1 µmol), concentrations of total isothiocyanate in spot urine samples were significantly associated with cruciferous vegetable intake and isothiocyanate intake, estimated from a semi-quantitative food-frequency questionnaire (Seow et al., 1998). In 34 post-menopausal women who provided 24-h dietary recalls, responded to a questionnaire on vegetable and fruit intake and collected a 24-h urine sample (Fowke et al., 2001), the urinary isothiocyanate correlated well with the 24-h consumption of cruciferous vegetables (Pearson correlation coefficient, 0.57; p < 0.01) and with an 'unknown but true intake' calculated from a structural equation (Ocké & Kaaks, 1997). Single-void urine samples are clearly less reliable markers than urine collected over 8 or 24 h (Seow et al., 1998; London et al., 2000). The former are useful mainly for assigning participants to reasonable categories of intake (e.g. negative, positive, low, high), while the latter, especially repeated 8- or 24-h urine collection, allow realistic assessments of consumption of cruciferous vegetables or isothiocyanates.

Indoles
Metabolism and disposition

The mildly acid environment of the stomach induces chemical modification of indole-3-carbinol, which is dehydrated in acidic solutions and is converted to its active derivates (Grose & Bjeldanes, 1992). Thus, indole-3-carbinol administered intraperitoneally does not exert metabolic change in the host (Bradfield & Bjeldanes, 1987a). The main products of this chemical reaction are 3,3′-diindolylmethane, triindolylmethane and indolo[3,2-b]carbazole (Figure 12). Many other indole-3-carbinol-derived compounds were detected in experimental animals exposed to this compound (Stresser et al., 1995a; Anderton et al., 2003).

Most of the information derives from studies in vitro in which condensation products were collected without ascorbic acid. When glucobrassicin and neoglucobrassicin are degraded in the presence of ascorbic acid, various ascorbigens are formed. It has been estimated that 20–60% of indolyl glucosinolates are converted to

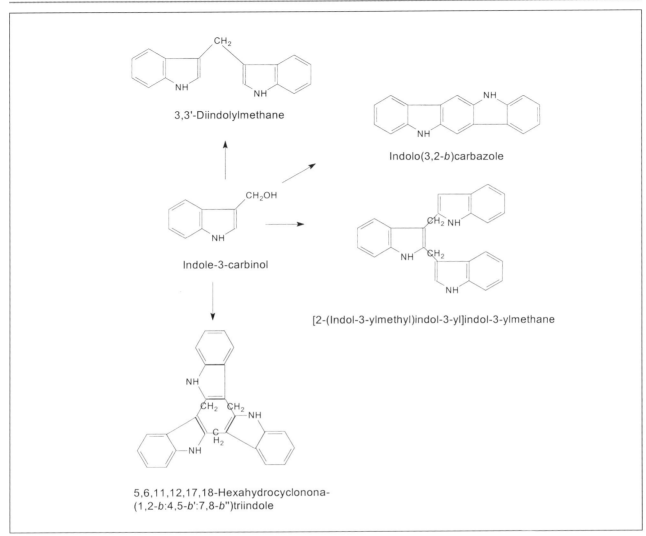

Figure 12   Indole-3-carbinol and its by-products

ascorbigens, depending on the pH (Buskov *et al.*, 2000; Hrncirik *et al.*, 2001).

Ascorbigen is unstable in acidic media (as in the stomach), giving rise to indolo[3,2-*b*]carbazole. About 20 times more indolo[3,2-b]carbazole was formed in vitro after incubation with ascorbigen than after incubation with indole-3-carbinol under identical conditions (Preobrazhenskaya *et al.*, 1993a).

3,3´-Diindolylmethane is the most common of derivative of indole-3-

carbinol, and it is the most stable, with the longest biological life (Broadbent & Broadbent, 1998a,b). pH affects the oligomerization process: only 5% of indole-3-carbinol was converted to 3,3´-diindolylmethane at neutral pH (Amat-Guerri *et al.*, 1984), but 80% was transformed at pH 4.5 (de Kruif *et al.*, 1991). As the pH falls, the production of indolo[3,2-*b*]carbazole and larger oligomers increases over that of 3,3´-diindolylmethane. Dilution of indole-3-carbinol favours the formation

of higher-order oligomers (Grose & Bjeldanes, 1992). In vitro at physiological pH, only 3,3´-diindolylmethane was detected after 48 h (Niwa *et al.*, 1994). In contrast, Staub *et al.* (2002) found that indole-3-carbinol was stable in cell-free medium or in cultured MCF-7 cells, with a half-life of about 40 h.

3,3´-Diindolylmethane can be extracted from the urine of volunteers given indole-3-carbinol. This assay has been used to estimate indole-3-carbinol intake, in order to correlate it with the severity of cervical dysplasia. In one volunteer given 150 mg of the indole, from whom urine was collected over the next 18 h, peak urinary excretion was observed after 7 h. In the same study, 10 women were treated with indole-3-carbinol for 4 weeks. In five treated with 200 mg/day, the mean urinary concentration of 3,3′-diindolylmethane was 12.1 ± 2.5 µg/mg creatinine; in the remaining five women, treated with 400 mg/day, the concentration was 15.6 ± 22.2 µg/mg creatinine (Sepkovic *et al.*, 2001). 3,3′-Diindolylmethane was also measured in plasma and blood of four women treated with 400 mg of indole-3-carbinol orally. The concentrations in plasma and serum were 0.1–0.4 µg/ml. No indole-3-carbinol was recovered in blood, confirming that it undergoes oligomerization in the stomach (Arneson *et al.*, 1999).

When indolo[3,2-*b*]carbazole was measured in two samples of faeces of volunteers eating controlled diets, both samples showed a chromatographic peak in the range 2–20 µg/kg (dry weight, w/w) (Kwon *et al.*, 1994).

The presence of other metabolites in human blood, urine or faeces has not been tested.

Induction and inhibition of metabolizing enzymes

Indoles modulate the activity of genes involved in the metabolism of both endogenous and exogenous compounds (Nho & Jeffery, 2001). Differences in dietary habits, in conjunction with metabolic gene polymorphisms, may partially explain ethnic differences in the ratio of 2-hydroxy-: 16-hydroxyestradiol in women's urine (Taioli *et al.*, 1996).

The metabolism of tobacco can also be influenced by dietary indole intake (Morse *et al.*, 1990a; Taioli *et al.*, 1997). Thirteeen healthy smokers treated with 400 mg of indole-3-carbinol for 5 days showed a change in the urinary levels of two metabolites of 4-(methylnitrosamino)-1-(3-pyridyl)-1-butanone (NNK): 4-(methylnitrosamino)-1-(3-pyridyl)-1-butanol and its glucuronide. These changes suggest that indole-3-carbinol increases NNK metabolism in smokers. It may also affect the metabolism of several other substances, including aflatoxins, alcohol and certain drugs (Fong *et al.*, 1990; Chung *et al.*, 1993; Manson *et al.*, 1997; Oganesian *et al.*, 1999).

In a study of structure–activity relationships of 3,3′-diindolylmethane analogues in human cells, substitutions at the 5 and 5′ positions induced the activity of both aromatase and ethoxyresorufin *O*-deethylase (EROD) activity, whereas analogues with a substitution in the bridging methylene carbon induced neither enzyme (Sanderson *et al.*, 2001)

Dimethyl 3,3′-diindolylmethane and tetramethyl 3,3′-diindolylmethane derivatives did not induce bacterial chloramphenicol acetyltransferase (CAT) reporter gene activity in T47D cell lines, and no aryl hydrocarbon (Ah) receptor antagonist activity was observed; however, no comparison was made with the induction ability of 3,3′-diindolylmethane under these conditions (McDougal *et al.*, 2001).

Experimental studies

Cruciferous vegetables
Metabolism and disposition
Few studies have been reported on the metabolism of isothiocyanates and indoles in experimental animals fed cruciferous vegetables.

Modulation of phase I and II enzymes[1]

The effects of cruciferous vegetables on phase I and II enzymes have been studied extensively (see also the section on intermediary biomarkers). Some of the studies addressed the effects of the vegetables themselves, while others focused on the effects of specific compounds in vegetables (e.g., glucosinolates, precursors of isothiocyanates and indoles). The vegetables studied were usually Brussels sprouts, cabbage, broccoli and cauliflower. The diets were often prepared by mixing lyophilized vegetables into the regular diet at concentrations of 2.5% up to 50% (w/w). In some studies, vegetables extracts were mixed into the regular diet after evaporation of the solvent, which was usually water, methanol or ethanol. Regardless of the study protocol and diet preparation, most of these studies showed that feeding cruciferous vegetables to animals generally induces phases I and II enzymes in the liver and intestinal tract.

Many biologically active compounds in cruciferous vegetables are likely to contribute to the effects on phase I and II activities, and the increased enzyme activities reflect a combined effect of these active compounds. Isothiocyanates and indoles are likely to have opposite effects on phase I enzymes, as indoles are strong inducers of cytochrome P450 enzymes, whereas isothiocyanates usually inhibit these enzymes (see below). Indoles also inhibit cytochrome P450 activity, however (Stresser *et al.*, 1995b; Takahashi *et al.*, 1995a). The induction of phase II enzymes such as GST by cruciferous vegetables is probably due to the concerted action of

---

[1]Usually, xenobiotic metabolizing enzymes are subdivided by toxicologists into phase I and phase II enzymes on the basis of whether they catalyse oxidation–reduction or conjugation reactions. Thus, NAD(P)H:quinone oxidoreductase 1 is sometimes classified as a phase I enzyme. In this Handbook, however, it is referred to as a phase II enzyme becuase it is coordinately regulated with xenobiotic conjugating enzymes through an antioxidant response element.

isothiocyanates and indoles. In all these studies, the contribution of isothiocyanates was difficult to assess quantitatively because of the presence of other active compounds in the vegetables (Loub et al., 1975; McDanell et al., 1989). Nevertheless, there is little doubt that the observed effects are due in part to isothiocyanates, as shown in studies with isothiocyanate as the only agent (see below).

Some reports have emphasized both the complexity of the phase I response to Brassica vegetables in rat models and the fact that it depends strongly on differences in the chemical composition of vegetables. Vang et al. (1991) studied the effects of broccoli on CYP1A1 and CYPIIB mRNA and proteins in rats fed freeze-dried vegetables for 7 days. In the colon, both CYP1A1 mRNA and protein were induced by the broccoli diet. CYPIA2 protein was present in the colon, but it was not altered by the diet, and the mRNA was not detectable. Paradoxically, CYPIIB mRNA was reduced, but the protein was increased. In the liver, CYPIIB and CYPIIE1 proteins were increased by the broccoli diet, but CYPIIB mRNA was not affected. In a later study in which different varieties of broccoli were fed to rats, it was also shown that modulation of cytochrome P450 and other phase I enzymes is critically dependent on the concentrations of glucosinolates and other biologically active phytochemicals in plant tissue (Vang et al., 2001). Various strategies have been used to overcome the problems due to the complexity of Brassica vegetables. Sorensen et al. (2001) fed rats a Brussels sprout extract containing a complex, incompletely characterized mixture of glucosinolates and their breakdown products for 4 days. No significant modulation of phase I enzymes but significant up-regulation of phase II enzymes was observed.

Bradfield and Bjeldanes (1984) fed rats a diet containing 25% (w/w) Brussels sprouts for 10 days and compared the effects on intestinal and hepatic GST activity with those of a diet containing indole-3-carbinol at 50–500 mg/kg. The Brussels sprouts diet increased GST activity by 1.9-fold in the gut and by 1.6-fold in the liver, but neither activity was significantly affected by purified indole-3-carbinol, even at the highest dose. The diet containing sprouts significantly increased the activities of Ah hydroxylase (by 3.6-fold) and ethoxycoumarin O-deethylase (by 3.2-fold). The same group (Bradfield et al., 1985) included hepatic GST in a study of the effects of 12 vegetables on phase I and phase II activity in mice. Diets containing 20% freeze-dried, powdered Brussels sprouts or cauliflower significantly increased the activities of GST (by 2.0- and 1.2-fold, respectively) and epoxide hydratase (both by 1.6-fold): the activity of ethoxycoumarin O-deethylase was increased significantly (by 2.2-fold) by cauliflower but that of Ah hydroxylase was not affected. The effects on enzyme activities were not confined to Brassica vegetables, although the high doses used make these results difficult to interpret.

Bogaards et al. (1990) studied the effects of dietary supplements of Brussels sprouts (2.5–30%), the sinigrin breakdown product allyl-ITC (0.03 and 0.1%) and goitrin (0.02%) on the GST subunit pattern in the liver and small intestinal mucosa of male rats. A statistically significant linear relationship was found between the amount of Brussels sprouts in the diet and induction of GST, with similar increases in the total amounts of GST subunits. When the average concentrations of sinigrin and progoitrin in the sprouts were 1835 µmol/kg and 415 µmol/kg, respectively, the subunit induction patterns in the liver and the small intestinal mucosa were similar to those

observed after feeding allyl-ITC, which caused stronger enhancement of subunit 2. When the average sinigrin concentration in the sprouts was as low as that of progoitrin (about 540 µmol/kg), however, a goitrin-like induction pattern was observed. The authors concluded that at least two compounds (probably allyl-ITC and goitrin) are responsible for the induction of GSTs in rat liver and small intestine by Brussels sprouts.

Thus, much of the induction of phase I and phase II enzymes by vegetables may be due to indoles. The vegetables studied, Brussels sprouts, cabbage, broccoli and cauliflower, have high concentrations of indole glucosinolates (glucobrassicin) and relatively little isothiocyanate glucosinolates (van Etten & Tookey, 1979; Fenwick & Heaney, 1983). Isothiocyanate-rich vegetables with a small amount of indoles might reduce phase I enzyme activity, as was observed in studies with pure isothiocyanate compounds (see below). The preparation of the vegetable diets for this type of experiment is an important consideration, as it might considerably alter the bioavailability of the hydrolysed products. The free isothiocyanates in freeze-dried broccoli samples are less bioavailable, as estimated from the mercapturic metabolite excreted in urine, and less effective in inducing quinone reductase activity in colon than freeze-dried broccoli samples containing intact glucosinolates (Keck et al., 2003). Equally important is the method of storage, which could have significant effects on the stability of compounds such as isothiocyanates.

A question of practical importance is whether cooked vegetables affect phase I and II enzymes. Cooked vegetables are devoid of myrosinase, the enzyme responsible for hydrolysing glucosinolates to release bioactive aglucones. In a study in which Wistar rats were fed a diet supplemented with cooked Brussels sprouts at 2.5–20% (w/w), various phase I and II enzymes were measured, including CYP1A1, CYP1A2 and CYP2B, GST, UDP-glucuronosyl transferases (UGTs) and NAD(P)H–quinone reductase (Wortelboer et al., 1992a). Almost all the enzymes were induced by the diet containing Brussels sprouts, and effects were seen as soon as 2 days after feeding. Although no direct comparison was made of the effects on these enzymes of cooked and uncooked vegetables, they appeared to have similar effects. This suggests that glucosinolates are hydrolysed to aglycones after ingestion of Brussels sprouts by a myrosinase-like microfloral activity in the rat intestinal tract. In a study of the influence of the intestinal microflora and dietary glucosinolates on hepatic cytochrome P450 enzymes (Nugon-Baudon et al., 1998), conventional rats and germ-free rats were fed a diet containing myrosinase-free rapeseed. While the effects of the glucosinolate-rich diet on these enzymes appeared to be complex, the rapeseed meal decreased total cytochrome P450 activity in conventional rats but not in germ-free rats, suggesting that the microflora present in the gut play a role.

The ability of nitriles to induce phase II enzymes was investigated in two studies. In a comparison of the effects of the major broccoli isothiocyanates and nitrile, groups of five 4-week-old male Fischer 344 rats were given 5-(methylsulfinyl)pentane nitrile in saline at 200, 500 or 1000 µmol/kg bw, sulforaphane in saline at 500 µmol/kg bw or saline, by gavage for 5 days. Controls and test animals given nitrile were pair-fed with semi-synthetic food throughout the study. The animals were killed 24 h after the last dose, and the activities of quinone reductase and GST were determined in cytosolic fractions from the liver, pancreas and colon mucosa. The nitrile had no effect,

while sulforaphane statistically significantly reduced both enzyme activities (Matusheski & Jeffery, 2001). In a subsequent study, groups of three male Fischer 344 rats [age not specified] were given the rapide seed nitrile crambene or sulforaphane at a dose of 50 mg/kg bw by gavage in corn oil for 7 days (515 µmol/kg bw for crambene, 282 µmol/kg bw for sulforaphane) (Keck et al., 2002). Controls were given corn oil only. Hepatic cytosolic quinone reductase activity was induced 1.5-fold by crambene and 1.7-fold by sulforaphane.

Isothiocyanates
Metabolism and disposition
The metabolism and tissue disposition of several isothiocyanates have been investigated extensively in rodents. These studies showed that the mercapturic acid pathway is the main route of metabolism of isothiocyanates, involving initial conjugation with GSH mediated by GSTs, followed by enzymatic degradation to its N-acetylcysteine conjugate (Meyer et al., 1995; Whalen & Boyer, 1998). Other, minor metabolites of isothiocyanates with an alkyl or aryl moiety have also been identified in animals. This section summarizes the data from these studies (Table 8).

Allyl isothiocyanate
In Wistar rats, the main urinary metabolite of allyl-ITC was the mercapturic acid N-acetyl-S-(N-allylthiocarbamoyl)-L-cysteine (allyl-ITC–N-acetylcysteine) (Mennicke et al., 1983). Studies of pharmacokinetics and metabolism were conducted after oral administration of [^{14}C]allyl-ITC labelled in the isothiocyanate moiety to Fischer 344 rats and B6C3F$_1$ mice (Bollard et al., 1997). Within 96 h, male and female mice had excreted ~80% of the ^{14}C in urine, and the rats had

excreted 50–55%. The rats had retained 20–25% of the dose in the carcass after 96 h. Faecal ^{14}C accounted for 6–12% and expired CO^2 for 4–7% of the dose. In this study, 67–85% of the ^{14}C in rat urine samples was identified as allyl-ITC–N-acetylcysteine by HPLC and positive-ion electrospray mass spectroscopy. Three metabolites were found in mice: 48–85% of the urinary ^{14}C was on thiocyanate, 7–52% on allyl-ITC–cysteine (Cys) conjugate and 8–12% on allyl-ITC–N-acetylcysteine (males only). In B6C3F$_1$ mice, allyl-ITC–N-acetylcysteine represented less than 20% of total urinary radioactivity; three other major and two minor unidentified urinary metabolites were also detected (Ioannou et al., 1984). In both rats and mice, 70–85% of the administered dose was collected in the urine by 72 h, while 13–15% was trapped as CO_2 (in rats only), and 3–6% of the ^{14}C, consisting of a single unidentified metabolite, was found in faeces. The urinary bladders of animals given [^{14}C]allyl-ITC showed sex and species differences, more ^{14}C being found in the bladder tissue of male rats. The amount of ^{14}C detected in bile from cannulated rats was greater than that in faeces, indicating possible enterohepatic circulation of metabolites and eventual urinary excretion (Borghoff & Birnbaum, 1986; Bollard et al., 1997). Biliary metabolites of allyl-ITC from Fischer 344 rats given [U-^{14}C]allyl-ITC by gavage were similar to urinary metabolites, as identified by HPLC, but the relative proportions differed considerably (Ioannou et al., 1984).

Benzyl isothiocyanate
Brüsewitz et al. (1977) identified the mercapturic acid of benzyl-ITC (benzyl-ITC–N-acetylcysteine) as its dicyclohexylamine salt after administration of benzyl-ITC and various thiol conjugates orally or by intraperitoneal or intravenous injection to rats. The

Table 8. Urinary metabolites in experimental animals after administration of isothiocyanates (ITCs)

Isothiocyanate	Route	Main metabolite(s)	Administered dose recovered (%)	Strain and species	Reference
Allyl-ITC	Oral	Allyl-ITC–NAC	40–50	Wistar rat	Mennicke et al. (1983)
		Allyl-ITC–NAC	75–82	Fischer 344 rat	Ioannou et al. (1984)
		Allyl-ITC–NAC	8–20	B6C3F$_1$ mouse	Ioannou et al. (1984)
		Allyl-ITC–NAC	67–85	Fischer 344 rat	Bollard et al. (1997)
		Allyl-ITC–NAC	8–12	B6C3F$_1$ mouse	Bollard et al. (1997)
		Allyl-ITC–Cys	7–52	B6C3F$_1$ mouse	Bollard et al. (1997)
		–SCN–	15–33	Fischer 344 rat	Bollard et al. (1997)
		–SCN–	48–85	B6C3F$_1$ mouse	Bollard et al. (1997)
		Allyl-ITC	0.3–0.4	Fischer 344 rat	Ioannou et al. (1984)
		Allyl-ITC	1.9	B6C3F$_1$ mouse	Ioannou et al. (1984)
Butyl-ITC	Oral	Butyl-ITC–NAC	10–20	Wistar rat	Mennicke et al. (1983)
Benzyl-ITC	Oral	Benzyl-ITC–NAC	Only metabolite	Wistar rat	Brüsewitz et al. (1977)
		Benzyl-ITC–NAC	Trace	Guinea-pig	Görler et al. (1982)
		4H4CBTT	23 ± 3	Guinea-pig	Görler et al. (1982)
Benzyl-ITC–Cys	Oral	Benzyl-ITC–NAC	62	Wistar rat	Brüsewitz et al. (1977)
		Benzyl-ITC	< 1	Wistar rat	Brüsewitz et al. (1977)
		Benzyl-ITC–Cys	< 1	Wistar rat	Brüsewitz et al. (1977)
		Hippuric acid	40	Beagle dog	Brüsewitz et al. (1977)
		4H4CBTT	33 ± 4	Guinea-pig	Görler et al. (1982)
Benzyl-ITC–NAC	Oral	Benzyl-ITC–NAC	Trace	Guinea-pig	Görler et al. (1982)
		4H4CBTT	4–9	Guinea-pig	Görler et al. (1982)
Phenethyl-ITC	Oral	Phenethyl-ITC–NAC	9–10	A/J mouse	Eklind et al. (1990)
		4H4CPETT	25	A/J mouse	Eklind et al. (1990)
		Phenethyl-ITC–NAC	> 90	Fischer 344 rat	Conaway et al. (1999)
		Phenethyl-ITC	< 1	Fischer 344 rat	Conaway et al. (1999)
Gluconasturtiin	Diet	Phenethyl-ITC–NAC	22± 8	A/J mouse	Chung et al. (1992)
6-Phenylhexyl-ITC	Oral	Unidentified	7 ± 1	Fischer 344 rat	Conaway et al. (1999)
		6-Phenylhexyl-ITC–NAC	Trace[a]	Fischer 344 rat	Conaway et al. (1999)
Sulforaphane	Intraperitoneal	Sulforaphane–NAC	~ 60	Sprague-Dawley rat	Kassahun et al. (1997)
		Erucin–NAC	~ 12	Sprague-Dawley rat	Kassahun et al. (1997)
Erucin	Intraperitoneal	Sulforaphane–NAC	~ 67	Sprague-Dawley rat	Kassahun et al. (1997)
		Erucin–NAC	~ 29	Sprague-Dawley rat	Kassahun et al. (1997)

NAC, N-acetylcysteine; Cys, cysteine; 4H4CBTT, 4-hydroxy-4-carboxy-3-benzylthiazolidine-2-thione; 4H4CPETT, 4-hydroxy-4-carboxy-3-phenylethylthiazolidine-2-thione
[a] Most metabolites found in faeces

thiol conjugates studied were GSH (benzyl-ITC–GSH), cysteinylglycine (benzyl-ITC–Cys–Gly) and cysteine (benzyl-ITC–Cys). The tissue disposi-tion of benzyl-ITC was studied with ^{14}C-labelled compound synthe-sized by radiolabelling the carbon adja-cent to the isothiocyanate group. When [^{14}C]benzyl-ITC–Cys was adminis-tered orally to fasted male and female rats, the mean peak plasma concentration of ^{14}C occurred within 45 min. The plasma radioactivity declined rapidly, with a half-time of 1–2 h. A total of 92.4% of the ^{14}C was collected in urine, while 5.6% appeared in faeces, and 0.4% was detected in expired air over 3 days. Metabolites in urine were analysed by mass spectrometry after isolation by thin-layer chromatography, and most of the recovered ^{14}C in the urine was identified as the mercapturic acid (see Figure 13A). Free [^{14}C]benzyl-ITC or [^{14}C]benzyl-ITC–Cys accoun-ted for less than 1% of the administered dose in urine. No other metabolite was iden-tified in rat urine after oral administra-tion of benzyl-ITC or its thiol conju-gates. Small amounts of free benzyl-ITC were recovered in urine after administration of the conjugates by the other routes, these presumably having been formed by dissociation of the conjugates in vivo. When the [^{35}S]Cys conjugate of benzyl-ITC was adminis-tered orally to the rats or unlabelled benzyl-ITC–Cys was given to rats pre-treated with [^{35}S]Cys to label the body sulfur pool, [^{35}S]mercapturic acid was recovered in the urine. Excretion of benzyl-ITC–[^{35}S]N-acetylcysteine after dosing with benzyl-ITC–[^{35}S]Cys indi-cates that the conjugate was at least partially absorbed unchanged, subse-quently acetylated and then excreted. The excretion of benzyl-ITC–[^{35}S]N-acetylcysteine after administration of unlabelled benzyl-ITC–Cys and –[^{35}S]Cys suggests that the benzyl-ITC–Cys was deconjugated and then reconjugated with [^{35}S]Cys or GSH.

The metabolism of benzyl-ITC in other species differs from that in the rat. When male guinea-pigs were given a single dose of benzyl-ITC or benzyl-ITC–Cys by gavage, 23.3 ± 2.8% and 33.1 ± 4.0 %, respectively, of the dose excreted in 24-h urine was identified as the cyclic 4-hydroxy-4-carboxy-3-benzylthiazolidine-2-thione, a mercaptopyruvic acid conjugate of benzyl-ITC (Görler et al., 1982; see

Figure 13B). The mechanism for its formation is thought to involve the cys-teine conjugate, which is transaminat-ed to the S-substituted mercaptopyru-vate, followed by enolysis and cycliza-tion to form the cyclic metabolite instead of the expected N-acetylated product. Benzyl-ITC–N-acetylcysteine was, however, also identified as a minor metabolite. Similar results were observed after administration of ben-zyl-ITC or benzyl-ITC–Cys to rabbits. Thus, guinea-pigs and rabbits excrete little mercapturic acid after isothio-cyanate metabolism and apparently do not readily form mercapturic acids after receiving other types of xenobiotic.

In beagle dogs given a single dose of [^{14}C]benzyl-ITC–Cys by gavage, absorption occurred more slowly than in rats, with a peak mean plasma concentration of ^{14}C within 1.5–6 h (Brüsewitz et al., 1977). After 3 days, 86.3% of the dose had been excreted in urine and 13.2% in faeces. Rather than the mercapturic acid metabolite, [^{14}C]hippuric acid (40% of the dose) was identified (see Figure 13C). Moreover, when benzyl-ITC–[^{35}S]Cys was administered, the radiolabelled metabolite was not recovered in urine, indicating that the conjugate had lost the cysteine moiety by dissociation. Components in dog urine with reten-tion times on thin-layer chromatogra-phy corresponding to the unchanged cysteine conjugate, free benzyl-ITC or other metabolites represented less than 5% of the administered dose. The fate of the free [^{35}S]Cys formed was not reported.

In summary, rats metabolized ben-zyl-ITC via the mercapturic acid path-way, and the major urinary metabolite formed was benzyl-ITC–N-acetylcys-teine. Guinea-pigs and rabbits excreted primarily the cyclic mercap-topyruvate conjugate 4-hydroxy-4-car-

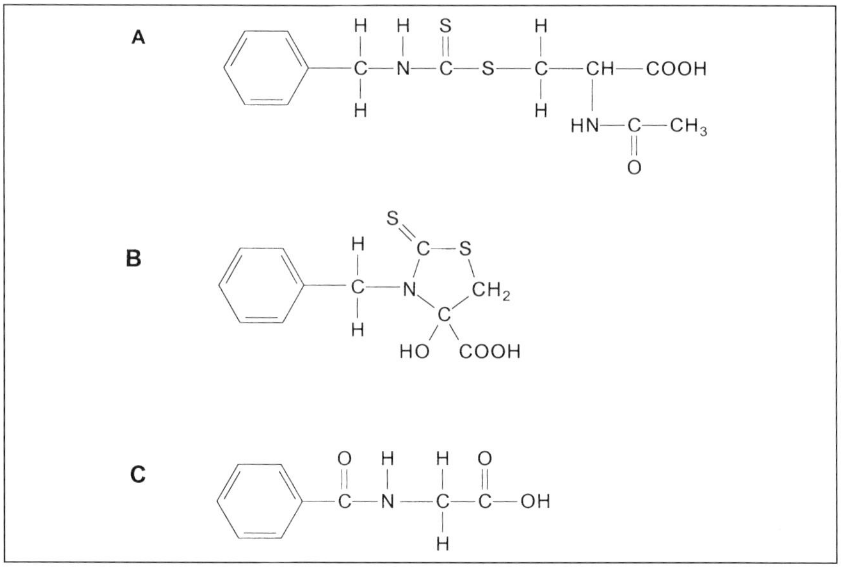

Figure 13 Variations in urinary metabolites of benzyl-isothiocyanate (ITC) and benzyl-ITC–cysteine
A) N-Acetyl-S-(N-benzylthiocarbamoyl)-L-cysteine (benzyl-ITC–N-acetylcysteine), the mercapturic acid of benzyl-ITC
B) 4-Hydroxy-4-carboxy-3-benzothiazolidine-2-thione, major benzyl-ITC–cysteine metabolite in urine of guinea-pigs and rabbits (Görler et al., 1982)
C) Hippuric acid, major metabolite in urine of beagle dogs (Brüsewitz et al., 1977)

boxy-3-benzythiozolidine-2-thione. In contrast, dogs excreted the glycine conjugate, hippuric acid, possibly because they readily hydroxylate the benzylic moiety of benzyl-ITC, which is subsequently oxidized to benzoic acid and conjugated.

Phenethyl isothiocyanate

The metabolism and tissue disposition of phenethyl-ITC was first investigated in A/J mice, a model of lung carcinogenesis (Shimkin & Stoner, 1975) widely used used to study the efficacy and mechanisms of action of chemopreventive agents (Eklind et al., 1990; Chung, 2001). When [^{14}C]phenethyl-ITC, synthesized from 2-phenyl[1-^{14}C]ethylamine hydrochloride, was administered by gavage (Eklind et al., 1990), 55.2% of the dose was excreted in urine within 72 h, and 23.3% appeared in faeces. Two major urinary metabolites were isolated in urine and identified by ^{1}H- and ^{13}C-nuclear magnetic resonance spectrometry and by HPLC co-chromatography with ultraviolet standards, as the cyclic mercaptopyruvic acid conjugate 4-hydroxy-4-carboxy-3-phenethylthiazolidine-2-thione (25% of the dose) and the mercapturic acid of phenethyl-ITC, N-acetyl-S-(N-phenethylthiocarbamoyl)-L-cysteine (phenethyl-ITC–N-acetylcysteine) (10% of dose) (see Figure 14). Radioactivity in major organs was determined up to 72 h after dosing: the maximum ^{14}C activity in liver and lung occurred within 2–8 h and 4–8 h, respectively. When gluconasturtiin, the glucosinolate precursor of phenethyl-ITC, was mixed into AIN-76 diet with myrosinase and fed to A/J mice, the same two metabolites were identified in urine, with only 22% recovery (Chung et al., 1992). These results indicate that gluconasturtiin is hydrolysed to phenethyl-ITC endogenously, presumably mediated by micro-flora in the gut, as described above.

The pharmacokinetics and metabolism of [^{14}C]phenethyl-ITC were investigated in Fischer rats. After receiving 10 μmol in corn oil by gavage, three rats were killed at various times over 48 h, and ^{14}C was evaluated in whole blood and in 13 major organs at each time, while ^{14}C in expired CO_2, urine and faeces was assayed at 8, 24 and 48 h. The ^{14}C in whole blood peaked at 2.9 h, with two compartments (α and β) with half-times of 2.4 and 21.7 h. The maximum activity of ^{14}C appeared in the liver at 2.5 h, the lungs at 4.5 h and brain at 6.5 h. The time course of absorption and elimination in selected tissues is presented in Figure 15. By 48 h, 88.7% of the ^{14}C was detected in urine, 9.9% in faeces and 0.1% trapped as CO_2. More than 90% of the urinary ^{14}C was identified by HPLC as phenethyl-ITC–N-acetylcysteine on the basis of co-chromatography with authentic standards, but less than 1% occurred as phenethyl-ITC in the urine. Measurement of radioactivity in homogenates of liver and lung by HPLC showed the presence of an additional major unidentified metabolite (other than phenethyl-ITC–GSH an phenethyl-ITC–Cys). A considerable amount of the

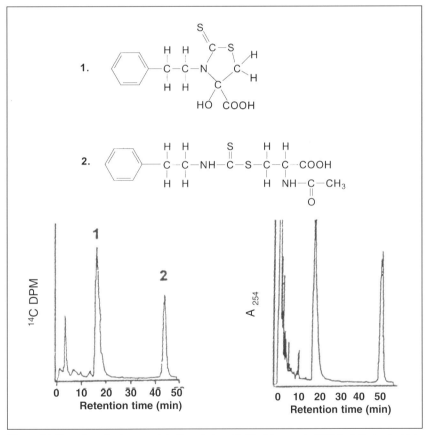

Figure 14 Detection of urinary metabolites of phenethyl-isothiocyanate (ITC) in A/J mice by high-performance liquid chromatography with radioflow and confirmation of the identities of metabolites by nuclear magnetic resonance and mass spectroscopy
1. 4-Hydroxy-4-carboxy-3-phenethylthiazolidine-2-thione, a cyclic mercaptopyruvic acid conjugate
2. N-Acetyl-S-(N-phenethylthiocarbamoyl)-L-cysteine (phenethyl-ITC–N-acetylcysteine, a mercapturic acid) (Eklind et al., 1990)

radioactivity was not extractable, sug-gesting covalent binding with proteins. Significant amounts of [^{14}C]phenethyl-ITC occurred in ethyl acetate extracts of faeces, indicating incomplete absorption from the intestinal tract (Conaway et al., 1999).

In beagle dogs given phenethyl-ITC, phenethylamine was identified in plasma by gas chromatography with mass spec-trometry and was proposed to be a degradation product of phenethyl-ITC formed at the low pH of the stomach (Negrusz et al., 1998). The urinary meta-bolites of phenethyl-ITC were not repor-ted, however. Therefore, as in humans, phenethyl-ITC is metabolized mainly via the mercapturic acid pathway in rats and appears in the urine as phenethyl-ITC–N-acetylcysteine; other pathways appear to predominate in mice and dogs.

Sulforaphane

Only one large study has been reported on the metabolism of sulforaphane in rodents (Kassahun et al., 1997). After intraperitoneal administration of sul-foraphane to male Sprague-Dawley rats, its metabolites were studied in urine and bile. Those identified in 24-h urine were the N-acetylcysteine conju-gates of sulforaphane and erucin, its reduction sulfur analogue, and accounted for ~60% and ~12% of the dose, respectively. When erucin was administered, the metabolites in 24-h urine consisted of ~67% sulfora-phane–N-acetylcysteine and ~29% erucin–N-acetylcysteine, indicating that oxidative metabolism of erucin was favoured over reductive metabolism of sulforaphane. Sulforaphane appeared to be metabolized by the phase I reac-tions of S-oxide reduction and dehydro-genation; the mercapturic acid pathway via GSH conjugation was the main route by which sulforaphane and its phase I metabolite erucin were elimi-nated. In another group of animals, bile was collected 0–4 h after administration of sulforaphane or [1,1-^{2}H$_2$]sulforaphane.

Biological fluids were analysed by liquid chromatogra-phy–mass spectroscopy. Five meta-bolites were detected in bile, two of which were identified as GSH conjugates of sulforaphane and erucin on the basis of synthesized standards. Two other metabolites were identified as the N-acetylcysteine conjugates of these compounds. A fifth biliary metabolite was tentatively identified as the GSH conjugate of a desaturated derivative of sulforaphane, Δ^1-sul-foraphane, on the basis of studies with deuterated [1,1-^{2}H$_2$]sulforaphane.

Modulation of phase I and phase II enzymes

Although the focus of this section is studies in experimental animals in vivo, the following section also briefly dis-cusses some in-vitro studies which should contribute to the interpretation of the in-vivo studies. Modulation of drug metabolizing enzymes by isothio-cyanates has been investigated exten-sively to determine the mechanism of their chemopreventive activity in ani-mal tumour bioassays (Zhang & Talalay, 1994; van Poppel et al., 1999;

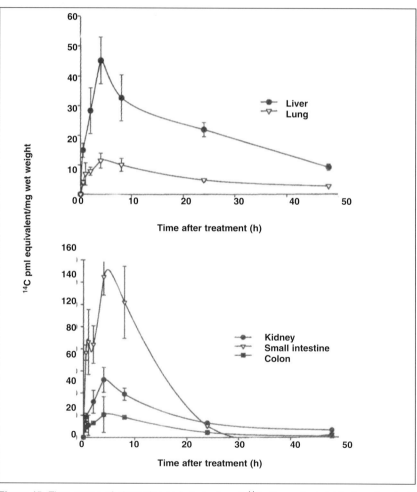

Figure 15 Time course of absorption and elimination of ^{14}C after oral administration of a single dose of 10 μmol of [^{14}C]phenethyl-isothiocyanate

Adapted from Conaway et al. (1999)

Hecht, 2000; Smith & Yang, 2000; Chung, 2001).

Phase I enzymes

Studies of structure–activity relationships in vivo and in vitro show that the length of the alkyl chain in arylalkyl isothiocyanates is critical for inhibition of cytochrome P450 enzymes, and increasing the alkyl chain length up to six carbons increases their chemopreventive efficacy (Morse et al., 1991; Guo et al., 1993; Jiao et al., 1994; Conaway et al., 1996). Considerable variability in the selectivity and potency of inhibition of cytochrome P450 enzymes by isothiocyanates has been found in vitro (Smith et al., 1993; Conaway et al., 1996; Jiao et al., 1996; Smith et al., 1996). Isothiocyanates are particularly strong inhibitors of CYP2B1, as determined by assays for pentoxyresorufin O-dealkylase (PROD). The inhibitory potency appeared to be positively correlated with the lipophilicity of the isothiocyanates. The most potent inhibitor of PROD was the synthetic 6-phenylhexyl-ITC. Morse et al. (1991) showed that it is also a remarkably effective inhibitor of lung tumorigenesis induced by NNK.

Oral administration of phenethyl-ITC to male Swiss-Webster mice inhibited the metabolism of acetaminophen by CYP2E1. Pretreatment with this isothiocyanate significantly reduced the amount of metabolites of acetaminophen in plasma and urine, prevented depletion of hepatic GSH and significantly reduced liver damage (Li et al., 1997).

Typically, administration of isothiocyanates to mice shortly before treatment with a carcinogen inhibits its metabolic activation (Chung et al., 1984a,b; Morse et al., 1989a, 1991). Nevertheless, isothiocyanates given 24 h before sacrifice as a single dose or in the diet sometimes enhanced cytochrome P450 activity measured at sacrifice (Guo et al., 1992, 1993; Smith et al., 1996). For example, an oral dose

of phenethyl-ITC to Fischer rats 24 h before death selectively inhibited CYP2E1-mediated N-nitrosodimethylamine demethylation by its demethylase, but the activity of PROD and the amount of CYP2B1 (measured by immunoblot analysis) were both markedly induced (Ishizaki et al., 1990). These results illustrate a complex mechanism in which regulation of cytochrome P450 enzymes by isothiocyanates is highly specific. In contrast to Fischer rats, mice given phenethyl-ITC in the diet showed induction of CYP2E1 activity in liver microsomes by a factor of 1.2 and of CYP2E1 activity in lung microsomes by a factor of 1.6 (Smith et al., 1993).

Phase II enzymes

Isothiocyanates induce phase II detoxification enzymes, including GSTs, quinone reductase, sulfatase and UGTs (Zhang & Talalay, 1994). GSTs catalyse the otherwise relatively slow conjugation reaction of GSH with electrophiles, including genotoxic chemicals and isothiocyanates. In vertebrates, GSTs are dimeric enzymes consisting of seven families: alpha, mu, kappa, pi, sigma, theta and zeta (Coles & Ketterer, 1990; Whalen & Boyer, 1998). Some isothiocyanates are readily conjugated by human GSTs M-1 (mu-1) and P1-1 (pi 1-1) but are slowly conjugated by other forms (Kolm et al., 1995; Meyer et al., 1995; Zhang et al., 1995). The rates of catalytic conjugation of isothiocyanates by various forms of GST apparently depend on the structure of the isothiocyanates. It is conceivable that isothiocyanate, as an inducer of GST, facilitates its own excretion by increasing its rate of conjugation with GSH.

Phenethyl-ITC is a tissue-specific inducer of phase II enzymes. In rats, a single administration of phenethyl-ITC by gavage induced quinone reductase and GST activity by 5.0- and 1.5-fold, respectively, in the liver, but the activi-

ties of these enzymes in lung and nasal mucosa were not significantly affected (Guo et al., 1992). Hepatic GST alpha and GST mu activity, protein levels and specific mRNAs were induced in a dose-dependent manner in rats given phenethyl-ITC orally for 3 days, and the hepatic GSH content increased twofold (Seo et al., 2000). In another study, administration of a relatively high concentration of phenethyl-ITC in the diet (1000 mg/kg) for 2 weeks induced both phase I and phase II enzymes in Fischer rats (Manson et al., 1997). The concentration of GST T1-1 in gastric mucosa was significantly increased after dietary administration of phenethyl-ITC at 450 mg/kg to male Wistar rats, but no such effect was observed in oesophagus, colon or liver (van Lieshout et al., 1998a).

Benzyl-ITC induced GST activity in the small intestine and liver of female ICR/Ha mice (Sparnins et al., 1982a). It was also the most potent component of papaya juice in inducing GST P1 in cultured rat liver epithelial cells. Subsequent investigations suggested that reactive oxygen intermediates are also involved (Nakamura et al., 2000a,b).

Sulforaphane was an extremely potent inducer of phase II enzymes in primary cultures of rat and human hepatocytes and in murine hepatoma cells (Prochaska et al., 1992; Zhang et al., 1992b; Mahéo et al., 1997). Related three- to eight-carbon (C3–C8) analogues of sulforaphane, the C3–C5 methyl sulfide isothiocyanates, C3–C5 methyl sulfone isothiocyanates and the methyl dithiocarbamyl analogue of sulforaphane, sulforamate, were also active inducers of a phase II detoxification enzyme (quinone reductase) in murine hepatoma cells (Zhang et al., 1992b; Gerhäuser et al., 1997; Rose et al., 2000). Northern blotting analysis of rat hepatocytes after treatment with sulforaphane showed dose-dependent induction of the mRNA of GST

Table 10. Cohort study of cruciferous vegetable consumption and risks for all cancers of the upper gastro-intestinal tract (including larynx)

Author, year, country	Years of follow-up	Cases/ cohort size, sex	Exposure assessment (no. of items)	Range contrast (no. of categories)	Relative risk (95% CI)	Statistical significance (p for trend when applicable)	Adjustment for confounding	Comments
Kjaerheim et al. (1998), Norway	25	71/10 960, male	FFQ (32), self-adminis-tered	≥ 6 times/month vs < monthly (3)	Cauliflower 0.8 (0.3–2.1)	> 0.5	Age, frequency of alcohol consumption, smoking level	Incidence
					Cabbage (0.8–4.1)	0.09		

FFQ, food frequency questionnaire

Table 11 Case-control studies of cruciferous vegetable consumption and risks for oral and pharynx cancers

Author, year, country	Cases (cancer sites)/controls, sex	Exposure assessment (no. of items)	Range contrast (no. of categories)	Relative risk (95% CI)	Statistical significance (p for trend when applicable)	Adjustment for confounding	Comments
McLaughlin et al. (1988), USA	871 (oral cavity and pharynx)/ 979 male, female	FFQ about usual adult diet (61), interview	Highest vs lowest (4)	Male: 0.6 Female: 0.8	0.006 0.83	Smoking and alcohol habits	Population-based Whites only Closest next of kin interviewed in 22% of cases
Gridley et al. (1990), USA	190 (pharynx, tongue and other parts of oral cavity)/201 male, female	FFQ about usual adult diet (61), interview	Highest vs lowest (4)	Male: 0.5 Female: 0.2	0.10 0.03	Smoking and alcohol habits and calories	Population-based Blacks only Interviews with next-of-kin in 56 cases and 3 controls
Franceschi et al. (1991a), Italy	302 (oral cavity and pharynx)/- 699 male, female	FFQ about recent diet (40)	Highest vs lowest (3)	1.0		Age, sex	Hospital-based No individual matching
Zheng et al. (1992a), China	204 (oral cavity and pharynx)	FFQ about usual diet in previous 10 years (41, 30 fruit and vegetables), interview	Highest vs lowest (3)	Male 0.76 Female 1.52		Smoking and education	Population-based
Garrote et al. (2001), Cuba	200 (oral cavity and pharynx)/ 200 male, female	FFQ about lifetime dietary habits, interview	≥ 4 vs 0 servings/ week(3)	1.11 (0.62–2.01)	0.54	Sex, age, area of residence, education, smoking and drinking habits	Hospital-based
Lissowska et al. (2003), Poland	122 (oral cavity, and pharynx)/ 124 male, female	FFQ (25), interview	≥ 1 vs < 1/week (2)	0.59 (0.33–1.06)		Sex, age, residence, smoking and drinking habits	Hospital-based
Sánchez et al. (2003), Spain	375 (cancer of oral cavity and oropharynx) / 375 male, female	FFQ (25), interview	≥ 2 vs 0 serving/- week (3)	1.33 (0.85–2.07)	0.19	Sex, age, centre, years of schooling, smoking and drinking habits	Hospital-based Three areas

FFQ, food frequency questionnaire

Table 12. Case–control study of cruciferous vegetable consumption and risk for salivary gland cancer

Author, year, country	Cases/ controls, sex	Exposure assessment (no. of items)	Range contrasts (no. of categories)	Relative risk (95% CI)	Statistical significance (p for trend when applicable)	Adjustment for confounding	Comments
Zheng et al. (1996) China	41/414 male, female	FFQ about usual frequency in previous 10 years (41, 30 fruit and vegetables), interview	Highest vs lowest (3)	0.6 (0.3–1.3)	> 0.10	Sex, age and income	Population-based

Table 13. Case–control study of cruciferous vegetable consumption and risk for nasopharynx cancer

Author, year, country	Cases/ controls, sex	Exposure assessment (no. of items)	Range contrasts (no. of categories)	Relative risk (95% CI)	Statistical significance (p for trend when applicable)	Adjustment for confounding	Comments
Armstrong et al. (1998), Malaysia	282/282 male, female	FFQ about diet 5 years before diagnosis and at age of 10 years (55), interview	Chinese flowering cabbage ≥ weekly vs < weekly (2)	0.64 (0.40–1.04)[a] 0.47 (0.29–0.77)[b]	0.02		Population-based (OR = 0.5 for lifetime consumption)
			Chinese kale ≥ weekly vs monthly (3)	0.63 (0.39–1.01)[b] 0.71 (0.46 1.09)[a]	0.07		

FFQ, food frequency questionnaire; OR, odds ratio
[a] Diet in recent 5 years
[b] Diet at age 10

Table 14. Case–control studies of cruciferous vegetable consumption and risk for oesophagus cancer

Author, year, country	Cases/controls, sex	Exposure assessment (no. of items)	Range contrasts (no. of categories)	Relative risk (95% CI)	Statistical significance (p for trend when applicable)	Adjustment for confounding	Comments
Gao et al. (1994), China	902 (624 male, 278 female)/ 1552 (851 male, 701 female)	FFQ on diet 5 years before interview (81), interview	Highest vs lowest (4)	Male: 0.8 Female: 1.1	0.51 0.28	Age, education, birthplace, tea drinking, cigarette smoking and alcohol drinking (only for men)	Population-based
Hu et al. (1994), China	196/392 male, female	FFQ about recent diet and diet in 1966 (32), interview (no mention which data used)	Chinese cabbage (fresh) > 54 vs < 18 kg/year (4)	0.8 (0.4–1.7)	0.38	Alcohol, smoking, income, occupation	Hospital-based
Brown et al. (1995), USA	174 adeno-carcinoma/ 750 white male	FFQ about usual adult diet (60), interview	Highest vs lowest (4)	0.3	< 0.001	Age, area, smoking, alcohol drinking, income, calories from food, body mass index	Population-based Included broccoli, cooked cabbage, coleslaw, cauliflower and 'southern greens'
Brown et al. (1998), USA	333 (114 white, 219 black) squamous-cell cancer / 1238 (681 white 557 black), male	FFQ about usual adult diet (60)	Highest vs lowest (4)	White: 0.7 Black: 0.8	0.33 0.50	Age, area, smoking, alcohol drinking, food calories	Population-based Included broccoli, cooked cabbage, coleslaw, cauliflower and 'southern greens'

FFQ, food frequency questionnaire

Table 15. Cohort studies of cruciferous vegetable consumption and risk for stomach cancer

Author, year, country	Years of follow-up	Cases/ cohort size, sex	Exposure assessment (no. of items)	Range contrasts (no. of categories)	Relative risk (95% CI)	Statistical significance (*p* for trend when applicable)	Adjustment for confounding	Comments
Chyou et al. (1990), Hawaii (Japanese)	18	111/361 (subcohort), male	24-h recall (54), interview	Consumer vs non-consumer (2)	0.7 (0.4–1.2)	0.07	Age, smoking	Case–cohort Incidence analysis Whole cohort: 8006
Kneller et al. (1991), USA	20	75/17 633, male	FFQ (35), self-administered	Highest vs lowest (4)	1.3 (0.67–2.68)	Not significant	Age, cigarette smoking	Mortality
Botterweck et al. (1998), Netherlands	6.3	281/3123 (subcohort), male, female	FFQ (150)	58 vs 10 g/day (5), median values	0.93 (0.61–1.43)	0.29	Age, sex, smoking, education, stomach disorders, family history of gastric cancer, total fruit consumption	Incidence Case–cohort analysis Whole cohort: 120 852

FFQ, food frequency questionnaire

Table 16. Case–control studies of cruciferous vegetable consumption and risk for stomach cancer

Author, year, country	Cases/ controls, sex	Exposure assessment (no. of items)	Range contrasts (no. of categories)	Relative risk (95% CI)	Statistical significance (p for trend when applicable)	Adjustment for confounding	Comments
Correa et al. (1985), USA	White: 94/99 Black: 52/72 male, female Matched by race, sex and age (within 5 years)	FFQ (59), interview	Broccoli Above vs below median (2)	White: 1.04 (0.66–1.65) Black: 0.50 (0.29–0.85)		Age, sex, race, respondent status, education, income, tobacco and alcohol use	Hospital-based
Risch et al. (1985), Canada	246/246 male, female Matched by sex, age, province of residence	Dietary history (94), interview	Increase of 100 g/day	0.65 (0.38–1.12)	0.11	Total food intake, ethnicity	Population-based
Boeing et al. (1991), Poland	741/741 male, female	FFQ (43), interview	Highest vs lowest (3)	Cabbage: 0.62 Cauliflower: 0.81	0.01 0.07	Age, sex, occupation, education, residence	Hospital-based Multicentre
Gonzalez et al. (1991), Spain	354/354 male, female Matched by age, sex and area of residence	Dietary history questionnaire (77), interview	Highest vs lowest (4)	0.9 (0.6–1.4)		Total calories and other vegetables	Hospital-based Multicentre
Hansson et al. (1993), Sweden	338/669 male, female	FFQ (45), interview, diet in adolescence	Broccoli, highest vs lowest (2) Cabbage. highest vs lowest (3)	0.63 (0.41–0.96) 0.64 (0.41–0.98)		Age, sex, socio-economic status	Population-based Slightly weaker associations for diet 20 years before interview
Lee et al. (1995), Republic of Korea	213/213 male, female	FFQ (64), interview	Cabbage ≥ 2–3 times/week vs none (3)	0.2 (0.02–0.3)	< 0.05	Age, sex, education, economic status, residence, other dietary factors	Hospital-based

Table 16 (contd)

Author, year, country	Cases/controls, sex	Exposure assessment (no. of items)	Range contrasts (no. of categories)	Relative risk (95% CI)	Statistical significance (p for trend when applicable)	Adjustment for confounding	Comments
Harrison et al. (1997), USA	91 (60 intestinal, 31 diffuse)/132 male, female	FFQ, self-administered	Increase in one standard deviation	Intestinal: 0.8 (0.5–1.5) Diffuse: 0.9 (0.5–1.7)		Calorie intake, age, sex, race, education, smoking, alcohol, body mass index	Hospital-based
Ji et al. (1998), China	770/819 male 354/632 female Matched by age and sex	FFQ (74), interview	≥ 60 vs ≤ 37.6 servings/month (4)	Male: 0.8 (0.6–1.1) Female: 0.8 (0.5–1.1)	0.07 0.20	Age, income, education, smoking, alcohol drinking	Population-based Response rate: 65.3% cases, 85.8% controls
Ekström et al. (2000), Sweden	Cardia 73, non-cardia 401/1052, male, female Matched by age, sex	FFQ (45), dietary habits 20 years before interview	≥ 2/week vs never or seldom (4)	Cardia: 0.7 (0.3–1.4) Non-cardia: 0.8 (0.6–1.2)	0.24 0.19	Age, sex, total calorie intake, smoking, body mass index, area, no. of siblings, socio-economic status, no. of meals/day, multi-vitamin supplements, table salt use, urban residence	Population-based Similar finding by histology Included broccoli, Brussels sprouts, kale and white cabbage
Huang et al. (2000), Japan	1111/26 996 male, female	FFQ, self-administered	Cabbage > 3 times/week vs < 3 times/month	Gastric cancer family history: (+) 0.73 (0.52–1.04) (–) 0.85 (0.70–1.04)		Age, sex	Hospital-based
De Stafani et al. (2001), Uruguay	160/320 male, female Matched for sex, age, residence and urban or rural status	FFQ (64), interview	> 16.0 g/day vs none (3)	1.72 (0.94–3.14)	0.21	Age, sex, residence, urban or rural status, education, body mass index, total energy intake	Hospital-based
Ito et al. (2003)	508/36 490 controls presenting at same centre at same time Female	FFQ, self-administered	Cabbage ≥ 5 vs < 1 times/week (4)	0.79 (0.55–1.13)		Age, year, season of first hospital visit, smoking habits, family history of gastric cancer	Hospital-based Findings similar for differentiated and undifferentiated gastric cancer

FFQ, food frequency questionnaire

Table 17. Cohort studies of consumption of cruciferous vegetables and risk for colorectal cancer

Author, year, country	Years of follow-up	Cases/ cohort size, sex	Exposure assessment (no. of items)	Range contrasts (no. of categories)	Relative risk (95% CI)	Statistical significance (p for trend when applicable)	Adjustment for confounding	Comments
Steinmetz et al. (1994), USA	5	212 colon/ 41 837, female	FFQ (127), at baseline, self-adminis-tered	> 4.0 vs < 1.5 servings/-week (4)	1.12 (0.74–1.70)	> 0.05	Age, energy	Incidence Iowa Women's Health Study
Platz et al. (1997), USA	9	690 (polyps)/ 16 448, male	FFQ (131), self-adminis-tered	1 vs 0.1 servings/day (5), median values	0.98 (0.71–1.35)	0.60	Age, endoscopy before 1986, family history of colorectal cancer, body mass index, pack–years smoked, use of multi-vitamins, physical activity, regular aspirin use, intake of energy, alcohol, red meat and methionine	Incidence Members of Health Professionals study who had left-sided adenomas and hyperplastic polyps at endoscopy
Hsing et al. (1998), USA	11.5	145 (colo-rectal)/17 633 male	FFQ (35), at baseline, self-adminis-tered	> 4.5 vs < 1.2 times/ month (4)	1.4 (0.9–2.2)	0.2	Age, energy, smoking, alcohol	Mortality Lutheran Brotherhood cohort; whites Risks for colon and colorectal cancer deaths almost identical
Pietinen et al. (1999), Finland	Mean = 8	185 colorectal/ 26 926, male	FFQ (276), at baseline, self-adminis-tered	39 vs 0 g/day (median values) (4)	1.6 (1.0–2.3)	0.04	Age, intervention group, years smoking, body mass index, alcohol, education, physical activity, calcium	Incidence Originally a vitamin supplement trial All smokers

Table 17 (contd)

Author, year, country	Years of follow-up	Cases/ cohort size, sex	Exposure assessment (no. of items)	Range contrasts (no. of categories)	Relative risk (95% CI)	Statistical significance (p for trend when applicable)	Adjustment for confounding	Comments
Michels et al. (2000), USA	16	569 colon, 155 rectum/ 88 764, female	FFQ (61 and then 127), at baseline, self-administered	≥ 5 vs < 1 servings/ week (5)	Colon: 0.89 (0.68–1.15) (RR for 1 additional serving/day: 1.00 (0.83–1.21)) Rectum: 1.29 (0.74–2.26) (RR for 1 additional serving/day: 1.08 (0.75–1.54))		Age, family history of colorectal cancer, sigmoidoscopy, height, body mass index, smoking, alcohol, physical activity, menopausal status, hormone replacement therapy, aspirin, vitamin supplements, energy (standard), red meat	Incidence Nurses Health Study cohort (female) and Health Professionals Follow-up Study (male) Pooled analysis of two cohorts
	10	368 colon, 89 rectum/ 47 325 male						
Voorrips et al. (2000a), Netherlands	6.3	313 colon, 201 rectum/ 58 279 male	FFQ (150), at baseline, self-administered	58 vs 11 g/day (median values) (5)	*Men* Colon: 0.76 (0.51–1.13)	0.11	Age, family history, alcohol	Incidence
					Rectum: 0.88 (0.56–1.39)	0.94		
		274 colon, 122 rectum/ 62 573 female			*Women* Colon: 0.51 (0.33–0.80)	0.004		
					Rectum: 1.66 (0.94–2.94)	0.05		
McCullough et al. (2003), USA	6	298/62 609 male 210/70 554 female Colon only	FFQ (68), self administered	Men: > 0.41 Vs < 0.08 Women: ≥ 0.5 vs < 0.11 (5)	Men: 0.74 (0.51–1.08)	0.15	Age, exercise, aspirin, smoking, family history of colorectal cancer, body mass index, education, energy, multivitamins, total calcium, red meat, hormone replacement therapy	Incidence Follow-up of American Cancer Society cancer prevention study II
					Women: 0.91 (0.58–1.44)	0.55		

FFQ, food frequency questionnaire; RR, relative risk

Table 18. Case–control studies of consumption of cruciferous vegetables and risk for colorectal cancer

Author, year, country	Cases/ controls, sex	Exposure assessment (no. of items)	Range contrasts (no. of categories)	Relative risk (95% CI)	Stastistical significance (p for trend when applicable)	Adjustment for confounding	Comments
Miller et al. (1983), Canada	Colon 348 (171 male, 177 female), rectum 194 (114 male, 80 female)/535 hospital and 542 population controls	FFQ (> 150), interview	Highest vs lowest (3)	*Male* Colon: 0.9 Rectum:0.9 *Female* Colon: 0.7 Rectum: 0.8	0.35 0.28 0.05 0.26	Age, saturated fat, other foods	Hospital-based and population-based
Kune et al. (1987), Australia	Colon 392, rectum 323/727 male, female	Dietary history (> 300)	Males: > 425 vs < 105 g/ week (5) Females: > 385 vs < 105 (5)	0.57 (0.44–0.75)	< 0.05	Age, sex	Population-based
Hoff et al. (1988), Norway	40/77 male, female	Dietician enquiry	Above and below median	Colorectal adenoma: 0.92	–	–	Endoscopy screening study; population-based; subjects aged 50–59 only
La Vecchia et al. (1988), Italy	Colon 339, rectum 236/778 male, female	FFQ (29)	Highest vs lowest (3)	Colon: 1.09 Rectum: 0.86		Age, sex	Hospital-based
Young & Wolf (1988), USA	Colon 353/ 618 male, female	FFQ (25), diet after age 35	8 times/month vs 1/month (4)	0.59 (0.41–0.85)		Age, sex and age × sex	Population-based Whites Similar findings for distal and proximal colon

Table 18 (contd)

Author, year, country	Cases/ controls, sex	Exposure assessment (no. of items)	Range contrasts (no. of categories)	Relative risk (95% CI)	Stastistical significance (p for trend when applicable)	Adjustment for confounding	Comments
Lee et al. (1989), Singapore (Chinese)	Colon 131, rectum 71/426 male, female	FFQ (116), interview	Highest vs lowest (3)	Colorectal: 0.50 (0.32–0.78)	< 0.01	Age, sex, dialect, education, occupation	Hospital-based Response: 82% cases, 87% controls
Benito et al. (1990), Spain	Colon 144, rectum 130/295 male, female	FFQ (99), interview	25 times/ month vs no consumption (4)	0.54	< 0.05	Age, sex, weight 10 years previously	Population-based
Bidoli et al. (1992), Italy	Colon 123, rectum 125/699 male, female	FFQ, interview	Highest vs lowest (3)	Colon: 0.6 Rectum: 0.6		Age, sex, social status	Hospital-based
Peters et al. (1992), USA	Colon 746/746 White male, female	Semi-quantitative FFQ (116), interview	Risk increase per 10 servings/ month	1.00 (0.99–1.01)		Age, sex, neighbourhood, fat, protein, carbo-hydrates, family history, weight, physical activity, pregnancy history, alcohol, calcium	Population-based
Steinmetz & Potter (1993), Australia	Colon 121/241 male, 99/197 female	FFQ (141), self-adminis-tered	Male: ≥ 5.8 vs ≤ 1.7 Female: ≥ 6.7 vs ≤ 2.2 servings/week (4)	Male: 1.10 (0.57–2.14) Female: 1.12 (0.51–2.46)		Age, occupation, Quetelet index, alcohol intake, protein intake, age at first live birth for women	Population-based
Witte et al. (1996), USA	488/488 male, female	Semi-quantitative FFQ (126)	7 vs 0.5 servings/week (5), median values	Colorectal adenomas 0.67 (0.41–1.09)	0.07	Race, body mass index, physical activity, smoking, calories, saturated fat, dietary fibre, folate, β-carotene, vitamin C	Subjects for screening sigmoidoscopy Analysis within matched pairs

Table 18 (contd)

Author, year, country	Cases/ controls, sex	Exposure assess- ment (no. of items)	Range contrasts (no. of categories)	Relative risk (95% CI)	Stastistical significance (p for trend when applicable)	Adjustment for confounding	Comments
Lin et al. (1998), USA	459/507, male, female	Semi- quantitative FFQ (126)	Highest vs lowest (4)	Colorectal adenoma: 0.66 (0.44–1.0)	0.04	Age, smoking, date of sigmoidoscopy, clinic, sex, saturated fat, energy, fruit and vegetable intake	Persons undergoing sigmoidoscopy at 2 clinics Significant inverse association with broccoli alone
Almendingen et al. (2001), Norway	87/35 hospital and 35 healthy controls, referred for sigmoidoscopy, male, female	5-day dietary record	≥ 61 vs ≤ 6 g/day (3)	Colorectal adenoma Hospital controls: 0.3 (0.1–1.1) Healthy controls: 0.9 (0.2–4.6)	0.06 0.8	Body mass index, colorectal cancer among first-degree relatives, energy, fat, fibre, smoking status	Hospital-based and population- based Subjects in a randomized trial, age- and sex- matched
Deneo- Pellegrini et al. (2002), Uruguay	Colon 260, rectum 224/1452 male, female	FFQ (64), interview	Highest vs lowest (4)	Colorectum 1.2 (0.8–1.6)	0.31	Age, sex, education, residence, urban or rural status, family history of colon cancer, body mass index, total energy, red meat intake	Hospital-based Response rate: cases 97%, controls 98%
Smith- Warner et al. (2002), USA	564/535 male, female	Semi- quantitative FFQ (153)	Highest vs lowest (3) Mean values: male, 4.9 vs 0.6, female, 6.7 vs 1.0 servings/ week	Colorectal adenomas Male: 0.84 (0.56–1.25) Female: 1.37 (0.83–2.25)	0.74 0.44	Age, energy intake, fat intake, body mass index, smoking, alcohol, use of NSAIDs, multi- vitamins, hormone replacement therapy	Population-based Cases from colonoscopy clinic, community controls (response rate: cases 68%, controls 65%)

FFQ, food frequency questionnaire; NSAID, non-steroidal anti-inflammatory drug

Table 19. Cohort study of cruciferous vegetable consumption and risk for pancreas cancer

Author, year, country	Years of follow-up	Cases/ control, sex	Exposure assessment (no. of items)	Range contrasts (no. of categories)	Relative risk (95% CI)	Statistical significance (*p* for trend when applicable)	Adjustment for confounding	Comments
Stolzenberg-Solomon et al. (2002), Finland	13	163 / 27 111 male smokers	FFQ (> 200), self-administered, portion size	Highest vs lowest (5)	0.82 (0.50–1.32)	0.44	Age, years of smoking, energy	Incidence Alpha-Tocopherol β-Carotene trial

FFQ, food frequency questionnaire

Table 20. Case–control studies of cruciferous vegetable consumption and risk for pancreas cancer

Author, year, country	Cases / controls, sex	Exposure assessment (no. of items)	Range contrasts (no. of categories)	Relative risk (95% CI)	Statistical significance (p for trend when applicable)	Adjustment for confounding	Comments
Olsen et al. (1989), USA	212/220 male	FFQ	≥ 9 vs ≤ 2 times/month (3)	0.57 (0.31–1.04)		Age, education, history of diabetes, cigarette smoking, alcohol and meat consumption	Population-based Data for 81% of cases ascertained Results similar in interviews with spouses
Baghurst et al. (1991), Australia	104/253 male, female	FFQ (179)		Significantly higher intake of Brussels sprouts, coleslaw, broccoli by controls than cases			Population-based Response rate: 62% for male and 63% for female cases, and 57% and 51% for controls
Bueno de Mesquita et al. (1991), Netherlands	164/480 male, female	Semi-quantitative FFQ (116)	Highest vs lowest (5)	0.32	< 0.05	Age, sex, response status (direct or proxy), smoking, energy	Population-based Overall response rate, 72% More than half the cases interviewed directly
Silverman et al. (1998), USA	436/2003 male, female	FFQ (60), interview	> 4 vs < 1.5 servings/ week (4)	0.5 (0.4–0.8)	0.004	Age, race, study area, calories from food, diabetes mellitus, cholecystectomy, body mass index, cigarette smoking, alcohol, income (men), marital status (women)	Population-based Multicentre study 1153 cases identified Only direct interviews of survivors performed (no proxy interviews) 78% of ascertained potential controls interviewed

FFQ, food frequency questionnaire

Table 21. Case–control studies of cruciferous vegetable consumption and risk for larynx cancer

Author, year, country	Cases / controls, sex	Exposure assessment (no. of items)	Range contrasts (no. of categories)	Relative risk (95% CI)	Statistical significance (*p* for trend when applicable)	Adjustment for confounding	Comments
Zheng, W. et al. (1992b), China	201/414 male, female	FFQ (41, 26 vegetables), interview, frequency, portion size	Highest vs lowest (3)	Male: 0.7 Female: 3.0 (1.0–9.2)	0.21	Age, education, smoking	Population-based No control for alcohol
De Stefani et al. (2000), Uruguay	148/444 male	FFQ (62, 11 vegetables), interview, frequency, portion size	Incremental risk: Cabbage 3.6 g/day Cauliflower 1.3 g/day	0.98 (0.74–1.30) 0.85 (0.63–1.16)		Age, residence, urban or rural, body mass index, smoking, intake of alcohol and energy	Hospital-based

FFQ, food frequency questionnaire

Table 22. Cohort studies of cruciferous vegetable consumption and risk for lung cancer

Author, year, country	Years of follow-up	Cases/ cohort size, sex	Exposure assessment (no. of items)	Range contrasts (no. of categories)	Relative risk (95% CI)	Statistical significance (p for trend when applicable)	Adjustment for confounding	Comments
Chow et al. (1992), USA	20	219/17 633 male	FFQ (35), self-administered, frequency	> 8 vs < 2 times/month (4)	0.8 (0.5–1.4)		Age, smoking status (six categories), occupation	Mortality Lutheran Brotherhood
Feskanich et al. (2000), USA	Female: 12 Male: 10	519/77 823 female 274/47 778 male	FFQ (116, 23 vegetables), self-administered, frequency, portion size; validated	Female: > 4.8 vs < 1.4 servings/-week (5) Male: > 5.0 vs < 1.4 servings/week (5)	0.74 (0.55–0.99) 1.11 (0.76–1.64)		Age, follow-up cycle, smoking status, years since quitting, cigarettes/day (current smokers), age at start of smoking, total energy intake, availability of data on diet after baseline measure	Incidence Nurses Health Study: risk for one additional serving/day 0.78 (0.59–1.04) Health Professionals Study: risk for one additional serving/day 1.20 (0.88–1.63)
Voorrips et al. (2000b), Netherlands	6.3	1010/2953 male, female	FFQ (150, 21 vegetables), self-administered, frequency, portion size; validated	58 vs 10 g/day (median values) (5) ≥ 3 times/-week vs ≤ 1 time/month (5)	0.7 (0.5–1.0) 0.5 (0.3–0.9)	0.009 0.003	Age, sex, family history of lung cancer, education, current smoker (yes/no), years of smoking, cigarettes/day	Incidence Total cohort, 120 852 Findings attenuated when adjusted for total vegetable consumption
Neuhouser et al. (2003), USA	12	414/7072 in intervention arm, 326 / 7048 in placebo arm, male, female	FFQ (45 fruits and vegetables), self-administered	≥ 3.5 vs ≤ 0.5 servings/week (5)	Intervention arm: 0.91 (0.65–1.28) Placebo arm 0.68 (0.45–1.04)	0.36 0.01	Sex, age, smoking status, total pack-years of smoking, asbestos exposure, race or ethnicity, enrolment centre	Incidence Follow up of participants in β-Carotene and Retinol Efficacy Trial (CARET) of smokers and asbestos workers

Table 22 (contd)

Author, year, country	Years of follow-up	Cases/ cohort size, sex	Exposure assessment (no. of items)	Range contrasts (no. of categories)	Relative risk (95% CI)	Statistical significance (p for trend when applicable)	Adjustment for confounding	Comments
Smith-Warner et al. (2003), North America and Europe	6–16	3206/430, 281 male, female	FFQ (study-specific, 9–54 fruits and vegetables)	≥ 1 vs no servings/ week (3)	Broccoli: 1.05 (0.89–1.24) Cabbage: 1.01 (0.88–1.02 1.17)	0.33 0.62	Age, education, body mass index, alcohol intake, calories, smoking status, amount, duration	Incidence Pooled analysis of eight cohort studies Only data from five cohorts included in each analysis
Miller et al. (2004), 10 European countries	0–14 (mean, 6 years)	860/478 021 male, female	FFQ (300), self-adminis-tered or interview, frequency, portion size; calibration study	Highest vs lowest (5)	1.21 (0.92–1.60)	0.25	Age, sex, weight, height, centre, smoking	Incidence No association in northern Europe, positive association in southern Europe

FFQ, food frequency questionnaire

Table 23. Case–control studies of cruciferous vegetable consumption and risk for lung cancer

Author, year, country	Cases/controls, sex	Exposure assessment (no. of items)	Range contrasts (no. of categories)	Relative risk (95% CI)	Statistical significance (p for trend when applicable)	Adjustment for confounding	Comments
Bond et al. (1987), USA	308 dead/308 dead controls/308 living controls male	FFQ (29, six vegetables), interview by telephone, frequency	Broccoli 4–6 times/week vs never (6)	0.33 (0.03–3.26)	0.001	Age, sex, centre, smoking, education, vitamin supplements	Analysis with living controls only
Koo (1988), China	88/137 female, never smokers	FFQ (three vegetables), interview, frequency	Highest vs lowest (3)	[0.96]	0.358	Age, no. of live births, schooling (yes/no)	Population-based
Le Marchand et al. (1989), USA	332/865 male, female	FFQ (> 130, 22 vegetables), interview, frequency, portion size; validated	Highest vs lowest (4)	Male: [0.6] Female: [0.4]	Male: 0.06 Female: 0.06	Age, ethnicity, smoking status, pack–years, cholesterol intake (males only), carrot, tomato, dark-green vegetable intake	Population-based Response rate: 67% cases, 70% controls
Alavanja et al. (1993), USA	429/1021 female non-smokers	FFQ (60, 28 vegetables), self-administered, frequency, portion size	≥ 4.0 vs ≤ 1.04 servings/week (5)	0.73	0.36	Age, smoking history (never, ex-smoker), previous lung disease, interview type, calories	Population-based Response rate: 70% cases, 68% controls, 58% of case interviews with proxies
Agudo et al. (1997), Spain	103/206 female	FFQ (33, 11 vegetables), interview, frequency, portion size	Highest vs lowest (3)	0.54 (0.26–1.13)	0.13	Age, residence, hospital, smoking status, pack–years	Hospital-based Response rate: 90% cases, OR = 1.01 for adenocarcinoma; OR = 0.59 for never smokers (only subgroups)

Table 23 (contd)

Author, year, country	Cases/ controls, sex	Exposure assessment (no. of items)	Range contrasts (no. of categories)	Relative risk (95% CI)	Statistical significance (p for trend when applicable)	Adjustment for confounding	Comments
Nyberg et al. (1998), Sweden	124/235 male, female (never smoked)	FFQ (19, four vegetables), interview, frequency	> 1/week vs < 1/week (3)	1.06 (0.58–1.92)	0.33	Age, sex, urban residence, occasional smoking, occupation, passive smoking, carrots, non-citrus fruits	Population-based
Brennan et al. (2000), 8 centres in Europe	506/1045 male, female (non-smokers)	Quantitative FFQ (varied by centre)	Several times/ week vs < 1/month (3)	1.1 (0.7–1.6)	0.76	Age, sex, centre	Hospital-based and population-based Part of large multicentre study, primarily designed to evaluate effects of passive smoking
Hu et al. (2002), Canada	161/483 female (never smoked)	FFQ (70), frequency, portion size	> 6 vs ≤ 0.9 servings/ week (4)	0.8 (0.4–1.4)	0.43	Age, province of residence, education, social class, total energy intake	Population-based
Seow et al. (2002b), Singapore	303/765 females	FFQ (39, 19 vegetables, interview, frequency, portion size	≥ 14.3 vs < 7.5 servings/week (3)	Smokers: 0.46 (0.22–0.96) Non-smokers: 0.89 (0.59–1.35)	0.06 / 0.6	Age, date admission, place of birth, family history of any cancer (yes/no) (for smokers: duration, no./day)	Hospital-based Non-smokers = lifetime non-smokers

FFQ, food frequency questionnaire; OR, odds ratio

Table 24. Cohort studies of cruciferous vegetable consumption and risk for breast cancer

Author, year, country	Years of follow-up	Cases/cohort size, age	Exposure assessment (no. of items)	Range contrasts (no. of categories)	Relative risk (95% CI)	Statistical significance (p for trend when applicable)	Adjustment for confounding	Comments
Zhang et al. (1999), USA	15	2697 (784 premeno-pausal, 1913 post-meno-pausal)/83 234 33–60 years	Semi-quantitative FFQ (61–126), past year, estimated frequency; validity and reliability assessed	≥ 1 vs < 0.25 servings/day	Premeno-pausal: 0.83 (0.52–1.32) Postmeno-pausal: 0.98 (0.77–1.25)	0.19 0.83	Age, length of follow-up, energy intake, parity, age at birth of first child, age at menarche, history of breast cancer in mother or sister, history of benign breast disease, alcohol intake, body mass index at age 18, weight change from age 18, height	Incidence Nurses Health Study
Smith-Warner et al. (2001), North America and Europe	5–10	7377/351 825 28–90 years	FFQ (study-specific, 9–54 fruits and vege-tables)	Increment, 100 g/day	0.96 (0.87–1.06)	0.95	Age at menarche, parity, age at birth of first child, oral contraceptive use, history of benign breast disease, menopausal status, hormone replacement therapy, family history of breast cancer, smoking, education, body mass index, height, alcohol and energy intake	Pooled analysis of seven cohort studies Study-specific RRs calculated from primary data and then combined in random-effects model
Frazier et al. (2003), USA	7	843/8430 40–65 years	FFQ (24, 6 fruits and vegetables), diet at high school, estimated frequency	Increment, 1 serving/day	Broccoli: 0.74 (0.39–1.41) Cabbage: 1.00 (0.64–1.57)		Age at diagnosis, age at menarche, menopausal status, family history, benign breast disease, adult height, parity or age at birth of first child, post-menopausal hormone use, body mass index at age 18, 1980 alcohol intake, 1980 vitamin A intake excluding supplements	Nested case–control study within Nurses' Health Study Number of cases = 64% of those diagnosed 1980–86 Similar relative risks for premenopausal and postmeno-pausal breast cancer

FFQ, food frequency questionnaire; RR, relative risk

Table 25. Case–control studies of cruciferous vegetable consumption and risk for breast cancer

Author, year, country	Cases/ controls, age	Exposure assessment (no. of items)	Range contrasts (no. of categories)	Relative risk (95% CI)	Statistical significance (p for trend when applicable)	Adjustment for confounding	Comments
Graham et al. (1982), USA	2024/1463	FFQ, year before symptoms, interview, estimated frequency; assessed reliability	≥ 20 vs ≤ 3/month (4)	1.00	> 0.05	Age	Hospital-based No association among women ≥ 55 years or women < 55 years studied separately
Katsouyanni et al. (1986), Greece	120/120 Mean age of cases, 55 years	FFQ (120), before onset of disease, interview, estimated frequency	Broccoli Cabbage, raw Cabbage, Cooked Cauliflower		Not significant < 0.05 Not significant Not significant	Age, interviewer, year of schooling	Hospital-based Response rate = 92% for cases
Young (1989), USA	277/372 35–89 years	FFQ, < 18 years, 18–35 years, > 35 years (but excluding past 5 years) (25), self-administered	8 vs 0/month	Age 18–35: 0.66 (0.42–1.02) Age > 35: 0.64 (0.41–1.00)		Age, alcohol consumption	Population-based Response rate = 64% for cases, 57% for controls
Ewertz & Gill (1990), Denmark	1474/1322 < 70 years	Semi-quantitative FFQ (21), year before diagnosis, estimated frequency and amount; included summary question on vegetables	Highest vs lowest (2)	0.94 (0.78–1.13)		Age, residence	Population-based Response rate: 88% for cases, 79% for controls Questionnaire completed 1 year after diagnosis
Levi et al. (1993a), Switzerland	107/318 ≤ 75 years	Questionnaire (50, 13 fruits and vegetables), estimated frequency	Highest vs lowest (3)	0.5	< 0.05	Age, education, energy intake	Hospital-based Response rate > 85%
Challier et al. (1998), France	345/345 30–78 years	Recalled 7-day food diary	> 3 vs ≤ 2/month (3)	1.45 (1.03–2.06)	0.03	Age, socio-economic status, energy intake, parity, weight, body surface	Population-based Response rate: 84% for cases, 70% for controls

Table 25 (contd)

Author, year, country	Cases/ controls, age	Exposure assessment (no. of items)	Range contrasts (no. of categories)	Relative risk (95% CI)	Statistical significance (*p* for trend when applicable)	Adjustment for confounding	Comments
Potischman *et al.* (1999), USA	568 (in situ or invasive localized disease; did not report chemotherapy/-1451 20-44 years	FFQ, past year (100, 25 fruits, 34 vegetables), estimated frequency and amount validated	> 3.5 vs < 1.4 times/week (4)	0.95 (0.7–1.3)		Age at diagnosis, study site, ethnicity, education, age at birth of first child, alcohol intake, years of oral contraceptive use, smoking status	Population-based Response rate: 84% for cases, 70% for controls
Ronco *et al.* (1999), Uruguay	400/405 20–89 years	FFQ (64, nine fruits, 15 vegetables), interview; reliability assessed	Highest vs lowest (3)	1.07 (0.72–1.60)	0.12	Age, residence, urban or rural status, history of breast cancer in a first-degree relative, body mass index, age at menarche, parity, menopausal status, energy intake	Hospital-based Response rate: 97% for cases, 94% for controls No effect of menopausal status
Rosenblatt *et al.* (1999), USA	220/291 male	FFQ (125), self-administered	Highest vs lowest (4)	0.8 (0.4–1.3)	0.32	Age, study site, energy intake	Population-based Response rate: 75% for cases, 45% for controls
Terry *et al.* (2001), Sweden	2832/2650 All post-menopausal	FFQ, past year (65, 19 fruits and vegetables), self-administered, estimated frequency	1.1 vs 0.1 servings/ day (4), median values	0.76 (0.62–0.93)	0.01	Age, height, body mass index, current smoking, socio-economic status, intake of alcohol, high-fibre grains and cereals, fatty fish, multivitamins, parity, hormone replacement therapy, history of benign breast disease, family history of breast cancer, type of menopause, age at menopause, age at menarche, age at birth of first child, non-*Brassica* vegetables, total fruit	Population-based Response rate: 84% for cases, 82% for controls
Fowke *et al.* (2003), China	337/337 28–64 years	FFQ, past 5 years, validated	Highest vs lowest (4)	0.8 (0.5–1.3)	0.79	Age, soya protein, fibro-adenoma, family history of breast cancer, leisure activities, waist:hip ratio, body mass index, age at menarche, no. of children	Population-based Selected from Shanghai Breast Cancer Study Overall response: 91% cases, 90% controls

Table 26. Case–control studies of cruciferous vegetable consumption and risk for invasive cervix cancer

Author, year, country	Cases/ controls	Exposure assessment (no. of items)	Range contrasts (no. of categories)	Relative risk (95% CI)	Statistical significance (p for trend when applicable)	Adjustment for confounding	Comments
Marshall et al. (1983), USA	513/490	FFQ (28), 100-g portion size assumed, interview	≥ 16 vs < 3 servings/ month (5)	1.9 (1.2–3.0) 1.14 for 1 SD increase in dietary factor	< 0.05	Marital history, parity Mean response, no. of marriages, marriage before and after age 25, cigarette smoking, beer drinking, interaction of no. of marriages and cigarette smoking	Hospital-based
Shannon et al. (2002), Thailand	134/384	FFQ (80), open-ended frequency, portion calculated from standard recipes, interview	> 1.2 vs ≤ 0.17 servings/day (4)	0.51 (0.25–1.06)	0.22	Age, total energy, interviewer	Hospital-based (excluded women with conditions associated with use of steroid contraceptives)

FFQ, food frequency questionnaire

Table 27. Case–control study of cruciferous vegetable consumption and risk for in situ cervix cancer

Author, year, country	Cases/ controls	Exposure assessment (no. of items)	Range contrasts (no. of categories)	Relative risk (95% CI)	Statistical significance (p for trend when applicable)	Adjustment for confounding	Comments
Shannon et al. (2002), Thailand	50/125	FFQ (80), open-ended, portion calculated from standard recipes, interview	> 0.39 vs ≤ 0.17 servings/day (3)	1.30 (0.51–3.30)	0.58	Age, total energy, interviewer	Hospital-based, age < 60, resident of Thailand for at least 1 year, screened controls, matched on region and age

FFQ, food frequency questionnaire

Table 28. Case–control studies of cruciferous vegetable consumption and risk for endometrium cancer

Author, year, country	Cases/ controls	Exposure assessment (no. of items)	Range contrasts (no. of categories)	Relative risk (95% CI)	Statistical significance (*p* for trend when applicable)	Adjustment for confounding	Comments
Levi *et al.* (1993b), Switzerland, northern Italy	274/572	Questionnaire (50), frequency interview	Highest vs lowest (3)	1.20	Not significant	Age, study centre	Hospital-based
Potischman *et al.* (1993), USA	399/296	FFQ (60), open-ended frequency of intake, one of three portion sizes, interview	> 3.1 vs < 1.0 time/ week (4)	0.8 (0.5–1.3)		Age group, body mass index, ever estrogen use, ever oral contraceptive use, no. of births, current smoking, education, total calories	Population-based Only controls with intact uterus Five regions Response: 87% of eligible cases, 66% of eligible controls
Shu *et al.* (1993), China	268/268	FFQ (63, three cruciferous vegetables), usual intake frequency, interview	Highest vs lowest (4)	1.1	0.67	Age, no. of pregnancies, body mass index, total calories	Population-based Response: cases 91%, controls 96%
Goodman *et al.* (1997), USA	332/511	FFQ (250), open-ended usual intake frequency, portion size from pictures of three different portions, interview	> 55.1 vs < 16.5 g/day (4)	0.8	0.26	Pregnancy history, oral contraceptive use, history of diabetes, body mass index, total calories	Population-based Response rate: cases 66%, controls 73%
Littman *et al.* (2001), USA	679/944	FFQ (98, five cruciferous vegetables), frequency 5 years previously, portion size relative to three categories, interview	> 0.8 vs < 0.3 servings/day (3)	0.71 (0.54–0.95)	0.03	Age, county of residence, total calories, unopposed oestrogen use, ever smoking, body mass index	Population-based Response rate: cases 72%, controls 73% among those eligible
Terry *et al.* (2002), Sweden	709/ 2887	FFQ, nine frequency categories, validated with four 7-day diet records, self-administered	> 7.4 vs < 0.8 servings/ week (4) (median values)	0.8 (0.6–1.1)	0.13	Age, body mass index, smoking, physical activity, prevalence of diabetes, fatty fish consumption, quintiles of total food consumption, other dietary factors	Population-based Post-menopausal women with intact uterus, no previous history of endometrial or breast cancer Response rate: 75% among cases, 80% among controls, 68% of eligible controls with usable FFQ

FFQ, food frequency questionnaire

Table 29. Case–control studies of cruciferous vegetable consumption and risk for ovary cancer

Author, year, country	Cases/ controls	Exposure assessment (no. of items)	Range contrasts (no. of categories)	Relative risk (95% CI)	Statistical significance (p for trend when applicable)	Adjustment for confounding	Comments
Shu et al. (1989), China	172/172	FFQ (63, four cruciferous vegetables), open-ended, usual intake frequency, portion per unit time, interview	Highest vs lowest (4)	1.2	0.55	Education	Population-based Response rate: for eligible cases 89%, for controls 100%
Cramer et al. (2001), USA	549/516	FFQ, frequency of consumption of fixed portion; validated, self-administered	Broccoli ≥ 5 times/ week vs < 1/month (5)	0.90 (0.42– 1.92)	0.76	Total calorie intake, age, site, parity, body mass index, oral contraceptive use, history of breast, ovarian or prostate cancer in a first-degree relative, tubal ligation, education, marital status	Population-based Cases in two states Response rate: cases 64%, controls 72% of those determined eligible by random-digit dialling, 31% for voter list controls
Zhang et al. (2002), China	254/652	FFQ (120), portion size from eight categories, cooking method, vitamin and mineral supplements; validated, interview	≥ 72.8 vs ≤ 34.22 kg/year (4)	0.67 (0.4– 1.3)	< 0.05	Age, education, area of residence, body mass index 5 years previously, smoking, alcohol, tea, family income, marital status, menopausal status, parity, tubal ligation, oral contraceptive use, physical activity, family history of ovarian cancer, total energy intake, other food groups	Hospital- and population-based Response rate: cases 99% controls > 92%

FFQ, food frequency questionnaire

Table 30. Cohort studies of cruciferous vegetable consumption and risk for prostate cancer

Author, year, country	Years of follow-up	Cases/ cohort size	Exposure assessment (no. of items)	Range contrasts (no. of categories)	Relative risk (95% CI)	Statistical significance (*p* for trend when applicable)	Adjustment for confounding	Comments
Hsing *et al.* (1990), USA	20	149/17 633	FFQ (35), self-administered	> 4.5 vs < 1.2 times/ month (4)	1.3 (0.8–2.0)		Age, tobacco use	Mortality
Giovannucci *et al.* (1995), USA	7	759/47 894	FFQ, past year (131), self-administered	Broccoli 2–4 servings/ week vs none (4)	1.05 (0.83–1.34)	0.17	Age, energy intake	Incidence Health Professionals Study
Schuurman *et al.* (1998), Netherlands	6.3	610/58 279	FFQ (150), self-administered	58.3 vs 10.7 g/day (5), median values	0.82 (0.59–1.12)	0.06	Age, family history of prostate cancer, socioeconomic status, total fruit consumption	Incidence

FFQ, food frequency questionnaire

Table 31. Case–control studies of cruciferous vegetable consumption and risk for prostate cancer

Author, year, country	Cases/controls	Exposure assessment (no. of items)	Range contrasts (no. of categories)	Relative risk (95% CI)	Statistical significance (p for trend when applicable)	Adjustment for confounding	Comments
Schuman et al. (1982), USA	240/223 hospital (H) and 223 neighbourhood (N) controls	FFQ, self-administered	Cabbage ≥ 6 times/month vs never (5) Cauliflower ≥ 3 times/month vs never (4) Rutabaga and kohlrabi ≥ once/month vs never (3)	H: [0.84] N: [0.72] H: [0.88] N: [0.83] H: [0.67] N: [1.03]			Hospital-based and population-based Response rates: 83% cases, 89% hospital, 90% neighbourhood controls
Ross et al. (1987), USA	Black: 142 pairs, population-based White: 142 pairs, retirement community	FFQ (20), interview	Cooked spinach, cabbage, collards Black: ≥ 3/week vs fewer (2) White: ≥ 2/week vs fewer (2)	0.6 1.3	< 0.05 > 0.05	Matched on age and race or length of residence in community	Population-based Response: cases 57%, controls 74% Retirement community Response: cases 75%, controls 71%
Le Marchand et al. (1991), USA	452/899	Diet history (> 100), interview	Highest vs lowest (4)	Age < 70 years: 0.8 Age ≥ 70 years: 1.1	0.27 0.40	Age, ethnicity	Population-based
Jain et al. (1999), Canada	617/636	Diet history (1129, summarized in 142 food groups), validated	> 44.6 vs < 8.7 g/day (4)	0.85 (0.64–1.13)		Age, total energy intake, area of study, vasectomy, ever smoked, marital status, study area, body mass index, education, vitamin supplements, other foods	Population-based Response: cases: 74% Ontario, 81% Quebec, 88% British Columbia Controls: 52% Ontario, 50% Quebec, 87% British Columbia

Table 31 (contd)

Author, year, country	Cases/con-trols	Exposure assessment (no. of items)	Range contrasts (no. of categories)	Relative risk (95% CI)	Statistical significance (p for trend when applicable)	Adjustment for confounding	Comments
Villeneuve et al. (1999), Canada	1623/1623	FFQ (60), self-administered	≥ 4 vs < 1 servings/week (4)	0.9 (0.7–1.1)	0.57	Age, province of residence, race, years since quitting smoking, cigarette pack–years, body mass index, alcohol, other foods, income, family history of cancer	Population-based Response: 69% for both cases and controls
Cohen et al. (2000), USA	628/602	FFQ (99), self-administered	≥ 3 vs < 1 serving/week (3)	0.59 (0.39–0.90)	0.02	Age, fat, energy, race, family history of prostate cancer, body mass index, PSA in previous 5 years, education, total fruit and vegetable consumption	Population-based Response rates: 82% cases, 75% controls
Kolonel et al. (2000), Canada and USA	1619/1618	Diet history (147), interview	> 72.9 vs ≤ 8.8 g/day (5)	0.78 (0.61–1.00) Advanced disease: 0.61 (0.42–0.88)	0.02 0.006	Age, education, ethnic group, geographical area, calories	Population-based Response rates: overall, cases 70%, controls 58%

FFQ, food frequency questionnaire; PSA, prostate-specific antigen

Table 32. Cohort studies of cruciferous vegetable consumption and risk for urinary bladder cancer

Author, year, country	Years of follow-up	Cases / cohort size, sex	Exposure assessment (no. of items)	Range contrasts (no. of categories)	Relative risk (95% CI)	Statistical significance (p for trend when applicable)	Adjustment for confounding	Comments
Michaud et al. (1999), USA	10	252/47 909 male	FFQ (131)	≥ 5 vs ≤ 1 serving/week (5)	0.49 (0.32–0.75)	0.008	Age, geographic region, smoking, fluid and caloric intake	Incidence Health Professionals Study Inverse association restricted to persons who had never smoked
Michaud et al. (2002), Finland	Median, 11	344/27 111 male, smokers	FFQ (276, 45 fruits and vegetables)	33 vs 0 g/day (5), median values	1.15 (0.83–1.60)	0.05	Age, duration of smoking, smoking dose, total energy, trial interventions	Incidence Follow-up of α-Tocopherol β-Carotene trial

FFQ, food frequency questionnaire

Table 33. Case–control study of cruciferous vegetable consumption and risk for urinary bladder cancer

Author, year, country	Cases / controls, sex	Exposure assessment (no. of items)	Range contrasts (no. of categories)	Relative risk (95% CI)	Statistical significance (p for trend when applicable)	Adjustment for confounding	Comments
Mettlin & Graham (1979), USA	377 male, 112 female/ 645 male, 257 female (white)	FFQ (29), interview	≥ 15 vs 0–4 /month	Male: [0.76 (0.50–1.15)] Female: [0.73 (0.36–1.45)]		Age, occupation, tobacco use	Hospital-based Controls had a wide variety of diseases other than cancer

FFQ, food frequency questionnaire

Table 34. Case–control studies of cruciferous vegetable consumption and risk for kidney cancer

Author, year, country	Cases/ controls, sex	Exposure assessment (no. of items)	Range contrasts (no. of categories)	Relative risk (95% CI)	Statistical significance (p for trend when applicable)	Adjustment for confounding	Comments
McLaughlin et al. (1984), USA	313/428 male, 182/269 female	FFQ (28), interview	Highest vs lowest (4)	Male 0.8 Female 1.0	Not significant Not significant	Age, cigarette smoking, relative weight	Population-based Response rate 98%
Maclure & Willett (1990), USA	203/605 male, female	Semiquanti- tative FFQ (57), interview	Cabbage: ≥ 113 g/week vs ≤ 85 g/month (3)	0.60 (0.35–1.1)	0.03	Age, sex	Population-based
			Broccoli: ≥ 85 g/week vs ≤ 57 g/month (3)	0.85 (0.57–1.3)	0.69		
			Brussels sprouts: ≥ 85 g/week vs ≤ 57 g/month (3)	0.95 (0.38–2.3)	0.94		
			Cauliflower: ≥ 85 g/week vs ≤ 57 g/month (3)	0.75 (0.43–1.3)	0.58		
McLaughlin et al. (1992), China	154/157 male, female	Structured question- naire, interview	Cabbage, cauliflower, Chinese cabbage	Not associated			Population-based Response rate: 87% cases, 100% controls
Chow et al. (1994), USA[a]	415/650 male, female	FFQ (65), self- administered	Male ≥ 1.5 vs ≤ 0.3, female ≥ 1.9 vs ≤ 0.5 servings/week (4)	1.0 (0.7–1.5)		Age, sex, smoking, body mass index	Population-based Response rate 79%
Mellemgaard et al. (1996), Denmark*	351 (216 male, 135 female)/ 340	FFQ (92), interview, validated	> 1/week vs rarely or never (4)	Male: 0.5 (0.2–1.0) Female: 1.4 (0.5–3.9)	0.09 0.41	Age, smoking, body mass index, socio- economic status	Population-based Response rate: 73% for cases, 68% for controls

Table 34 (contd)

Author, year, country	Cases/ controls, sex	Exposure assessment (no. of items)	Range contrasts (no. of categories)	Relative risk (95% CI)	Statistical significance (p for trend when applicable)	Adjustment for confounding	Comments
Wolk et al. (1996), Australia, Denmark, Sweden, USA[a]	1185/1526 male, female	FFQ (63–205, depending on study centre), interview or self-adminis- tered	Highest vs lowest (4)	0.83 (0.65–1.05) Non-smokers 0.6 (0.4–0.9)	0.07	Age, sex, study centre, body mass index, smoking, total calories	Population-based Multicentre analysis Response rate: 54–72% for cases, 53–78% for controls
Lindblad et al. (1997), Sweden*	378/350 male, female	FFQ (63), interview	≥ 138 vs < 41.2 g/week (4)	0.87 (0.57–1.32) Non- smokers: 0.64 (0.35–1.16) Smokers: 1.12 (0.61–2.07)	0.25 0.10 0.99	Age, sex, body mass index, smoking, education	Population-based Response rate: 70% for cases, 72% for controls
Yuan et al. (1998), USA	1204/1204 male, female	FFQ (40), interview	≥ 21.6 vs ≤ 4.2 times/month (5)	0.53 (0.39–0.72)	< 0.001	Age, sex, education, body mass index, hypertension, smoking, analgesics, amphetamines	Population-based Response rate: 74% for cases, 69% of controls

FFQ, food frequency questionnaire
[a]Substudy in multicentre analyses (Wolk et al., 1996)

Table 35. Case–control studies of cruciferous vegetable consumption and risk for childhood brain cancer

Author, year, country	Cases/ controls, sex	Exposure assessment (no. of items)	Range contrasts (no. of categories)	Relative risk (95% CI)	Statistical significance (*p* for trend when applicable)	Adjustment for confounding	Comments
Bunin et al. (1993), Canada, USA	166/166 Interviews of mothers about their diet during pregnancy	FFQ (designed to evaluate nitrosamine hypothesis)	Weekly vs less (2)	Cabbage 0.91 (0.45–1.81) Kale, collards, greens 1.50 (0.36–7.22)		Age, race, residence	Population-based Study of primitive neuroectodermal tumours (mostly medulloblastomas) 74% first eligible controls contacted
Cordier et al. (1994), France	75/113 male, female	Interview about maternal diet during pregnancy	Cabbage Weekly vs less (2)	0.7	> 0.05	Child's age and sex, maternal age, no. of years of schooling of mother	Population-based Response: 69% of identified cases, 71.5% of eligible controls contacted

FFQ, food frequency questionnaire

Table 36. Case–control studies of cruciferous vegetable consumption and risk for thyroid cancer

Author, year, country	Cases / controls, sex	Exposure assessment (no. of items)	Range contrasts (no. of categories)	Relative risk (95% CI)	Statistical significance (*p* for trend when applicable)	Adjustment for confounding	Comments
Ron et al. (1987), USA	159/285 male, female	FFQ (12), interview	Frequent (a few times a week or daily) vs infrequent (never or a few times a year) (3)	0.77	0.17 (one-sided test)	Age, sex, prior radiotherapy to head and neck, thyroid nodules, goitre	Population-based
Kolonel et al. (1990), USA	191/441 male, female	Diet history (150), questionnaire interview	Goitrogenic vegetables Highest vs lowest (4)	Male: 1.0 (0.3–3.0) Female: 0.6 (0.3–1.2)	0.63 0.10	Age, ethnic group	Population-based
Franceschi et al. (1991b), Italy and Switzerland	385/798 male, female	FFQ (30–38)	Highest vs lowest (3)	0.8	> 0.05	Centre, age, sex, education	Hospital-based Pooled analysis of three studies in northern Italy and one in Switzerland
Wingren et al. (1993), Sweden	93 (papillary)/187, female	FFQ related to diet at > 20 years, self-administered	Several times/week vs seldom or never (4)	[0.2 (0.06–0.8)]	0.05	Univariate	Population-based
Hallquist et al. (1994), Sweden	171/325 male, female	FFQ about diet at two age periods, self-administered	Several times/week vs less than some times/week (3)	Cabbage: age ≤ 20: 1.0 (0.5–2.0) age > 20: 1.1 (0.6–1.8)		Age, sex	Population-based

Table 36 (contd)

Author, year, country	Cases / controls, sex	Exposure assessment (no. of items)	Range contrasts (no. of categories)	Relative risk (95% CI)	Statistical significance (p for trend when applicable)	Adjustment for confounding	Comments
Galanti *et al.* (1997), Norway and Sweden	246 / 440 male, female	FFQ (56), self-administered	> 6 vs < 2 portions/month (3)	0.9 (0.6–1.4)	> 0.05	Univariate	Population-based
Memon *et al.* (2002) Kuwait	313 / 313 male, female	Frequency of 13 habitual dietary items, interview	≥ 2 days/week vs never or occasionally (3)	Cabbage: 1.9 (1.1–3.3) Cauliflower: 1.8 (1.0–3.2) Brussels sprouts: 0.7 (0.1–4.3) Broccoli: 0.9 (0.2–3.6)	0.08 0.16 0.44 0.90	Education	Population-based Cases from cancer register (66 known to have died excluded)
Pooled estimate Bosetti *et al.* (2002) (see text)	2241 / 3716 male, female		Highest vs lowest (3)	0.94 (0.80–1.10) Weighted mean of ORs from each study		Age, sex, history of goitre, thyroid nodules and adenomas, history of irradiation	Collaborative re-analysis of 11 case–control studies Test for heterogeneity between studies: *p* = 0.016

FFQ, food frequency questionnaire; OR, odds ratio

Table 37. Cohort studies of cruciferous vegetable consumption and risk for malignant lymphoma

Author, year, country	Years of follow-up	Cases / cohort size, sex	Exposure assessment (no. of items)	Range contrasts (no. of categories)	Relative risk (95% CI)	Statistical significance (p for trend when applicable)	Adjustment for confounding	Comments
Chiu et al. (1996), USA	7	104/35 156, female	Semi-quantitative FFQ (126), self-administered	> 12 vs < 8 servings/month (3)	1.01 (0.63–1.62)	0.97	Age and total energy intake	Incidence Iowa Women's Health Study
Zhang et al. (2000), USA	14	199/88 410, female	Semi-quantitative FFQ (61), self-administered	≥ 5–6/week vs < 2/week (3)	0.69 (0.41–1.15)	0.04	Age, total energy, length of follow-up, geo-graphical region, cigarette smoking, height, beef, pork or lamb as a main dish	Incidence Nurses' Health Study

FFQ, food frequency questionnaire

were measured gave promising results. Those available are reviewed below.

The few published epidemiological studies on the relationship between exposure to isothiocyanates and cancer risk are summarized in Table 38. Four of the five studies were conducted in Asian populations who have a high intake of cruciferous vegetables. In three studies, intake of isothiocyanates was measured from food-frequency questionnaires about usual intake and from food composition databases. In one prospective study (London *et al.*, 2000) and one case–control study (Fowke *et al.*, 2003), urinary isothiocyanate was used as a biomarker of exposure.

Colorectal cancer

Dietary intake of isothiocyanate was evaluated in a nested case–control study conducted within the Singapore Chinese Health Study (Seow *et al.*, 2002a). The mean energy-adjusted intake of cruciferous vegetables was 26 g/1000 kcal among cases and 28.9 g/1000 kcal among controls, corresponding to isothiocyanate intakes of 5.4 µmol/1000 kcal and 6.0 µmol/1000 kcal, respectively. While the risk estimates (above median versus at or below median consumption) indicated an inverse association, they were not statistically significant for smokers, non-smokers or both combined (Table 38).

Lung cancer

London *et al.* (2000) conducted a nested case–control study on a cohort of 18 244 men in Shanghai, China, each of whom provided a sample of blood and a single-void urine sample [no details given] and responded to a structured questionnaire covering 45 dietary items. Of the 232 patients with lung cancer and 710 controls, 81.5% and 47.5% were smokers, respectively; 77.6% of the patients and 84.4%

of the controls had detectable isothiocyanates in their urine, with a median concentration of 1.71 (range, 0.04–77.7) µmol/mg creatinine. The OR for lung cancer was 0.65 for persons with detectable urinary isothiocyanate in comparison with those without, although no dose–response relationship was observed for persons with detectable urinary isothiocyanate (Table 38).

Spitz and colleagues (2000) examined the effect of isothiocyanate intake from food-frequency questionnaires in a case–control study, in which controls were recruited from a large managed care organization. When the association was examined separately for current and ex-smokers, a significant inverse relationship was found with intake among current smokers [OR, 0.58; 95% CI, 0.38–0.88]. The authors observed that this finding was consistent with the effects of isothiocyanate against lung cancer induced by NNK and benzo[*a*]pyrene (Hecht, 1999).

Similarly, Zhao *et al.* (2001) conducted a hospital-based case–control study among Singapore Chinese women, with isothiocyanate intake estimated from a food-frequency questionnaire, and reported an inverse association, which appeared to be greater among smokers (OR, 0.31) than among women who had never smoked (OR, 0.70).

Breast cancer

Fowke *et al.* (2003) collected first morning urine specimens from a subset of 337 case–control pairs in the Shanghai Breast Cancer Study. The response rate in the overall study was 98.7% for patients and 99.8% for controls. A small, non-significant difference in dietary intake of *Brassica* vegetables was found between women with breast cancer and controls (median intake, 77.4 g/day for patients and 81.5 g/day for controls, *p* = 0.16), and a significant inverse relationship (OR, 0.5)

was found with quartile of urinary isothiocyanate concentration for all women and for premenopausal women. [The Working Group noted that the concentration of the biomarker might have been affected by the disease status of the women at the time of specimen collection.]

Studies of Mendelian randomization

Genes that are polymorphic in a population and that code proteins which metabolize specific environmental (including nutritional) factors may act as determinants of response to an environmental exposure. Furthermore, studies of associations with such genes might, under certain assumptions, obviate confounding as an explanation for an association between an environmental factor and disease. This phenomenon, known as 'Mendelian randomization', arises from Mendel's 'principle of independent inheritance', whereby a genetic variant is unlikely to be related to other lifestyle characteristics or even to the vast majority of other genes (Davey Smith & Ebrahim, 2003).

Several assumptions are required for a Mendelian randomization comparison to be valid:

- the gene does not influence behaviour,
- there is no linkage disequilibrium with other genes that influence disease, and
- the gene does not have other functions that influence disease susceptibility.

Effect of glutathione S-transferase genotype on the association between intake of isothiocyanates and cancer

The GSTM1 null genotype, which affects 50% of most populations (Garte *et al.*, 2001), has been hypothesized to increase cancer risk by reducing the capacity to detoxify activated carcinogens. This relationship has not been

Table 38. Observational epidemiological studies on the association between dietary isothiocyanate (ITC) intake and risk for cancer

Author, year, country	Cancer site	Type of study	No. of cases/ controls	Exposure variable; contrast, stratification	Relative risk (95% CI)[a]	Adjustment for confounding	Comments
Seow et al. (2002a), Singapore	Colo-rectum	Cohort (nested case-control)	213/1194	Average daily ITC intake from semi-quantitative FFQ[b]; high (> 5.16 µmol/1000 kcal, cohort median) vs low All Never smokers Ever smokers	 0.81 (0.59–1.12) 0.89 (0.58–1.36) 0.77 (0.44–1.36)	Sex, year of birth, year of recruitment, dialect group (matching factors), education, body mass index, smoking, strenuous sports or vigorous work, alcohol, saturated fat	Dietary information collected at recruitment
London et al. (2000), Shanghai, China	Lung	Cohort (nested case-control)	232/710 (all men)	Urinary ITC; detectable vs undetectable All Smokers only	 0.65 (0.43–0.97) 0.60 (0.39–0.93)	Age, age started to smoke, cigarettes/day, years since quitting	Dietary information and urine specimens collected at recruitment
Spitz et al. (2000), USA	Lung	Case-control, population-based	503/465	ITC intake from semi-quantitative FFQ[c]; high (> 0.39 mg/1000 kcal) vs low Current smokers Ex-smokers	 [0.58 (0.38–0.88)] [0.77 (0.53–1.11)]		Controls recruited from a large managed care organization
Zhao et al. (2001), Singapore	Lung	Case-control, hospital based	233/187 (all women)	ITC intake from semi-quantitative FFQ[b]; high (> 53 µmol/week) vs low All women Smokers Never smokers	 0.63 (0.41–0.95) 0.31 (0.10–0.96) 0.70 (0.45–1.11)	Age, smoking at recruitment, years of smoking, cigarettes/day	Frequency matching for age, date of admission, hospital
Fowke et al (2003), Shanghai, China	Breast	Case-control, population-based	337/337	Urinary ITC; highest vs lowest quartile All subjects Postmenopausal Premenopausal	 0.5 (0.3–0.8) $p_{trend} < 0.01$ 0.6 (0.2–1.7) $p_{trend} = 0.38$ 0.5 (0.2–0.9) $p_{trend} = 0.01$	Matched by age, menopausal status, date of sample collection and interview. ORs adjusted for soya protein, fibroadenoma, family breast cancer, leisure activity, waist:hip ratio, body mass index, age at menarche, number of children	Individually matched case–control pairs within the Shanghai Breast Cancer Study

FFQ, food frequency questionnaire; OR, odds ratio

[a] Estimates and confidence intervals in square brackets were calculated by the Working Group from data presented in the paper. In reports in which odds ratios for low vs high intake were given, the inverse was calculated.

[b] Cruciferous vegetables listed in questionnaire, from which ITC intake was derived: Chinese white cabbage, Chinese mustard, Chinese flowering cabbage, watercress, Chinese kale, head cabbage, celery cabbage, broccoli, cauliflower

[c] Cruciferous vegetables listed in questionnaire, from which ITC intake was derived: broccoli, cauliflower, Brussels sprouts, coleslaw, cabbage, sauerkraut, mustard greens, turnip greens, collard greens, kale

found in all studies, but a recent meta-analysis showed an overall risk for lung cancer of 1.17 (95% CI, 1.07–1.27) with the null genotype (Benhamou *et al.*, 2002). Some authors have suggested that, if GST plays a role in the metabolism of isothiocyanate, differences in isothiocyanate-related risk would be expected between individuals who are null and non-null for these enzymes.

Five of the epidemiological studies summarized in Table 38 included stratification by *GST* genotype. Three more studies in which the frequency of intake of cruciferous vegetables was used as an exposure variable also included stratification by *GST* genotype. Fowke *et al.* (2003) examined the effect of genetic polymorphisms in NAD(P)H:quinone oxidoreductase (NQO1), another phase II detoxifying enzyme. The results of studies on cancer risk and intake of cruciferous vegetables or isothiocyanates according to GST genotype are summarized in Table 39.

With respect to GST, the assumption that the gene does not have other functions that influence disease susceptibility is particularly relevant, given that both GSTM1 and GSTT1 are responsible for deactivating highly reactive polycyclic aromatic hydrocarbon substrates, which are ubiquitous in the diet. An overall analysis of GSTs and lung cancer might therefore not distinguish between the potentially increased risk due to greater exposure to these compounds and the decreased risk associated with higher isothiocyanate concentrations. If there is a real effect associated with higher isothiocyanate concentrations, the pleiotropic effects of GSTM1 and GSTT1 would either dilute or negate this effect, instead of resulting in a false-positive result.

Colon and colorectal cancer
A case–control study conducted by Lin et al. (1998) of 966 persons showed a significant interaction between broccoli intake and GST genotype in the risk for adenomatous polyps of the colon, which are considered to be precursors to cancer. A statistically significant trend in an inverse relationship with broccoli and cruciferous vegetable intake was restricted to individuals with the GSTM1 null genotype. This interaction was more marked for intake of broccoli alone than for intake of all cruciferous vegetables. After stratification by GSTT1 genotype alone, however, the inverse relationship with intake of both broccoli and all cruciferous vegetables was stronger for persons with the GSTT1 non-null genotype (Lin *et al.*, 2002).

Slattery and colleagues (2000) examined the relationship between cruciferous vegetable intake and incident colon cancer in a study of members of a large medical care programme and population controls. They reported an effect of age, an inverse relationship between cruciferous vegetable intake and risk for colon cancer being observed only in persons aged 55 years or less. The relationship was once again strongest among GSTM1-null individuals (OR for four or more servings per week versus none: 0.23 compared with 0.59 for GSTM1 non-null persons). [The number of individuals in the study who were aged 55 years and below was not reported.] When people under 65 years of age were stratified by smoking, the inverse relationship was more consistent for smokers than for non-smokers (smokers, 0.36 versus 0.80; non-smokers, 0.96 versus 0.50 for GSTM1 null and non-null individuals, respectively).

A nested case–control study among Singapore Chinese (Seow *et al.*, 2002a) showed a significant reduction in the risk for colorectal cancer associated with isothiocyanate intake, only among persons null for both GSTM1 and GSTT1 (OR, 0.43; 95% CI, 0.20–0.96). The authors also examined the role of the GSTP1 polymorphism, this isoform being the most abundant in the colon, and found no evidence that absence of the high activity (A) allele interacts with isothiocyanate intake to influence risk.

Lung cancer
In the study of London and colleagues (2000), described earlier, 60% of the controls were null for GSTM1, and a similar percentage were null for GSTT1. These genotypes were not associated with an elevated risk for lung cancer. When the isothiocyanate–lung cancer relationship was examined by GST genotype, the reduction in risk associated with detectable urinary isothiocyanate was restricted to individuals with the GSTM1-null or GSTT1-null genotype, or both. The difference in relative risks was significant ($p < 0.01$) for GSTM1 and the combined null genotype, but not for GSTT1 ($p = 0.15$).

Among men and women in the USA (Spitz *et al.*, 2000), the effect of GSTM1 and GSTT1 genotypes was inconsistent. The ORs for current smokers were 0.47 for GSTM1 non-null and 0.70 for GSTM1 null; for GSTT1, the corresponding figures were 0.58 and 0.41. There appeared to a stronger inverse association for individuals null for both GSTM1 and GSTT1 than for persons who were non-null for either genotype (OR, 0.20 and 0.60, respectively).

Zhao *et al.* (2001) conducted a study in a population containing a high proportion (72.9%) of non-smokers who were known to have a relatively high isothiocyanate intake. The inverse association with isothiocyanate intake was evident in all groups and was particularly marked among smokers, but the interaction with GST could not be examined among smokers because of small numbers. No main effects were

Table 39. Epidemiological studies on intake of cruciferous vegetables or isothiocyanates (ITCs) and cancer risk, by glutathione _S_-transferase (GST) genotype

Author, year, country Type of study	Cancer site	No. of cases/controls	Exposure variable; comparison	Stratification	Relative risk (95% CI) by urinary ITC or ITC / cruciferous vegetable intake[a]		Adjustment for confounding	Comments
					Non-null	Null		
Lin et al. (1998, 2002), USA Case–control with sigmoidoscopy controls	Colorectal adenomas	459/507	Weekly servings of cruciferous vegetables from semi-quantitative FFQ; highest vs lowest quartile	GSTM1 GSTT1 GSTM1/ T1	[0.77] p_{trend} = 0.71; p_{int} = 0.26 [0.55] p_{trend} = 0.003; p_{int} = 0.45 [0.64] p_{trend} = 0.20 p_{int} = 0.66	0.52 (0.29–0.93) p_{trend} = 0.02 0.89 (0.41–1.96) p_{trend} = 0.46 0.57 (0.34–0.90) p_{trend} = 0.017	Smoking, age, date of sigmoid-oscopy, clinic, sex, saturated fat, energy intake, intake of other fruit and vegetables	Cruciferous vegetables: broccoli, cabbage or coleslaw, cauliflower, Brussels sprouts, kale or mustard or chard greens
Slattery et al. (2000), USA Case–control, population-based	Colon	1579/1898	Intake in servings per week from FFQ (≥ 4 vs none)	GSTM1 ≤ 55 years 55–64 years ≥ 65 years	[0.59] [0.87] [1.05]	0.23 (0.10–0.54) 1.31 (0.60–2.87) 1.47 (0.94–2.30)	Age, sex, body mass index, long-term vigorous physical activity, total energy intake, smoking	Cruciferous vegetables: broccoli, Brussels sprouts, cabbage, cauliflower, greens, kale, mustard, turnip, rutabaga
Seow et al. (2002a), Singapore Cohort (nested case–control)	Colo-rectum	213/1194	Average daily ITC intake from semi-quantitative FFQ; high (> 5.16 mmol/ 1000 kcal, cohort median) vs low	GSTM1 GSTT1 GSTM1/T1	0.71 (0.45–1.1) 0.97 (0.64–1.47) 0.92 (0.64–1.32)	0.85 (0.54–1.35) 0.63 (0.37–1.07) 0.43 (0.20–0.96)	Sex, year of birth, year of recruitment, dialect group (matching factors), educa-tion, body mass index, smoking, strenuous sports or vigorous work, alcohol, saturated fat	Dietary information collected at recruitment
London et al. (2000), Shanghai, China Cohort (nested case–control)	Lung	232/710, men	Urinary ITC, detectable vs undetectable	GSTM1 GSTT1 GSTM1/T1	1.22 (0.67–2.24) 0.95 (0.50–1.80) 1.04 (0.60–1.67)	0.36 (0.20–0.63) 0.51 (0.30–0.86) 0.28 (0.13–0.57)	Age, age started to smoke, cigarettes/day, years since quitting	Age- and smoking-adjusted relative risks were similar, restriction to smokers (89.7%) gave similar results

Table 39 (contd)

Author, year, country Type of study	Cancer site	No. of cases / controls	Exposure variable; comparison	Stratification	Relative risk (95% CI) by urinary ITC or ITC/ cruciferous vegetable intake[a] Non-null	Null	Adjustment for confounding	Comments
Spitz et al. (2000), USA Case–control, population-based	Lung	503/465	ITC intake from semi-quantitative FFQ; high vs low	Current smokers GSTM1 GSTT1 GSTM1/T1	0.47 (0.26–0.87)] [0.58 (0.35–0.96)] [0.60 (0.38–0.93)]	[0.70] [0.41] [0.20]	Age, sex	Controls recruited from a large managed care organisation
Zhao et al. (2001), Singapore Case–control, hospital-based	Lung	233/187 (all women)	ITC intake from semi-quantitative FFQ; high (> 53 mmol/-week) vs low	All GSTM1 GSTT1 GSTM1/T1 Non-smokers GSTM1 GSTM1 GSTM1/T1	0.78 (0.39–1.59) 0.75 (0.40–1.40) 0.69 (0.41–1.17) 1.07 (0.50–2.29) 0.82 (0.41–1.62) 0.83 (0.47–1.46)	0.5 (0.33–0.93) 0.54 (0.31–0.95) 0.47 (0.23–0.95) 0.54 (0.30–0.95) 0.62 (0.33–1.13) 0.50 (0.23–1.08)	Age, smoking at recruitment, years of smoking, cigarettes/day	
Lewis et al. (2002), Europe and South America Case–control, multicentre	Lung	122/123	Cruciferous vegetable intake from FFQ (high vs low)	All GSTM1	0.64 (0.25–1.67) p_{trend} = 0.35 0.65 (0.16–2.66) p_{trend} = 0.57	0.27 (0.06–1.33) p_{trend} = 0.12	Age, sex, centre	
Fowke et al. (2003), Shanghai, China Case–control, population-based	Breast	337/337	Urinary ITC; highest vs lowest quartiles	GSTM1 GSTT1	0.6 (0.3–1.4) p_{trend} = 0.20; p_{int} = 0.82 0.6 (0.3–1.3) p_{trend} = 0.20; p_{int} = 0.44	0.5 (0.2–0.9) p_{trend} = 0.05 0.4 (0.2–0.9) p_{trend} = 0.03	Matched by age, menopausal status, date of sample collection and interview. ORs adjusted for soya protein, fibroadenoma, family breast cancer, leisure activity, waist:hip ratio, body mass index, age at menarche, number of children	Individually matched case–control pairs within the Shanghai Breast Cancer study

GSTM1/T1 non-null indicates non-null for either or both genotypes; FFQ, food frequency questionnaire
[a] Estimates and confidence intervals in square brackets were calculated by the Working Group from data in the paper. When odds ratios for low vs high intake were given, the inverse was calculated. When separate reference groups were not used for the null and non-null genotypes, the odds ratio for the other genotype was computed empirically from the ratio of the highest to lowest intake in that stratum.

observed for the GSTM1 and GSTT1 genotypes. When the population was stratified by GST genotype, the inverse association with high isothiocyanate intake was consistently greater and statistically significant only among persons with the null or combined null genotypes. For non-smokers, a significant inverse association with high isothiocyanate was restricted to persons with the GSTM1-null genotype.

Lewis *et al.* (2002) examined the association between GSTM1 genotype, cruciferous vegetable intake and lung cancer among non-smokers recruited at nine centres throughout Europe and South America. The majority were women. The risk for lung cancer among non-smokers who were of the GSTM1-null genotype was 1.53 (95% CI, 0.87–2.71) relative to those who were non-null. Although the study was limited by a small sample size, a dose–response pattern for reduction in risk with increasing intake of cruciferous vegetable was observed only among GSTM1-null individuals.

Breast cancer

Among women in Shanghai, China (Fowke *et al.*, 2003), the inverse relationship with isothiocyanate intake was more consistent among those who were null for GSTM1 and GSTT1. Inverse relationships by quartile of urinary isothiocyanate concentration were significant for women who were GSTT1 null (quartile 4 versus quartile 1: OR, 0.4; *p* for trend = 0.03), marginally significant for those who were GSTM1 null and not significant for non-null genotypes. The interaction terms were not statistically significant. There was no apparent effect of the GSTP1 or NQO1 genotype on the isothiocyanate-related risk for breast cancer in this study. The OR for women with the GSTP1 high-activity (AA) genotype was 0.6 (95% CI, 0.4–1.3) whereas that of women with the AG/GG geno-

type was 0.5 (0.2–1.2). Similarly for NQO1, the ORs were 0.6 (0.3–1.1) for women with the CC/CT genotype and 0.5 (0.1–1.8) for those with the TT genotype.

Studies of intermediate effect biomarkers

The biological effects of cruciferous vegetables, indoles and isothiocyanates can be studied by means of biomarkers. Intermediate biomarkers include:

- detectable precancerous changes in an organ (confirmed by histology);
- alteration of a gene that is considered to play a causative role;
- DNA damage;
- other indicators of carcinogenesis, such as the expression of a marker of an exposure known to be a cause of a cancer (e.g. positivity for human papilomavirus [HPV] DNA); and
- effects on metabolic factors thought to be involved in cancer etiology, e.g. effects on phase I and II enzymes, antioxidant pathways and steroid hormone metabolism (IARC, 2003).

Cruciferous vegetables

The mechanisms of the chemopreventive effects of cruciferous vegetables might include alterations to the metabolism of carcinogens and reduction of oxidative DNA damage. These mechanisms can be studied by short-term intervention studies in limited numbers of healthy persons by measuring intermediate effect biomarkers, as listed in Table 40 (see also section 3). Most of the studies included only biomarkers related to metabolism of substrates, including some carcinogens, by phase I and II enzymes, whereas three studies included DNA damage as a biomarker. None of the studies therefore included biomarkers that can be directly related to cancer risk. In none was an assessment made of the con-

tent of glucosinolates, isothiocyanates or indoles in the diets of controls or those receiving the diets enriched with cruciferous vegetables, although urinary excretion of phenethyl-ITC, the putative active principle of watercress, and the glucosinolate content of the diet of the general population were each assessed in one study.

Cruciferous vegetables and CYP1A2 activity

The activity of CYP1A2 in humans eating diets rich in cruciferous vegetables was assayed in a number of studies. As demethylation of caffeine at the 3 and 7 positions is catalysed mainly by CYP1A2, various indices of caffeine metabolism, e.g. clearance and urinary metabolic ratios, are used as biomarkers of CYP1A2 activity. Similarly, antipyrine and phenacetin, which have been used to assess the effects of cruciferous vegetables, are at least partly metabolized by CYP1A2. 2-Hydroxylation of estradiol and estrone is also partly catalysed by CYP1A2, whereas 16α-hydroxylation is catalysed mainly by other enzymes. The six published studies on CYP1A2 activity consistently showed that its activity is moderately enhanced by diets containing relatively large amounts of cruciferous vegetables.

The importance of the GSTM1 genotype in the effect of *Brassica* vegetables on CYP1A2 activity was investigated in one study, which found no effect (Lampe *et al.*, 2000a). An interaction with the GSTM1 genotype had been suggested by an observational study showing higher caffeine metabolic ratios in frequent consumers of cruciferous vegetables who had the GSTM1 null genotype than among persons with the non-null genotype (Probst-Hensch *et al.*, 1998).

The elimination rate of the anticoagulant warfarin was increased by 29% after a diet containing 400 g of Brussels sprouts per day (Ovesen *et al.*, 1988). Warfarin is a racemic

Table 40. Studies of intermediate effect biomarkers of the biological effects of cruciferous vegetables

Author, year, country	Intervention	Study sample	Biomarker	Effect during diet rich in cruciferous vegetables	Comment
Pantuck et al. (1979), USA	Supplementation with 200 g of cabbage and 300 g of Brussels sprouts for 7 days	10 healthy volunteers	AUC for phenacetin / Antipyrine clearance	49% decrease / 11% increase	
Vistisen et al. (1992), Denmark	Supplementation with 500 g of cooked broccoli or non-cruciferous vegetables per day for 10 days	9 healthy, non-smoking persons (five women)	Caffeine metabolic ratio	12% increase	
Kall et al. (1996), Denmark	12-day periods on a diet supple-mented with 500 g of broccoli, habitual diet and a diet free of known inducers and inhibitors of cytochrome P450 enzymes	16 healthy non-smoking persons (two women)	Caffeine metabolic ratio / 2-/16α-hydroxyestrone ratio in urine / Plasma ratio of chlorzoxazone and its 6-hydroxylated metabolite	19% increase / 29.5% increase / No effect	
Lampe et al. (2000a), USA	16 g of fresh radish sprouts, 150 g of frozen cauliflower, 200 g of frozen broccoli and 70 g of fresh shredded cabbage per day for 6 days	36 healthy persons (19 men)	Caffeine metabolic ratio	18–37% increase / No influence of GSTM1 genotype	
Murray et al. (2001), United Kingdom	250 g each of broccoli and Brussels sprouts per day for 12 days or no cruciferous vegetables / Known amounts of heterocyclic amines present in cooked meal	20 healthy, non-smoking men	Caffeine clearance / Excretion of MeIQx and PhIP in 10-h urine / Urinary mutagenicity with/ without metabolic activation / Adducts of PhIP to DNA in lymphocytes	7% increase / 23% and 21% decrease / 64% / 52% increase / Undetectable	12 days after stopping the diet, excretion of MeIQx and PhIP was still decreased by 17% (not significantly) and 30%, respectively, whereas urinary mutagenicity was still increased with metabolic activation
Fowke et al. (2000), USA	Increased consumption of Brassica vegetables for 5 weeks; average consumption reached 193 g/day	34 healthy women	2-:16α-hydroxyestrone ratio in urine	Increased by ~ 3.5% per 10 g/day increase in Brassica vegetable consumption (regression analysis)	

Table 40 (contd)

Author, year, country	Intervention	Study sample	Biomarker	Effect during diet rich in cruciferous vegetables	Comment
DeMarini et al. (1997), USA	6-week exposure to heterocyclic amines from various well-cooked meat products, comparable to 300 g of well-cooked hamburger per day. Four persons also ate undescribed amounts of cauliflower, Brussels sprouts and cabbage	Eight healthy non-smoking subjects (five women)	Mutagenicity of 24-h urine with and without enzymatic hydrolysis	No significant difference in mutagenicity of urine from women also eating cruciferous vegetables	
Knize et al. (2002), USA	At least one cup of broccoli for 3 days before well-cooked chicken	6 healthy persons	Excretion of PhIP metabolites in 6-h urine	Increased in five persons	
Ovesen et al. (1988), Denmark	400 g of Brussels sprouts per day for 2 weeks	10 healthy persons	Warfarin clearance	27% increase	
Hecht et al. (1995, 1999), USA	56.8 g of watercress at each meal for 3 days	11 healthy smokers	Urinary excretion of non-toxic NNK metabolites Oxidative nicotine metabolites	34% increase No effect	Significant correlation between excretion of phenethyl-ITC and NNK metabolites Increased excretion of glucuronidated metabolites of cotinine
Hecht et al. (2004), Singapore	Cross-sectional study of habitual intake of cruciferous vegetables	84 smokers	Urinary excretion of non-toxic NNK metabolites	Inverse association with calculated glucobrassicin intake	
Caporaso et al. (1994); United Kingdom and USA	50 g of watercress 2 h before measurement	29 healthy persons	Debrisoquine metabolite ratio	No effect	
Pantuck et al. (1984), USA	200 g of cabbage and 300 g of Brussels sprouts per day for 10 days	10 healthy persons	Oxazepam elimination Acetaminophen glucuronidation clearance	19% increase 17% increase 13% decrease	

Table 40 (contd)

Author, year, country	Intervention	Study sample	Biomarker	Effect during diet rich in cruciferous vegetables	Comment
Bogaards et al. (1994), Netherlands	300 g of cooked glucose-nolate-free vegetables per day for 6 weeks; 300 g of Brussels sprouts for last 3 weeks	10 healthy male non-smokers	GSTA1-1 protein in plasma	40% increase	
Nijhoff et al., (1995a) Netherlands	300 g of Brussels sprouts or non-cruciferous vegetables for consecutive periods of 1 week in random order	5 male and 5 female non-smokers	GSTA1-1 protein in rectal mucosa GSTA1, M1 and P1 protein in duodenum GSTP1 and M1 protein in lymphocytes GST activity in duodenum, rectum, lymphocytes	30% and 15% increase No effect No effect No effect	
Nijhoff et al., (1995b) Netherlands	300 g of Brussels sprouts or non-cruciferous vegetables for consecutive periods of 1 week in random order	5 male and 5 female non-smokers	GSTA1-1 protein in plasma GSTP1-1 in plasma GSTA1 and P1 in urine	50% increase in men; no effect in women No effect	
Verhagen et al. (1995), Netherlands	300 g of cooked glucosinolate-free vegetables per day for 6 weeks; 300 g of Brussels sprouts for five persons for last 3 weeks	10 healthy male non-smokers	8-oxodG excretion in 24-h urine	28% increase	
Verhagen et al. (1997), Netherlands	300 g of Brussels sprouts or non-cruciferous vegetables for consecutive periods of 1 week in random order	5 male and 5 female non-smokers	8-oxodG excretion in 24-h urine	No significant effect	Decrease in four men and two women
Lampe et al. (2000b), USA	16 g of fresh radish sprouts, 150 g of frozen cauliflower, 200 g of frozen broccoli and 70 g of fresh shredded cabbage per day for 6 days	43 healthy persons (21 men)	GSTA1-1 protein in serum GST activity in serum GSTM1 activity in lymphocytes	26% increase in GSTM1 null No change 36% increase in non-null women	No change in GSTM1 non-null

AUC, area under the time plasma concentration curve; CYP, cytochrome P450 enzymes; GST, glutathione S-transferase; ITC, isothiocyanate; PhIP, 2-amino-1-methyl-6-phenylimidazo[4,5-b]pyridine; MeIQx, 2-amino-3,8-dimethylimidazo[4,5-f]quinoxaline; NNK, 4-(methylnitrosamino)1-(3-pyridyl)-1-butanone; 8-oxodG, 8-oxo-7,8-dihydro-2'-deoxyguanosine mixture, the pharmacological action of which is due mainly to the S isomer and which is eliminated mainly by the action of the genetically polymorphic CYP2C9 enzyme (Takahashi & Echizen, 2001). It is not known whether the effect of cruciferous vegetables on warfarin elimination is related to the R or the S enantiomer, and the clinical consequence of this effect is therefore also unknown.

Cruciferous vegetables and metabolism of cooked food mutagens

Consumption of cruciferous vegetables may affect the metabolism and effects of heterocyclic amines in cooked food, partly because CYP1A2 is involved in bioactivation of these compounds to the pre-ultimate mutagens. Such interactions were investigated in three studies.

Eight healthy non-smokers (five women) received a diet containing heterocyclic amines from various well-cooked meat products, comparable to 300 g of well-cooked hamburger per day, for 6 weeks (DeMarini et al., 1997). In addition, four of the persons ate undescribed amounts of cauliflower, Brussels sprouts and cabbage, whereas the other four ate non-cruciferous vegetables. The mutagenicity of urine collected for 24 h every week was measured with and without enzymatic hydrolysis. Excretion of free urinary mutagens increased significantly during meat consumption, whereas the excretion of conjugated mutagens was unchanged. Excretion of free mutagens increased non-significantly in both vegetable groups. [The small number of persons and the relatively wide variation appear to preclude any conclusions.]

The metabolism of the heterocyclic amines 2-amino-3,8-dimethylimidazo-[4,5-*f*]quinoxaline (MeIQx) and 2-amino-1-methyl-6-phenylimidazo[4,5-*b*]pyridine (PhIP) was investigated in 20 healthy non-smokers who had eaten 250 g each of broccoli and Brussels sprouts per day for 12 days and had had two periods without cruciferous vegetables (Murray et al., 2001). The heterocyclic amines were present in known amounts in a cooked meal during each period. Excretion of MeIQx and PhIP in 10-h urine decreased by 23% and 21%, respectively, during cruciferous vegetable intake. Similarly, urinary mutagenicity was increased by 52% and 64% in the absence and presence, respectively, of a metabolic activation system during consumption of cruciferous vegetables. Interestingly, 12 days after the diet was discontinued, the excretion of MeIQx and PhIP was still decreased by 17% (not significantly) and 30%, respectively, and urinary mutagenicity was still increased when assessed in the presence of metabolic activation. No adducts of PhIP to DNA in lymphocytes could be detected during the study. MeIQx and to a lesser extent PhiP are metabolized by CYP1A2 as a first step in activation to the ultimate mutagens. The metabolism of the CYP1A2 substrate caffeine was increased only during cruciferous vegetable consumption, as described above. Accordingly, the transient decrease in MeIQx excretion and the increase in urinary mutagenicity without metabolic activation are consistent with increased CYP1A2-catalysed bioactivation. The prolonged changes in PhIP excretion and mutagenicity with metabolic activation, however, appear to be related to other alterations in metabolizing enzymes.

Increased bioactivation of PhIP after ingestion of well-cooked chicken was shown in a study of six healthy persons who ate broccoli for 3 days (Knize et al., 2002)

Cruciferous vegetables, metabolism of tobacco-specific carcinogens and CYP2E1, CYP2A6 and CYP2D6 activity

In an intervention study, the effect of eating watercress (56.8 g at each meal for 3 days) rich in phenethyl-ITC on the metabolism of NNK, catalysed by CYP1A2, was investigated in 11 healthy smokers (Hecht et al., 1995). The participants were asked not to change their smoking habits during the intervention. Urine was collected over 24-h periods at baseline, during the intervention and during follow up. Urinary excretion of 4-(methyl-nitrosamino)-1-(3-pyridyl)-1-butanol (NNAL) and NNAL glucuronides, which are detoxification products or alternative metabolites of the putative carcinogenic metabolites, increased by 34% on average during watercress consumption but returned to baseline during follow up. There was a significant correlation between excretion of the N-acetyl metabolite of phenethyl-ITC and excretion of the two NNK metabolites. Nicotine is 5-hydroxylated, forming cotinine, after an intermediate step, mainly by CYP2A6. In the intervention described above, there was no effect on the excretion of oxidative nicotine metabolites, although excretion of the glucuronides of cotinine and trans-3´-hydroxycotinine increased significantly (Hecht et al., 1999).

The metabolism of NNK was investigated in a cross-sectional study in relation to habitual dietary intake of cruciferous vegetables, assessed from a structured questionnaire including nine relevant items, in 84 smokers in Singapore (Hecht et al., 2004). Sam-ples of these vegetables obtained on markets at three times of the year were analysed, and glucobrassicins were found to be the main glucosinolates (70–93%) in seven of the nine vegetables studied. Urine was analysed for NNAL and its glucuronides. A significant inverse association (p = 0.01) was found between increased consumption of glucobrassicins and concentrations of NNAL in urine, after adjustment for the number of cigarettes smoked per day; similar trends were observed for NNAL glucuronides (p = 0.08) and all NNAL (p = 0.03).

The effect of eating 50 g of watercress on the activity of CYP2D6, which is important for elimination of many drugs used in psychiatric and cardiovascular diseases, was assessed in 29 healthy persons. No effects were found (Caporaso et al., 1994).

Acetaminophen is metabolized by conjugation and to a minor extent by oxidation to the reactive N-acetyl-para-aminobenzoquinone imine, catalysed by CYP2E1, CYP3A4 and CYP1A2, the first appearing to be most important in metabolism by human microsomes in vitro (Thummel et al., 1993). The imine is detoxified by glutathione conjugation, and the products cysteine and mercapturate acetaminophen can be measured in plasma and urine. In a cross-over study, the elimination and metabolism of acetaminophen (1 g as an oral tablet) were studied in 10 healthy, non-smoking volunteers, half of whom had received 50 g of a homogenate of watercress the previous evening (Chen, L. et al., 1996). The area under the plasma concentration–time curve (AUC) for the cysteine and mercapturate metabolites were decreased by 28% and 20%, respectively, after watercress ingestion, whereas the kinetics of the parent compound and the other metabolites were unchanged. Similarly, urinary excretion of the two metabolites was decreased by 30% and 24%. In a similar experiment, with only urine collection, the excretion of the cysteine and mercapturate metabolites was decreased by 40% and 38%, respectively, after watercress ingestion. Excretion of cysteine conjugates of acetaminophen was reduced by only 13% after a diet containing 500 g of Brussels sprouts or cabbage per day for 10 days (Pantuck et al., 1984).

Chlorzoxazone is metabolized through 6-hydroxylation, mainly by CYP2E1, and various metabolic indices of chlorzoxazone have been used as biomarkers of CYP2E1 activity. The oral pharmacokinetics of this compound was studied in 10 healthy volunteers before and after a single ingestion of 50 g of watercress homogenate (Leclercq et al., 1998). During watercress ingestion, the AUC of chlorzoxazone was increased by 56%.

Sixteen healthy non-smokers (two women) were studied after 12 days of eating a diet supplemented with 500 g of broccoli, after their usual diet or after a diet free of known inducers and inhibitors of cytochrome P450 enzymes (Kall et al., 1996). The ratio of chlorzoxazone to its 6-hydroxylated metabolite in plasma was not significantly affected by these diets.

Cruciferous vegetables and metabolism by phase II enzymes

The activity of GSTs, assessed from oxazepam and acetaminophen metabolism, was found to be moderately increased after ingestion of large amounts of cabbage and Brussels sprouts (Pantuck et al., 1984).

The effects of a diet rich in Brussels sprouts on GST activity and protein levels were investigated in two intervention studies (Bogaards et al., 1994; Nijhoff et al., 1995a,b). Ten healthy non-smoking men were given a diet containing 300 g of cooked vegetables per day for 6 weeks (Bogaards et al., 1994). During the first 3 weeks, all the vegetables were non-cruciferous. During the following 3 weeks, five men continued with non-cruciferous vegetables (controls), whereas the other five ate 300 g of Brussels sprouts per day. In the last group, the amount of GSTA1-1 protein in plasma, determined by radioimmunoassay, was increased by 40%. In a cross-over study, five male and five female non-smokers ate a diet containing 300 g of Brussels sprouts or non-cruciferous vegetables for consecutive periods of 1 week in random order. The amounts of GSTA1 and GSTP1 protein in rectal mucosa increased by 30% and 15% after consumption of Brussels sprouts (Nijhoff et al., 1995a). No change was found in the amounts of GSTA1, GSTM1 or GSTP1 protein in duodenum or of GSTP1 or GSTM1 protein in lymphocytes. The GST activity in cells was unchanged by the diet. In the men, the amount of GSTA1-1 protein in plasma increased by 50% while they were eating the Brussels sprouts diet, whereas there was no significant effect in women. The amounts of GSTP1 protein in plasma and GSTA1 and GSTP1 protein in urine were unchanged (Nijhoff et al., 1995b).

The effect of a diet rich in Brassica vegetables on GST protein and activity and modification by the GSTM1 genotype was investigated in 43 healthy persons (21 men) (Lampe et al., 2000b). In a random cross-over design, a basal vegetable diet was supplemented with 16 g of fresh radish sprouts, 150 g of frozen cauliflower, 200 g of frozen broccoli and 70 g of fresh shredded cabbage per day for 6 days. During the intervention with Brassica vegetables, the concentration of GSTA1 in serum increased by 26% in persons with the GSTM1-null genotype, whereas there was no change in persons with the non-null GSTM1 type. GST enzyme activity towards 1-chloro-2,4-dinitrobenzene and 7-chloro-4-nitrobenzo-2-oxa-1,3-diazole in plasma was unchanged. GSTM1 activity towards trans-stilbene oxide in lymphocytes increased significantly in women with the non-null genotype, but there was no change in men. The activity of this enzyme was low in all persons with the GSTM1-null genotype.

Biomarkers of oxidative DNA damage

Oxidative modification of DNA may be mutagenic, although many lesions are efficiently repaired. Measurement of 8-oxoguanine or its corresponding nucleoside 8-oxo-7,8-dihydro-2′deoxy-guanosine (8-oxodG) is one of the most widely used markers of oxidative DNA damage. The level of 8-oxodG in DNA isolated from cells or tissues is believed to reflect steady-state damage to DNA resulting from damage and repair, whereas excretion of 8-oxodG and 8-oxo-7,8-dihydro-2′-deoxyguanine in urine provides an estimate of the rate of damage to DNA in the whole body (Loft & Poulsen, 2000). 8-oxodG in urine may originate from nucleotide excision repair but also from removal of oxidized 2′-deoxyguanosine phosphate from the cellular pool of GTP by the MT1 enzyme and from turnover of mitochondria and cells. The effect of a diet rich in Brussels sprouts on 8-oxodG excretion was investigated in two studies.

Ten healthy non-smoking men were given a diet containing 300 g of cooked vegetables per day for 6 weeks (Verhagen et al., 1995). During the first 3 weeks, the vegetables were all non-cruciferous. During the next 3 weeks, five men continued with non-cruciferous vegetables (controls), whereas the other five ate 300 g of Brussels sprouts per day. Urinary excretion of 8-oxodG was measured on days 12 and 33. The group eating Brussels sprouts had a 28% decrease in 8-oxodG excretion (95% CI, 2–54%; $p = 0.039$, paired t test), whereas there was no significant change in the control group (95% CI, 46% decrease to 35% increase). No test of significance between the two groups was reported.

In a cross-over study, five male and five female non-smokers ate a diet containing 300 g of Brussels sprouts or non-cruciferous vegetables for consecutive periods of 1 week in random order (Verhagen et al., 1997). 8-oxodG excretion was measured at the end of each week. Excretion decreased in four of five men, whereas it increased

by about fourfold in a man who already had an excretion rate that was higher (> 5000 pmol/kg bw per 24 h) than any found by others using HPLC-based analytical methods. Two of the women showed decreased excretion while eating sprouts, whereas the other three women showed increased excretion.

The two studies suggest that a diet rich in Brussels sprouts might decrease the rate of oxidative damage to DNA and/or deoxynucleotides.

Isothiocyanates
No data were available.

Indoles
Ratio of 2-:16α-hydroxylation of estrogens
Seven volunteers were given 500 mg of indole-3-carbinol in a capsule daily for 1 week and then a dose of [2-^{3}H]estradiol. The dose of indole-3-carbinol was equivalent to 300–500 g of cabbage per day. The extent of 2-hydroxylation was measured by determining the amount of tritium released into the medium after hydroxylation at the C2 position. All seven persons showed increased 2-hydroxylation after treatment (Michnovicz & Bradlow, 1990). In a second study, groups of 20 persons received 400 mg of indole-3-carbinol, pure fibre (α-cellulose) or a placebo daily for 3 months. Increased 2-hydroxylation was observed only in those given indole-3-carbinol, and the response was stable over 3 months (Bradlow et al., 1994).

To determine the minimum effective dose of indole-3-carbinol, groups of 10 persons were given increasing doses, from 50 mg/day to 100 mg/day, 200 mg/day, 300 mg/day and finally 400 mg/day. Clinical chemical parameters were normal in all persons at all times. No increase in 2-hydroxylation of estradiol was observed at doses up to 200 mg/day, but significant increases

were seen at 300 mg/day and 400 mg/day (Wong et al., 1997).

Cervical intra-epithelial neoplasia is a premalignant lesion associated with HPV infection, and malignant progression has been linked to particular subtypes, including HPV16, 18, 33 and 35. In a placebo-controlled trial involving 30 patients with cervical intra-epithelial neoplasia, the group given indole-3-carbinol orally at 200 or 400 mg/day showed a higher tendency to regression of their lesions than the placebo group, in a dose-dependent pattern (Bell et al., 2000). [The Working Group noted that the period of observation in this study might not have been long enough to detect the extent of spontaneous regression that might have occurred.]

Cervical tissue and foreskin tissue have a high rate of 16α-hydroxylation, which is further increased by HPV infection. In addition, 16α-hydroxy-estrone has been shown to promote viral proliferation, resulting in a positive feedback loop. Indole-3-carbinol and 2-hydroxyestrone have been shown to inhibit viral proliferation by blocking exons E6 and E7 of the virus, which are diminished (Yuan et al., 1999). As a result, further growth of the virus is inhibited. Recurrence in a case of laryngeal papillomatosis was blocked (Auborn et al., 1998) (Figure 16).

Less oncogenic types of HPV are believed to cause benign tumours, including recurrent respiratory papillomatosis, which, while rare, is the commonest benign laryngeal tumour of childhood. Indole-3-carbinol has been investigated for use as a non-invasive means of treating this condition. A case report (Coll et al., 1997) and the preliminary results of a phase I trial (Rosen et al., 1998) indicated cessation of papilloma growth in children given indole-3-carbinol. In the trial, clinical response correlated well with changes in urinary 2-:16α-hydroxy-estrone ratios. [The Working Group

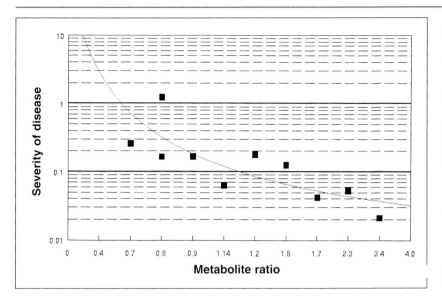

Figure 16 Relationship between ratio of 2-:16α-hydroxyestradiol and severity of laryngeal papillomatosis

noted that a high proportion of the patients in complete remission were adults and had presumably had the condition for a long time, so that there may have been substantial age-related confounding in the study.] Positive treatment responses were associated with an increase in 2-hydroxylation. Failure of treatment to raise the 2-:16α metabolite ratio was associated with absence of a therapeutic response.

Dietary supplementation with 3,3′-diindolylmethane given to one breast cancer patient treated after surgery with tamoxifen resulted in a significant increase in the 2-:16 α-hydroxyestrone metabolite ratio (Zeligs et al., 2003).

Discussion

Few studies were available for evaluating the relationship between intake of cruciferous vegetables or their constituents and cancers at several sites; for others, the findings with regard to intake of cruciferous vegetables were inconsistent. The sites investigated include the oropharynx, oesophagus, pancreas, larynx, cervix,

endometrium, ovary, prostate, urinary bladder, kidney and brain, and malignant lymphoma. Studies on associations with cancers at these sites are summarized in Handbook 8 (IARC, 2003), and the findings are therefore not further discussed here. With regard to cancers of the thyroid and stomach, data were available only from studies in which food frequency questionnaires were used. For cancers of the colorectum, lung and breast, however, at least one study was available in which an exposure marker or assessment of genetic polymorphism had been used.

Studies were considered in the evaluation of cancer preventive activity only if the reports provided estimates of risk for estimated consumption of all or individual cruciferous vegetables (e.g. broccoli) and 95% confidence intervals.

Figures 17–24 show the estimated weighted means of the reported relative risks (represented as diamonds) for cancers at some sites. In the figures, the width of the confidence interval is represented by the horizontal

line, and the relative size of the study is shown by the size of the squares. If a study report included estimates for different sub-groups, e.g. males and females, both were included. In interpreting weighted means, it should be recognized that they do not represent the result of a formal meta-analysis and that contrasts of high versus low consumption were not consistent among studies.

Figures 17 and 18 summarize the evaluable data for stomach cancer. Two of the three cohort studies were based on incident cases, but one, which reported a positive association with cruciferous vegetable intake, was based on deaths. The lack of information on incident cases in that study is, however, probably not critical, as stomach cancer is usually fatal. The overall OR was 0.91 (95% CI, 0.67–1.23). This value is similar to the overall OR from five studies on intake of all vegetables (IARC, 2003). The results of the case–control studies were more consistent, resulting in an overall significant inverse association with cruciferous vegetable intake (OR, 0.81; 95% CI, 0.73–0.90). It is impossible, however, to exclude recall bias and confounding from unmeasured confounders (including other dietary factors) in the case–control studies, and it is relevant that the overall OR for intake of all vegetables was 0.66 (0.61–0.71) (IARC, 2003).

Figures 19 and 20 summarize the evaluable data for colorectal cancer. Overall, there was no association with cruciferous vegetable intake in the cohort studies. In the case–control studies (Figure 20), a significant inverse association was found (OR, 0.73; 95% CI, 0.63–0.84). A large case–control study (Peters et al., 1992) could not be included in Figure 20, however, as findings were reported only for a small increment in consumption, and this showed no association with cruciferous vegetable intake.

Table 41. Studies of prevention of carcinogen-induced tumours of preneoplastic lesions by cruciferous vegetables in experimental animals

Organ site, species, strain (sex)	Age at start (weeks)	No. of animals per group	Carcinogen, dose, route, duration	Cruciferous vegetables, amount, duration	Timing of treatment	Preventive efficacy by tumour incidence (TI) or multiplicity (TM)	Summarized effect	Reference
Stomach								
Rat Wistar WKY (M)	8	30	MNNG, 50 μg/ml drinking-water, killed at 40 weeks	*Wasabi*, 10% diet, 40 weeks	Through-out	Glandular stomach TI (%): MNNG alone, 20[b], + *wasabi*, 0[a]; Gastroduodenal TI (%): MNNG alone, 30[b], + *wasabi*, 3[a]	*Wasabi* suppressed glandular stomach tumours	Tanida et al. (1991)
Colon								
Mouse CF1 (M)	Weanling	20–22	DMH, 20 mg/kg bw × 20 s.c., killed at 20 and 34 weeks. Control diet: soya bean meal extract, 44% protein	Cruciferous seed meals and hulls (crambe, rapeseed and canola), 12% diet, 20 or 34 weeks	Initiation or throughout	Colon TI (%) at 20 weeks: DMH alone, 70[b]; + commercial crambe, 14[a], + autolysed crambe, 50; + crambe hulls/soya bean, 42; + rapeseed, 15[a], + canola, 32[a]. Colon TI (%) at 34 weeks: DMH alone, 100[b]; + commercial crambe, 67[a], + autolysed crambe, 25[a] (high mortality); + crambe hulls/soya bean, 79[a], + rapeseed, 80[a]; + canola, 67[a]	Cruciferous seed meals and hulls reduced incidence of colon tumours	Barrett et al. (1998)
Rat Fischer 344 (M)	6	20	DMH: 20 mg/kg bw × 4 s.c. + PhIP: 0.02% diet; killed 36 weeks after first DMH. Control diet: commercial powdered diet (Labo MR stock)	Red cabbage colour, 5% diet, 32 weeks	Post-initiation (DMH) or through-out (PhIP)	Adenoma incidence: DMH + PhIP, 16[b], + red cabbage colour, 8[a]. Adenocarcinoma incidence: DMH + PhIP, 11[b], + red cabbage colour, 4[a]. Total tumours/rat: DMH + PhIP, 2.7[b], + red cabbage colour, 1.0[a]. ACF/rat: PhIP, 2.5[b], + red cabbage colour, 0.9[a]. AC/ACF: PhIP, 1.75[b], + red cabbage colour, 0.73[a]	Red cabbage colour diet suppressed both colorectal tumours and ACFs	Hagiwara et al. (2002)

Table 41 (contd)

Organ site, species, strain (sex)	Age at start (weeks)	No. of animals per group	Carcinogen, dose, route, duration	Cruciferous vegetables, amount, duration	Timing of treatment	Preventive efficacy by tumour incidence (TI) or multiplicity (TM)	Summarized effect	Reference
Rat Sprague-Dawley (M)	8	15	AOM, 15 mg/kg bw × i.p., killed after 14 weeks Control diet: AIN-93M	Sprouts, 10% diet Broccoli, 10% diet	Throughout or post-initiation	ACF multiplicity reduced (23%) by sprouts ($p < 0.05$)	Sprouts reduced ACFs	Rijken et al. (1999)
Rat Fischer 344 (M)	250 g	8	IQ, 100 mg/kg bw × 10 gavage, killed 16 weeks after the last IQ Control diet: modified AIN-76	Garden cress juice, 5%, drinking-water	Initiation	ACF/ rat: IQ alone, 8.16[b], + garden cress, 3.90[a] ACF with 4 or more crypts: IQ alone, 2.27[b], + garden cress, 1.00[a]	Garden cress reduced ACFs	Kassie et al. (2002)
Rat Fischer 344 (M)	4	8	IQ, 100 mg/kg bw × 10, gavage, killed 16 weeks after last IQ Control diet: modified AIN-76	Brussels sprouts and red cabbage juice, 5%, drinking-water 5 days before and during IQ treatment	Initiation	ACF/rat: IQ alone, 10.33[b]; + Brussels sprouts (Cyrus, raw), 5.50[a], + Brussels sprouts (Cyrus, cooked), 5.00[a], + brussels sprouts (Maximus, raw), 6.00[a], + brussels sprouts (Maximus, cooked), 6.14[a], + red cabbage (Roxy, raw), 8.25; + red cabbage (Roxy, cooked), 9.66; + red cabbage (Reliant, raw), 8.25; + red cabbage (Reliant, cooked), 8.57	Brussels sprouts reduced ACFs	Kassie et al. (2003a)
Rat Wistar (M)	7	7	DMH, 30 mg/kg bw × 2 s.c., killed 42 days after second DMH Control diet: semi-synthetic basal diet appropriate for growing rats	Freeze-dried, raw or blanched Brussels sprouts, 10% juice or diet, 4 weeks	Post-initiation	ACF/colon: DMH alone, 24.1; + raw sprout, 15.3; blanched sprout, 21.6	Brussels sprouts reduced ACFs	Smith et al. (2003)

Table 41 (contd)

Liver

Organ site, species, strain (sex)	Age at start (weeks)	No. of animals per group	Carcinogen, dose, route, duration	Cruciferous vegetables, amount, duration	Timing of treatment	Preventive efficacy by tumour incidence (TI) or multiplicity (TM)	Summarized effect	Reference
Rat Fischer 344 (M)	Weanling	10	AFB_1, 2 mg/kg diet for 26 weeks, killed at 41 weeks Control diet: purified diet	Freeze-dried cauliflower head, 20% diet, 26 weeks	Throughout	Survival (%): AFB, alone, 0; + cauliflower, 100 Hepatic TI (%): AFB_1 alone, 100; + cauliflower, 100 Histopathology of hepatic tumours: AFB_1 alone, very large and metastasized; + cauliflower, small and localized	Cauliflower reduced mortality from and progression of hepatic tumours	Stoewsand et al. (1978)
Rat Fischer 344 (M)	Weanling	8–11	AFB_1, 1 mg/kg diet for 26 weeks, killed at 42 weeks Control diet: modified AIN-76	Freeze-dried cabbage, 25% diet, 26 weeks	Throughout	Liver tumours/rat: AFB_1 alone, 30[b]; + cabbage, 13[a]	Dried cabbage decreased liver tumours	Boyd et al. (1982)
Toad *Bufo viridis* (M, F)	40 g	50/50	DMBA, 0.5 mg per toad × 36 injected into dorsal lymph sac, killed after 12 weeks Control diet: earthworms	Ground cabbage, 1–2 ml, 12 weeks	Initiation or post-initiation	Liver-cell TI: DMBA, 29[b]; + 1 ml cabbage diet before, 15[a]; + 2 ml cabbage diet before, 12[a]; + 2 ml cabbage diet after, 27	Cabbage inhibited liver tumours	Sadek et al. (1995)
Rat Fischer 344 (M)	Weanling	7–8	AFB_1, 250 µg/kg bw per day, gavage × 10, killed after 6 and 12 weeks Control diet: purified diet	Brussels sprouts, glucosinolate extract and non-glucosinolate residue, 20% diet, 5 weeks	Initiation	Liver GGT foci (no./cm²) after 6 weeks: AFB, alone, 13.1[b]; + Brussels sprouts, 5.9[a], + extract, 6.0[a], + residue, 13.1 Liver GGT foci (no./cm²) after 12 weeks: AFB_1 alone, 12.5[b], + Brussels sprouts, 8.6[a], + extract, 7.9[a]; + residue, 11.3	Brussels sprouts and its extract inhibited hepatic GGT foci	Godlewski et al. (1985)

Table 41 (contd)

Organ site, species, strain (sex)	Age at start (weeks)	No. of animals per group	Carcinogen, dose, route, duration	Cruciferous vegetables, amount, duration	Timing of treatment	Preventive efficacy by tumour incidence (TI) or multiplicity (TM)	Summarized effect	Reference
Rat Fischer 344 (M)	4	8	IQ, 100 mg/kg bw × 10 gavage, killed 16 weeks after last IQ Control diet: modified AIN-76	Brussels sprouts and red cabbage juice, 5%, drinking-water, 5 days before and during IQ treatment	Through-out	GST-P$^+$ foci/ cm^2: IQ alone, 13.00[b]; + Brussels sprouts (Cyrus, raw), 4.32[a]; + Brussels sprouts (Cyrus, cooked), 7.01; + Brussels sprouts (Maximus, raw), 9.45; + Brussels sprouts (Maximus, cooked), 5.38[a]; + red cabbage (Roxy, raw), 10.26; + red cabbage (Roxy, cooked), 7.47[a]; + red cabbage (Reliant, raw), 6.52[a]; + red cabbage (Reliant, cooked), 10.51 GST-P$^+$ foci area (mm^2/cm^2): IQ alone, 0.0903[b]; + Brussels sprouts (Cyrus, raw), 0.0079[a]; + Brussels sprouts (Cyrus, cooked), 0.0105[a]; + Brussels sprouts (Maximus, raw), 0.0137[a]; + Brussels sprouts (Maximus, cooked), 0.0078[a]	Brussels sprouts and red cabbage reduced GST-P$^+$	Kassie et al. (2003a)
Mammary gland								
Rat Sprague-Dawley (F)	7	16	DMBA, 12 mg, gavage, killed 18 weeks after DMBA Control diet: semi-purified diet (casein 27%, starch 59%, corn oil 10%, salt mix 4%, vitamins)	Dehydrated powdered cabbage, 10% diet, 17 weeks Cauliflower, 10% diet, 17 weeks	Post-initiation (1 week after DMBA)	TI (%): DMBA alone, 94[b]; + cabbage diet, 63[a]; + cauliflower diet, 63[a] No. of tumours/rat: DMBA alone, 3.4[b]; + cabbage diet, 1.1[a], + cauliflower diet, 1.4[a]	Cabbage and cauliflower inhibited mammary tumours	Wattenberg (1983)

Table 41 (contd)

Organ site, species, strain (sex)	Age at start (weeks)	No. of animals per group	Carcinogen, dose, route, duration	Cruciferous vegetables, amount, duration	Timing of treatment	Preventive efficacy by tumour incidence (TI) or multiplicity (TM)	Summarized effect	Reference
Rat Sprague-Dawley (F)	6	15	DMBA, 60 mg/kg bw, gavage, observed 15 weeks after DMBA Control diet: semi-purified (sucrose 18.7%, fibre 1.3%)	Freeze-dried Brussels sprouts, 20% diet, 4 weeks	Initiation	Palpable mammary TI (%): DMBA alone, 77[b], + Brussels sprouts, 13[a]	Brussels sprouts reduced mammary tumours	Stoewsand et al. (1988)
Rat Sprague-Dawley (F)	6	16–20	DMBA, 50 mg/kg bw, gavage, killed 27 weeks after DMBA Control diet: AIN-76, except glucose 25%, sucrose 25%	Freeze-dried Brussels sprouts, 20% diet, 4 weeks	Initiation	Papillary carcinoma incidence (%): DMBA alone, 50; + Brussels sprouts, 35 Adenocarcinoma incidence (%): DMBA alone, 35; + Brussels sprouts, 10 Fibroadenoma incidence (%): DMBA alone, 10; + Brussels sprouts, 5 No statistical evaluation	Brussels sprouts reduced mammary tumours	Stoewsand et al. (1989)
Rat Sprague-Dawley (F)	50 days	25–35	MNU, 50 mg/kg bw, i.v., killed when palpable tumours reached 0.5 cm Control diet: American Institute of Nutrition, except dextrin/dextrose substituted for sucrose	Dried cabbage, 5% diet and 10% diet; collards, 5%; cabbage residue, 3.2% diet	Post-initiation	TI (%): MNU alone, 84[b], + 5% cabbage, 63[a], 10% cabbage, 70; 5% collards, 80 MNU alone, 85[b], + 5% cabbage, 53[a], 3.2% cabbage residue, 56[a]	Cabbage diets reduced tumours	Bresnick et al. (1990)

Table 41 (contd)

Organ site, species, strain (sex)	Age at start (weeks)	No. of animals per group	Carcinogen, dose, route, duration	Cruciferous vegetables, amount, duration	Timing of treatment	Preventive efficacy by tumour incidence (TI) or multiplicity (TM)	Summarized effect	Reference
Rat Sprague-Dawley (F)	50 days	20	DMBA, 10 mg, gavage, killed 18 weeks after DMBA. Control diet: Emulphor 620P and water	Dried broccoli sprouts extract (25 or 100 μmol glucosinolates; 25, 50 or 100 μmol ITC), gavage × 5	Initiation	All treatments markedly reduced total number of tumours: DMBA alone, 34; + treatments, 11–19	Broccoli sprout extracts reduced mammary tumours	Fahey et al. (1997)
Skin								
Mouse Swiss albino (M)	7–8	8	DMBA, 100 μg + croton oil topically × 48, killed at week 16	Mustard seed), 800 mg/kg bw, gavage, 18 weeks	Throughout	TI (%): DMBA alone, 100[b]; treatment, 50[a] Cumulative number of papillomas: DMBA alone, 71[b]; treatment, 9[a] Latency of tumours (weeks): DMBA alone, 7.8[b]; treatment, 11.3[a]	Brassica compestris reduced skin tumours	Qiblawi & Kumar (1999)
Transplacental and lactational								
Mouse Swiss albino (M, F)	Pregnant (13–14 weeks)	6–8	DMBA, 5 mg, gavage, days 15–17 of gestation, F1 progeny killed at 56 weeks of age	Mustard seed oil, 0.05 and 0.1 ml, gavage, days 13–19 of gestation	Initiation	TI of F1 (%): DMBA alone, 65[b]; 0.05 mustard oil, 29[a]; 0.1 mustard oil, 16[a]	Mustard seed oil inhibited transplacental and translactational carcinogenesis	Hashim et al. (1998)
	Lactating	6–8	DMBA, 3 mg, gavage, days 3, 6, 9, 12 and 15 of lactation, F1 progeny killed at 56 weeks of age	Mustard seed oil, 0.05 and 0.1 ml, gavage, days 1–15 of lactation	Initiation	TI of F1 (%): DMBA alone, 70[b]; 0.05 mustard oil, 32[a]; 0.1 mustard oil, 18[a]		
Metastasis								
Mouse BALB/c (F)	6	15	BALB/c mammary tumour cells (410.4), 5 × 10^4, i.v., killed 3 weeks later	Dried cabbage and collards, 9.1% and 4.8% diet, 9 weeks	Throughout	Pulmonary colonies in experiment 1: Control, 100; diet, 60 Pulmonary colonies in experiment 2: Control, 200; diet, 125	Cabbage and collards decreased pulmonary metastasis	Scholar et al. (1989)

[a,b], statistically significant when letters are different

AC, aberrant crypts; ACF, aberrant crypt foci; GGT, γ-glutamyl transferase; GST-P[+], glutathione S-transferase placental positive; AFB, aflatoxin B₁; AOM, azoxymethane; DMBA, 7,12-dimethylbenz[a]anthracene; DMH, 1,2-dimethylhydrazine; F, female; M, male; MNNG, N-methyl-N'-nitro-N-nitrosoguanidine; MNU, N-methyl-N-nitrosourea; PhIP, 2-amino-1-methyl-6-phenylimidazo[4,5-b]pyridine; IQ, 2-amino-3-methylimidazo-[4,5-f]quinoline; s.c., subcutaneously; i.p., intraperitoneally; i.v., intravenously juice. The total numbers of IQ-induced aberrant crypts and crypt foci and the number of foci with four or more aberrant crypts were significantly reduced in the group that received IQ plus garden cress juice compared with the group that was given IQ only.

Kassie et al. (2003a) also reported the preventive effects of widely eaten cruciferous vegetables such as Brussels sprouts and red cabbage against IQ-induced aberrant crypt foci. Male Fischer 344 rats were given IQ on 10 alternate days and received drinking-water supplemented with Brussels sprouts and red cabbage juice (5% v/v) before and during carcinogen treatment. Two cultivars of each vegetable were tested. Brussels sprouts reduced the frequency of IQ-induced aberrant crypt foci by 41–52%, but no protection was seen in the colon after treatment with red cabbage. Cooking of the vegetables at 100 °C for 10 min had no influence on their protective effect. The stronger effects of the Brussels sprouts may be due to the fact that the overall glucosinolate content was substantially higher than that of the cabbage cultivars, but it was not possible to attribute the reduction in preneoplastic lesions to specific glucosinolates.

Smith et al. (2003) explored the effects of both raw and thermally processed Brussels sprout tissue on the frequency of aberrant crypt foci induced by 1,2-dimethylhydrazine in rat colon. Oral administration of uncooked Brussels sprouts as a freeze-dried powder reduced the number of foci, significantly enhanced the level of apoptosis and reduced mitosis in colonic crypts. There was little evidence of these effects when intact glucosinolates were administered in blanched sprout tissue, which lacked active myrosinase. [The Working Group concluded that glucosinolate breakdown products derived from Brassica vegetables can affect the balance of colorectal cell proliferation and death.]

Liver

Diets containing cruciferous vegetables such as cauliflower, cabbage and Brussels sprouts consistently inhibited liver tumorigenesis induced in rats and toads by aflatoxin B_1, IQ or DMBA.

Stoewsand et al. (1978) reported that a cauliflower diet attenuated the toxic effects of aflatoxin B_1 in Fischer 344 rats, preventing death and internal haemorrhage and consequently reducing liver tumour size and metastasis.

Boyd et al. (1982) reported the inhibitory effects of cabbage on hepatocarcinogenesis in weanling male Fischer 344 rats fed a purified diet or diets containing 25% (w/w) freeze-dried cabbage with or without aflatoxin B_1 at 1 mg/kg for 26 weeks. Within 3–7 weeks, the cabbage diet had diminished the aflatoxin B_1-induced increase in plasma α-fetoprotein. When the experiment was extended to 42 weeks by maintaining the animals on the basal diet for a further 16 weeks, the rats given the control diet had 30 tumours per liver, whereas those receiving the cabbage diet had 13 tumours per liver.

Sadek et al. (1995) induced hepatocellular carcinoma in 29 of 100 toads (Bufo viridis) by administering 0.5 mg of DMBA 3 times per week for 12 weeks. Toads treated with 1 or 2 ml of cabbage slurry 3 h before the carcinogen every day for 12 weeks had a lower incidence of liver tumours, but administration of 2 ml of cabbage 3 h after DMBA treatment was ineffective in 27 of 100 toads.

Godlewski et al. (1985) determined whether the liver detoxication enzymes GST-P+ and GGT induced in foci by aflatoxin B_1 were changed by feeding weanling rats a diet containing Brussels sprouts, a glucosinolate fraction of Brussels sprouts (extract) or a non-glucosinolate fraction (residue). All three of these diets induced high levels of hepatic GST-specific activity as compared with purified basal diet fed to control rats. The Brussels sprouts and the extract, but not the residue, inhibited hepatic GGT foci induced by aflatoxin B_1.

Kassie et al. (2003a) reported the preventive effects of Brussels sprouts and red cabbage against IQ-induced liver GST-P+ foci. Male Fischer 344 rats were given IQ at 100 mg/kg bw per day on 10 alternate days and received drinking-water supplemented with Brussels sprouts and red cabbage juice (5% v/v) before and during carcinogen treatment. The size of the liver GST-P+ foci was reduced by 85–91% with Brussels sprouts and by 41–83% with the red cabbage, whereas the frequency of foci was only moderately decreased (by 19–50%). Cooking of the vegetables at 100 °C for 10 min had no effect on their protective effects.

Mammary gland

Diets containing cruciferous vegetables such as cabbage, cauliflower, Brussels sprouts and broccoli consistently inhibited mammary tumorigenesis in rats induced by 7,12-dimethylbenz[a]anthracene (DMBA) or N-methyl-N-nitrosourea.

Wattenberg (1983) reported that several plant materials, including cabbage and cauliflower, inhibited mammary carcinogenesis when fed after carcinogens. Female Sprague-Dawley rats were given 12 mg of DMBA by gavage and 1 week later were fed a basal diet or a diet supplemented with 10% (w/w) cabbage or cauliflower. The experiment was terminated 18 weeks after DMBA administration. The incidences and multiplicity of mammary tumours were significantly reduced in the groups fed cabbage or cauliflower as compared with the group fed the basal diet.

Stoewsand et al. (1988) examined the effect of dietary Brussels sprouts on mammary carcinogenesis induced by DMBA in female Sprague-Dawley rats. The animals fed a 20% Brussels sprouts diet only during the initiation period of carcinogenesis had a palpable mammary tumour incidence of 13%, while those fed a semi-purified diet during this period had a tumour incidence of 77% 15 weeks after the dose of DMBA.

Stoewsand *et al.* (1989) also reported on the preventive effect of Brussels sprouts cultivated with the addition of inorganic selenium to the plant growth medium. Groups of female Sprague-Dawley weanling rats were fed diets containing 20% Brussels sprouts supplemented with 0.03, 0.58, 1.29 or 6.71 mg/kg of naturally occurring selenium 2 weeks before and 2 weeks after a single dose of DMBA. The rats were then placed on a low selenium basal diet for an additional 25 weeks. All the Brussels sprouts diets reduced the incidence of DMBA-induced mammary carcinogenesis. Differences in selenium content did not further influence mammary tumorigenesis.

Bresnick *et al.* (1990) examined the effects of cruciferous vegetables in combination with high dietary fat on mammary tumorigenesis. Mammary cancer was induced in female Sprague-Dawley rats by a single injection of *N*-methyl-*N*-nitrosourea, and the rats were then randomized to control fat (5%) or high fat (24.6%) diets. Dried cabbage (5% and 10%) and collards (5%) were included in the diets of some animals. The rats on the control fat diet containing 5% cabbage had a significantly lower incidence of mammary cancer than rats fed the control fat diet without cabbage. This effect was not observed in comparable rats on the high-fat diet. The inhibitory effect on mammary tumorigenesis was also found with a residue obtained from cabbage by exhaustive extraction with methanol, methylene chloride and petroleum ether.

Fahey *et al.* (1997) reported that extracts of 3-day-old broccoli sprouts containing either glucoraphanin or sulforaphane were highly effective in reducing the incidence, multiplicity and rate of development of mammary tumours in DMBA-treated rats. The sprouts of many broccoli cultivars contain negligible quantities of indole glucosinolates, which predominate in the mature vegetable and may give rise to degradation products that can enhance tumorigenesis. The authors concluded that small quantities of cruciferous sprouts can protect against mammary tumours as effectively as much larger quantities of mature vegetables of the same variety.

Skin

Qiblawi and Kumar (1999) reported the preventive properties of an ethanol extract of the seeds of *Brassica compestris* var. *sarason* (mustard seed) on DMBA-induced skin tumorigenesis in male Swiss albino mice. Significant reductions in tumour incidence, tumour burden and the cumulative number of papillomas were observed in mice treated orally with the seed extract, continuously before and after the initiation stages of tumorigenesis, compared with the control groups. The latency in the experimental group increased significantly (to 11.3 weeks) compared with the control group (7.8 weeks).

Transplacental and translactational carcinogenesis

Hashim *et al.* (1998) reported the chemopreventive potential of mustard seed oil on DMBA-induced transplacental and translactational carcinogenesis in Swiss albino mice. As the mustard oil was a lipid component, the diet is unlikely to have contained significant quantities of isothiocyanates. Mice were treated with mustard oil at a concentration of 0.05 or 0.10 ml per day on days 13–19 of gestation, each also

receiving 5 mg of DMBA on days 15–17 of gestation. The tumour incidence in the F_1 progeny was significantly reduced at both concentrations, from 65% in the control group to 29% and 16%, respectively, in the experimental groups. The mean number of tumours per effective F_1 progeny was reduced from 1.56 in the control group to 0.93 and 0.41 in the animals treated with lower and higher doses of mustard oil, respectively. When lactating dams were given the mustard oil at 0.05 or 0.10 ml per day for the first 15 days of lactation, in addition to 3 mg of DMBA on days 3, 6, 9, 12 and 15, the tumour incidence at multiple sites was significantly reduced, from 70% in controls to 32% and 18%, respectively, at the lower and higher doses. The mean number of tumours in F_1 mice was reduced from a control value of 1.71 to 0.96 at the lower dose and 0.34 at the higher dose.

Lung metastasis

Six-week-old female BALB/c mice were fed diets supplemented with dried cabbage or dried collards at a concentration of 9.1% or 4.8% for 6 weeks, and then received an injection of BALB/c mammary tumour cells into the lateral tail vein. The mice continued to receive the diets for another 3 weeks. The incidence of surface metastases on the lungs was reduced from the control value by about 50% at both doses (Scholar *et al.*, 1989).

Selenium-enriched broccoli

In the studies with selenium-enriched broccoli summarized below, the main objective was to study the effects of selenium and not those of broccoli. These studies are summarized in Table 42.

Finley *et al.* (2000) examined the effects of high-selenium broccoli on aberrant crypt focus formation. Fischer 344 rats were given diets supplemented with selenium at 0.1 or 1.0

Table 42. Studies of prevention of carcinogen-induced colon preneoplastic lesions by selenium-rich broccoli

Organ site, species, strain (sex)	Age at start (weeks)	No. of animals per group	Carcinogen, dose, route, duration	Cruciferous vegetables, amount, duration	Timing of treatment	Preventive efficacy by tumour incidence (TI) or multiplicity (TM)	Summarized effect	Reference
Rat Fischer 344 (M)	Weanling	18	DMABP, 100 mg/kg bw × 2 s.c., killed 8 weeks after second DMABP DMH, 25 mg/kg bw × 2 s.c., killed 8 weeks after second DMH Control diet: low-selenium torula yeast	High selenium broccoli (1 mg/kg selenium), diet, 11 weeks High selenium broccoli (2 mg/kg selenium), diet, 11 weeks	Throughout	AC/rat: DMABP + selenate, 8.6[b], DMABP + high-selenium broccoli, 4.3[a] ACF/rat: DMABP + selenate, 3.4[b], DMABP + high-selenium broccoli, 2.1[a] AC/rat: DMH + selenite > DMH + high-selenium broccoli ACF/rat: DMH + selenite > DMH + high-selenium broccoli	Selenium from broccoli reduced ACFs in colon	Finley et al. (2000)
Rat Fischer 344 (M)	Weanling	18	DMH, 25 mg/kg bw × 2 s.c., killed 8 weeks after second DMH Control diet: selenium-deficient torula yeast	High-selenium broccoli florets (2 mg/kg selenium), diet, 11 weeks; High-selenium broccoli sprouts (2 mg/kg selenium), diet, 11 weeks	Throughout	Total ACFs: DMH alone, 137[b]; + high-selenium broccoli, 68[a],+ high-selenium sprouts, 71[a]	Selenium-enriched broccoli decreased ACFs in colon	Finley et al. (2001)
Rat Sprague-Dawley (F)	7	30	MNU, 50 mg/kg bw, killed at 22 weeks Control diet: AIN76A + 0.1 mg/kg selenium	High-selenium broccoli (3 mg/kg selenium), diet, 22 weeks	Throughout	Mammary TI: MNU alone, 90[b]; + high selenium broccoli, 37[a]	Selenium-enriched broccoli decreased mammary tumours	Finley et al. (2001)
Rat Fischer 344 (M)	Weanling	18	DMABP, 100 mg/kg bw × 2 s.c. or DMH, 25 mg/kg bw × 2 s.c, killed 8 weeks after second treatment Control diet: selenium-deficient torula yeast	High-selenium broccoli (1 mg/kg selenium), diet, 11 weeks High-selenium broccoli (2 mg/kg selenium), diet, 11 weeks	Through-out	AC/rat: DMABP alone, 9.7[b]; + 0.1 mg/kg selenium as broccoli, 8.4; + 1.0 mg/kg selenium as broccoli, 4.3[a] ACF/rat: DMH alone, 95; + 2.0 mg/kg selenite + low-selenium broccoli, 102[b]; + 2.0 mg/kg selenite as high-selenium broccoli, 56[a] ACF/rat: DMH alone, 239; + 2.0 mg/kg selenite + low-selenium broccoli, 299[b]; + 2.0 mg/kg selenite as high-selenium broccoli, 153[a]	Selenium from broccoli reduced ACFs in colon	Finley & Davis (2001)

AC, aberrant crypts; ACF, aberrant crypt foci; DMABP, 3',2'-dimethyl 4-aminobiphenyl; DMH, 1,2-dimethylhydrazine; s.c., subcutaneously; MNU, N-methyl-N-nitrosourea µg/g as selenized broccoli. In another experiment, rats were given the same diet supplemented with selenium at 2.0 µg/g diet as selenite plus low-selenium broccoli or as selenized broccoli. The rats received the diets for 3 weeks and were then injected with 3′,2′-dimethyl-4-aminobiphenyl or 1,2-dimethylhydrazine. Supranutritional amounts of selenium supplied as high-selenium broccoli significantly decreased the incidences of aberrant crypts and aberrant crypt foci compared with other dietary treatments.

Finley et al. (2001) examined the ability of high-selenium broccoli or high-selenium broccoli sprouts to protect against 1,2-dimethylhydrazine-induced aberrant crypt foci in the colon. Fischer 344 rats fed diets containing selenium at 2.0 µg/g as either high-selenium broccoli florets or high-selenium broccoli sprouts had significantly fewer aberrant crypt foci than rats fed a diet containing selenium at 0.1 or 2 µg/g supplied as selenite with or without the addition of low-selenium broccoli. In another experiment (Finlay & Davis, 2001), weanling Fischer 344 rats were fed diets containing various amounts of selenium from broccoli and were injected with 3′,2′-dimethyl-4-aminobiphenyl or 1,2-dimethylhydrazine. After 11 weeks on the diets, the animals were killed and their colons examined for aberrant crypt foci. The incidence was significantly reduced in animals fed high-selenium broccoli.

Finley et al. (2001) also reported that Sprague-Dawley rats given diets containing either low- or high-selenium broccoli had significantly fewer mammary tumours induced by N-methyl-N-nitrosourea (MNU) than rats fed 0.1 mg of selenium as selenite without the addition of broccoli. High-selenium broccoli was more protective than low-selenium broccoli.

Glucosinolates

The first study on inhibition of carcinogenesis by glucosinolates was described by Wattenberg et al. (1986). When glucotropaeolin, glucosinalbin and glucobrassicin were administered to rats before benzo[a]pyrene, glucobrassicin inhibited the occurrence of forestomach tumours and pulmonary adenomas, whereas glucotropaeolin and glucosinalbin inhibited only forestomach tumours.

Tanaka et al. (1990) observed a significant reduction in the incidences of hepatic tumours and preneoplastic foci in rats fed a diet containing sinigrin at 1200 mg/kg and treated with NDEA at 40 mg/l in drinking-water for 5 weeks compared with controls treated only with NDEA. They also observed a significant reduction in preneoplastic lesions and carcinomas of the tongue in rats fed a diet containing sinigrin at 1200 mg/kg during or after administration of 4-nitroquinoline 1-oxide at 10 mg/l in drinking-water for 12 weeks (Tanaka et al., 1992).

Sinigrin, which yields the breakdown product allyl-ITC, increased apoptosis and decreased aberrant crypt foci in the colon of Wistar male rats initiated with 1,2-dimethylhydrazine (Smith et al., 1998). For the studies of apoptosis, rats received two subcutaneous injections of 1,2-dimethylhydrazine at 30 mg/kg bw 5 days apart; sinigrin was given in the diet at 400 µg/g after 6 h. Colons were harvested at intervals of 18, 24, 38, 48, and 72 h, and the frequency of apoptosis was determined in isolated crypts. Apoptotic cells were not observed in control rats, but their frequency was significantly increased in rats initiated with 1,2-dimethylhydrazine; e.g., after 18 h on the sinigrin-free diet, rats had approximately 4.5 and 2.5 apoptotic cells per crypt in the mid- and distal colon. The number of apoptotic cells was significantly increased by sinigrin at all times

except 72 h, the most substantial difference being seen at 48 h. In a second experiment, the number of apoptotic cells per crypt increased from 0.28 to 0.61 in the mid-colon of rats initiated with two subcutaneous doses of 1,2-dimethylhydrazine at 30 mg/kg bw given 5 days apart, and given a diet containing sinigrin at 400 µg/g after 22 h. Colons harvested after 42 days from rats treated with 1,2-dimethylhydrazine alone had a mean of 25.3 aberrant crypt foci per colon, whereas those from rats treated with sinigrin had 15 aberrant crypt foci per colon; however, the numbers of crypts per focus were not significantly different with 1,2-dimethylhydrazine and with 1,2-dimethylhydrazine plus sinigrin (2.1 versus 2.33).

Isothiocyanates

The numerous studies on the prevention of cancer in animals by isothiocyanates stem from early work by Lopez and Mazzanti (1955) and McLean and Rees (1958), who, in the 1950s, observed no liver cancers in the presence of bile-duct hyperplasia induced by the same isothiocyanate compound. Later, Sasaki (1963) and Sidransky et al. (1966) demonstrated the inhibitory effects of α-naphthyl-ITC on liver cancer induced by several carcinogenic agents given in various regimens.

After these early demonstrations of the inhibitory activity of isothiocyanates, various compounds (principally phenethyl-ITC and benzyl-ITC) were tested for their capacity to inhibit oesophagus, lung, stomach, pancreas, colon, liver, mammary and bladder tumour formation in rats, mice and hamsters. Comprehensive reviews on the preventive activity of isothiocyanates in animal models have been reported by Hecht (1995, 2000) and by Zhang and Talalay (1994). This section presents the experimental evidence for the prevention of cancer in rats (Table 43), mice (Table 44) and hamsters

(Table 45) by isothiocyanates and the relationship between prevention and dose, alkyl chain length and time and duration of treatment.

Rats

Oesophagus: Male Fischer 344 rats aged 7 weeks were given AIN-76A diet containing phenethyl-ITC at 3 or 6 μmol/g for 2 weeks before *N*-nitrosomethylbenzylamine (NMBA; 0.5 mg/kg bw by subcutaneous injection once a week for 15 weeks), during treatment with the carcinogen and for the remaining 8 weeks of the study. In rats treated with 3 or 6 μmol/g in the diet, phenethyl-ITC reduced the tumour incidence from 100% in control rats to 13% and 0% and reduced tumour multiplicity from 11.5 in controls to 0.1 and 0, respectively, preventing hyperkeratosis and the formation of preneoplastic (leukoplakia and leuko-keratosis) and neoplastic (papilloma and carcinoma) lesions (Stoner *et al.*, 1991).

In view of the almost complete inhibition of oesophageal tumours in rats by phenethyl-ITC at 3 and 6 μmol/g in the diet, Morse *et al.* (1993) studied the dose–response relationship with concentrations ranging from 0.325 to 3 μmol/g of diet. Rats were fed phenethyl-ITC in the diet for 2 weeks before, during and for 8 weeks after NMBA (0.5 mg/kg bw subcutaneouly, once a week for 15 weeks). Control animals developed 9.3 ± 0.9 oesophageal tumours per rat with 100% incidence, whereas the tumour multiplicity in rats treated with phenethyl-ITC at 0.75, 1.5 and 3 μmol/g of diet were reduced by 39%, 90% and 100%, respectively, and the tumour incidences were reduced by 0, 40% and 100%. The concentration of 0.325 μmol/g was ineffective in inhibiting either tumour multiplicity or incidence. When a single dose of NMBA at 0.5 mg/kg bw was given 2 weeks after the beginning of phenethyl-ITC treatment and oesophagi were harvested 24 h

later, the inhibition of tumorigenesis correlated in a dose-dependent manner with the percentage inhibition of N^7- and O^6-methylguanine adducts.

These findings indicated that the inhibitory effect of phenethyl-ITC on oesophageal cancer occurs during tumour initiation or induction. In order better to define this period, Siglin *et al.* (1995) gave male Fischer 344 rats a diet containing phenethyl-ITC at 500 mg/kg for 2 weeks before NMBA given at 1 mg/kg bw three times a week for 5 weeks and throughout the 25 weeks of the experiment or 1 week after completion of dosing with NMBA. The tumour incidence and multiplicity were reduced from 100% to 46.7% and from 2.9 to 0.9, respectively, when phenethyl-ITC was given before and during carcinogen treatment. When it was administered in the diet from 1 week after the final injection of NMBA, there was no significant effect on either tumour incidence or multiplicity (93.3% incidence and 2.7 tumours per animal), showing that phenethyl-ITC inhibits tumour induction but not progression.

The strong inhibitory effect of phenethyl-ITC prompted Stoner and Morse (1997) and Wilkinson *et al.* (1995) to investigate the inhibitory properties of other arylalkyl isothiocyanates, in the expectation that longer-chain compounds, including synthetic ones, might be more potent than phenethyl-ITC in inhibiting oesophageal cancer. In addition to the naturally occurring phenethyl-ITC, benzyl-ITC and 3-phenylpropyl-ITC, the synthetic homologues 4-phenylbutyl-ITC, 5-phenylpentyl-ITC and 6-phenylhexyl-ITC were also evaluated in the NMBA model in rat oesophagus. Male Fischer 344 rats were given diets containing the isothiocyanates at 2.5, 1.0 or 0.4 μmol/g 2 weeks before and during the experimental period of 25 weeks. Neither benzyl-ITC nor 4-phenylbutyl-ITC affected tumour incidence, and they had little effect on mul-

tiplicity, with values similar to those with NMBA alone, whereas 3-phenylpropyl-ITC had a stronger effect than phenethyl-ITC, reducing the incidence by 93–100% at all three doses and reducing multiplicity by 99–100%. In contrast, 6-phenylhexyl-ITC at 2.5, 1.0 or 0.4 μmol/g of diet increased tumour multiplicity at all three doses by 69%, 61% and 21%, respectively. The inhibitory effects on tumour multiplicity were in good agreement with inhibition of O^6-methylguanine adducts: the rank order for inhibition of oesophageal DNA adducts was 3-phenylpropyl-ITC > phenethyl-ITC > 4-phenylbutyl-ITC > benzyl-ITC.

Colon: Sugie *et al.* (1994) evaluated the preventive activity of benzyl thiocyanate and benzyl-ITC in the colon of female ACI/N rats in relation to administration of the carcinogen methylazoxymethanol. Rats aged 5 weeks were given diets containing benzyl-ITC (400 mg/kg) or benzyl thiocyanate (400 and 100 mg/kg) for 1 week before and during injection of methylazoxymethanol at 25 mg/kg bw intraperitoneally once a week for 3 weeks. Control animals received three intraperitoneal injections of methylazoxymethanol alone. After treatment, the rats were given basal diet for 45 weeks. Another group of animals received methylazoxymethanol first, at the same dose and schedule as above; 1 week after the last injection, the rats were given diets containing benzyl-ITC or benzyl thiocyanate or control diet for 45 weeks. The incidence of tumours (adenomas and adenocarcinomas) was 89% in controls, 53% with benzyl-ITC given in the diet before and during carcinogen treatment and 95% when benzyl-ITC was given 1 week after the last injection. Treatment with benzyl thiocyanate, whether given before or after methylazoxymethanol, resulted in no significant decrease in tumour incidence

Table 43. Effects of isothiocyanates (ITCs) on carcinogen-induced tumours in rats

Oesophagus

Organ site, strain (sex)	Age at start (weeks)	No. of animals per group	Carcinogen, route, dose, duration	ITC, dose, route	Length and timing of ITC treatment	Preventive efficacy by tumour incidence (TI) or multiplicity (TM) (low to high dose)	Summarized effect	Reference
Fischer 344 (M)	7	15	NMBA, s.c., 0.5 mg/kg bw, once a week, 15 weeks	Phenethyl-ITC, 3 or 6 μmol/g, diet	25 weeks, 2 weeks before, during and after NMBA	TI reduced by 100% and 87% TM reduced by 99% and 100%	Phenethyl-ITC prevented tumour formation when given before and during NMBA	Stoner et al. (1991)
Fischer 344 (M)	6–7	13–27	NMBA, s.c., 0.5 mg/kg bw, once a week, 15 weeks	Phenethyl-ITC, 0.325, 0.75, 1.50 or 3.0 μmol/g, diet	25 weeks, 2 weeks before, during and after NMBA	TI reduced by 0, 40% and 100% TM reduced by 39%, 90% and 100% at 0.75, 1.5 and 3.0 μmol/g	Phenethyl-ITC prevented tumours when given before and during NMBA	Morse et al. (1993)
Fischer 344 (M)	6	15	NMBA, s.c., 1.0 mg/kg bw, three times a week, 5 weeks	Phenethyl-ITC, 3.1 μmol/g, diet	25 weeks, 2 weeks before during and after NMBA	TI reduced by 53% when given with NMBA and 7% when given after NMBA TM reduced by 69% when given with NMBA and 7% when given after NMBA	Phenethyl-ITC prevented tumours when given before but not after NMBA	Siglin et al. (1995)
Fischer 344 (M)	6–8	15	NMBA, s.c., 0.5 mg/kg bw, once a week, 15 weeks	Benzyl-ITC, phenethyl-ITC, 3-phenyl-propyl-ITC, 4-phenyl-butyl-ITC and 6-phenyl-hexyl-ITC at 0.4, 1.0 and 2.5 μmol/g, diet	25 weeks, 2 weeks before, during and after NMBA	TI reduced by 43%, 60%, 93% with phenethyl-ITC; 93%, 93%, 100% with 3-phenyl-propyl-ITC TM reduced by 83%, 94%, 99% with phenethyl-ITC; 93%, 99%, 100% with 3-phenyl-propyl-ITC; 41%, 24%, 40% with 4-phenylbutyl-ITC; increased by 21%, 61%, 69% with 6-phenylhexyl-ITC	Benzyl-ITC, 4-phenylbutyl-ITC and 6-phenyl-hexyl-ITC did not inhibit incidence. TM inhibited by phenethyl-ITC, 3-phenylpropyl-ITC and 4-phenylbutyl-ITC. Inhibition correlated with chain length	Wilkinson et al. (1995); Stoner & Morse (1997)

Table 43 (contd)

Organ site, strain (sex)	Age at start (weeks)	No. of animals per group	Carcinogen, route, dose, duration	ITC, dose, route	Length and timing of ITC treatment	Preventive efficacy by tumour incidence (TI) or multiplicity (TM) (low to high dose)	Summarized effect	Reference
Colon ACI/N (F)	5	19–21	Methylazoxymethanol, i.p., 25 mg/kg bw, once a week, 3 weeks	Benzylthiocyanate 400 and 100 mg/kg Benzyl-ITC, 400 mg/kg diet	4 weeks, 1 week before and during methylazoxymethanol 45 weeks, 1 week after methylazoxymethanol	TI reduced by 47% (intestine) with benzyl-ITC in both small intestine and colon; tumour size not affected	Tumours inhibited by benzyl-ITC in both small intestine and colon; tumour size not affected	Sugie et al. (1994)
Fischer 344 (M)	6	6	Azoxymethane, s.c., 15 mg/kg bw, twice at 7-day interval	Phenethyl-ITC or phenethyl-ITC–N-acetylcysteine, 20 or 50 µmol, once a day (pre-initiation) and 5 µmoles or 20 mmol, three times a week (post-initiation), gavage	3 days, 2 h before azoxy-methane (pre-initiation), repeated during second week 8 weeks, 2 days after azoxy-methane (post-initiation)	ACF Reduced by 25% with phenethyl-ITC, increased by 29% with phenethyl-ITC–N-acetylcysteine Reduced by 35% with phenethyl-ITC and by 26% with phenethyl-ITC–N-acetylcysteine	Phenethyl-ITC inhibited total number of aberrant crypt foci and no. of foci with multiple crypts when given before or after azoxymethane; phenethyl-ITC–N-acetylcysteine inhibited when given after but not before	Chung et al. (2000)
Sprague-Dawley (M)	8	7–10	Azoxymethane, s.c., 15 mg/kg bw, twice at 7-day interval	Phenethyl-ITC, 0.65 g/kg diet	5 weeks, 1 week before and 4 weeks after first azoxymethane	228 ACF per animal in controls, 191 with phenethyl-ITC	Phenethyl-ITC did not significantly alter number of ACF	Pereira & Khoury (1991)
Liver Sprague-Dawley (M)	~ 228 g	11–22	D,L-Ethionine, 0.25% diet	α-Naphthyl-ITC, 0.1% diet	4 or 8 weeks before D,L-ethionine or in combination	TI, 67% with D,L-ethionine, 47% and 18% after 4 and 8 weeks pretreatment with α-naphthyl-ITC, 0 with combination	α-Naphthyl-ITC inhibited hepato-cellular carcinomas when given either before or with carcinogen	Sidransky et al. (1996)
Wistar (M)	~ 200 g	6–20	FAA, 0.04% diet	α-Naphthyl-ITC, 0.1% diet	FAA 4 months FAA + α-naphthyl-ITC 2 months and FAA 2 months α-Naphthyl-ITC 2 months + FAA 2 months	TI, 62% TI, 25% TI, 24%		

Table 43 (contd)

Organ site, strain (sex)	Age at start (weeks)	No. of animals per group	Carcinogen, route, dose, duration	ITC, dose, route	Length and timing of ITC treatment	Preventive efficacy by tumour incidence (TI) or multiplicity (TM) (low to high dose)	Summarized effect	Reference
Wistar (M)	150–180 g	6–9	*Meta*-Toluylene-diamine, 0.1%, diet	α-Naphthyl-ITC, 0.1% in diet	35 weeks, during *meta*-toluylene-diamine	TI reduced by 100% in 36 weeks	α-Naphthyl-ITC inhibited cancer and nodular hyperplasia	Ito *et al.* (1969)
Lung Fischer 344 (M)	8	20–40	NNK, s.c., 1.76 mg/kg bw three times a week, 20 weeks	Phenethyl-ITC, 3 µmol/g, diet	21 weeks, 1 week before and during NNK	TI at 104 weeks reduced from 80% to 43%	Phenethyl-ITC reduced liver but not other tumours	Morse *et al.* (1989a)
Fischer 344 (M)	6	36	NNK, s.c., 1.5 mg/kg bw. three times a week, 20 weeks	6-Phenyl-hexyl-ITC, 2 or 4 µmol/g, diet Phenethyl-ITC, 4 or 8 µmol/g, diet	22 weeks, 1 week before and 1 week after NNK	TI reduced by 72%, 64% with 6-phenyl-hexyl-ITC TI reduced by 75%, 87% with phenethyl-ITC	Phenethyl-ITC and 6-phenyl-hexyl-ITC had equal activity; no dose–response relationship	Chung *et al.* (1996)
Fischer 344 (M)	7	20–60	NNK, 2 mg/l in water, 111 weeks	Phenethyl-ITC, 3 µmol/g, diet	112 weeks, 1 week before and during NNK	TI reduced by 93% in lung, 100% in pancreas (malignant exocrine)	Phenethyl-ITC inhibited lung tumours and malignant tumours in pancreas. No effect on liver or nasal cavity	Hecht *et al.* (1996a)
Fischer 344 (M)	7	60	NNK, 2 mg/l in water, 111 weeks	6-Phenyl-hexyl-ITC, 1 µmol/g, diet	112 weeks, 1 week before and during NNK	TI reduced by 63% in lung TI reduced by 59% for leukaemia and lymphoma	Phenethyl-ITC inhibited lung tumours, leukaemia and lymphoma. No effect on other tumours	Hecht *et al.* (1996b)
Sprague-Dawley (F)	7	16–27	DMBA, 12 mg once, oral	Benzyl-ITC, 17 µmol/g, diet	15 weeks, 1 week after DMBA	TI reduced by 37% TM reduced by 59%	Benzyl-ITC inhibited mammary TI and TM	Wattenberg (1981)

113

Table 43 (contd)

Organ site, strain (sex)	Age at start (weeks)	No. of animals per group	Carcinogen, route, dose, duration	ITC, dose, route	Length and timing of ITC treatment	Preventive efficacy by tumour incidence (TI) or multiplicity (TM) (low to high dose)	Summarized effect	Reference
Mammary gland								
Sprague-Dawley (F)	7	20	DMBA, 50 mg/kg bw once, oral	Phenethyl-ITC, 0.1%, diet	35 weeks, 1 week after DMBA	TI not reduced TM not significantly different Size reduced by 51%	Phenethyl-ITC had no effect on TI or TM but reduced size of tumours	Futakuchi et al. (1998)
Sprague-Dawley (F)	7	20–25	DMBA, 8 mg once, oral	Sulfora-phane, 75 and 150 µmol, oral	3 h before DMBA	After 152 days, TI reduced by 49% and 61% and TM reduced by 71% and 85%	Sulforaphane reduced tumour incidence and multiplicity	Zhang et al. (1994)
Urinary bladder								
Wistar (M)	8	30–40	BBN, 0.025% for 15 week, water	Phenethyl-ITC and 6-phenylhexyl-ITC, 0.5 µmol/g, diet	16 weeks, 1 week before BBN	TI not significantly reduced TM reduced by 47% with 6-phenylhexyl-ITC Phenethyl-ITC ineffective	6-Phenyl-hexyl-ITC but not phenethyl-ITC reduced no. of papillomas per rat	Nishikawa et al. (2003)
Fischer 344 (M)	6	20	BBN, 50 mg/l, 40 weeks, water	Benzyl-ITC, 10, 100 and 1000 mg/kg, diet	40 weeks, during BBN	TI and TM of dysplasia, papillomas and carcinoma inhibited in dose-response relationship	Benzyl-ITC reduced tumour incidence and multiplicity induced by BBN, but alone it increased epithelial hyperplasia at 100 and 1000 mg/kg	Okazaki et al. (2002)

ACF, aberrant crypt foci; BBN, N-butyl-N-(4-hydroxybutyl)nitrosamine; DMBA, 7,12-dimethylbenz[a]anthracene; FAA, N-2-fluorenylacetamide; NMBA, N-nitrosomethylbenzylamine; NNK, 4-(methylnitrosamino)-1-(3-pyridyl)-1-butanone; PhIP, 2-amino-1-methyl-6-phenylimidazo[4,5-b]pyridine; i.p., intra-peritoneally; s.c., subcutaneously

(81% and 92% when given before and 83% and 95% when given after methylazoxymethanol). Nevertheless, both benzyl-ITC and benzyl thiocyanate at 400 mg/kg given in the diet before and during carcinogen treatment significantly decreased tumour multiplicity in the intestine (2.56 with methylazoxymethanol alone versus 1.11 and 1.29, respectively). Neither agent had a significant effect on multiplicity when given after the carcinogen. Both benzyl-ITC and benzyl thiocyanate inhibited cell proliferation in the colon when given during the initiation phase of methylazoxymethanol-induced tumorigenesis, but were ineffective when given after carcinogen treatment.

Chung et al. (2000) evaluated the efficacy of phenethyl-ITC and its N-acetylcysteine conjugate, given either before or after initiation, in inhibiting azoxymethane-induced aberrant crypt foci. Male Fischer 344 rats were given two weekly subcutaneous injections of azoxymethane at 15 mg/kg bw. They were also given phenethyl-ITC (5 µmol) or its N-acetylcysteine conjugate (20 mmol) three times a week by gavage for 8 weeks after the carcinogen (post-initiation) or once a day for 3 days (20 or 50 µmol) before azoxymethane (inhibition of initiation). Ten weeks after the last azoxymethane injection, the animals were killed and the aberrant crypt foci were counted. When given post-initiation, phenethyl-ITC and its conjugate inhibited the formation of aberrant crypt foci by 35% and 26%, respectively, and inhibited the formation of foci with more than four crypts by 48% and 27%. When given for 3 days before azoxymethane, phenethyl-ITC reduced the number of foci and the number with multiple crypts by 25% and 33%, whereas the N-acetylcysteine conjugate increased the number of aberrant crypt foci by 29% and the number with multiple crypts by 42%. In contrast, Pereira and Khoury (1991) found that the numbers of azoxymethane-induced aberrant crypt foci in the colons of Sprague-Dawley rats were unaffected by previous administration of phenethyl-ITC, ellagic acid or diallyl sulfide but were inhibited 93% and 30% by N-acetylcysteine and α-difluoromethylornithine, respectively.

Liver. Sidransky et al. (1966) showed that a diet containing 0.1% α-naphthyl-ITC given before or with DL-ethionine or N-2-fluorenylacetamide inhibited the formation of hepatocellular carcinoma. In the first set of experiments, male Sprague-Dawley rats were given the α-naphthyl-ITC diet for 4 or 8 weeks before addition of 0.25% DL-ethionine or both α-naphthyl-ITC and DL-ethionine. The tumour incidence was 67% with ethionine alone and 47% and 18%, respectively, after pretreatment with α-naphthyl-ITC for 4 or 8 weeks; the combined regimen did not cause tumours. In the second set of experiments, male Wistar rats were given 0.04% N-2-fluorenylacetamide in the diet for 4 months; N-2-fluorenylacetamide plus 0.1% α-naphthyl-ITC for 2 months followed by N-2-fluorenylacetamide for 2 months; or α-naphthyl-ITC in the diet for 2 months followed by N-2-fluorenylacetamide in the diet for 4 months. The tumour incidences were 62% with N-2-fluorenylacetamide alone for 4 months, 25% with the combined treatment and 24% after pretreatment with α-naphthyl-ITC. N-2-Fluorenylacetamide induced a small number of ear-duct tumours and myelogenous leukaemia, which were apparently inhibited by α-naphthyl-ITC when given before or during dosing with the carcinogen.

Ito et al. (1969) showed that 0.1% α-naphthyl-ITC given in the diet for 35 weeks at the same time as 0.1% *meta*-toluylenediamine completely inhibited the development of liver tumours in male Wistar rats, from 100% in six controls given the carcinogen to 0%. All animals given diets containing *meta*-toluylenediamine failed to gain weight. Although there were relatively few animals per group, there was a marked reduction in the number of nodular hyperplasias.

Ogawa et al. (2001) presented evidence that phenethyl-ITC promoted liver tumours (see section 6) when given post-initiation. This finding and those for oesophagus, lung and liver indicate that the preventive activity of phenethyl-ITC is most evident when it is given before or during carcinogen treatment.

Lung: In studies designed to identify agents that prevent the development of lung cancer, Morse et al. (1989a) and Hecht et al. (1996a) evaluated phenethyl-ITC for its ability to prevent lung tumours induced in rats by NNK. In the first study (Morse et al., 1989a), male Fischer 344 rats aged 8 weeks were given a diet containing phenethyl-ITC at a concentration of 3 µmol/g, beginning 1 week before subcutaneous injection of NNK at a dose of 1.76 mg/kg bw three times a week for 20 weeks and during NNK treatment. The experiment was terminated after 104 weeks, and the total numbers of tumours in the lungs (adenomas and carcinomas), liver and nasal cavity were evaluated. The dose of phenethyl-ITC, estimated to be 8.8 mg/day per rat, did not cause significant differences in body weight, food consumption or survival. Nevertheless, there were adverse effects in the liver, consisting of centrilobular and midzonal fatty metamorphosis. Dietary phenethyl-ITC reduced the incidence of lung tumours from 80% in controls to 43%, but the numbers of tumours in the liver and nasal cavity were unaffected. In addition, the treatment resulted in no significant differences in NNK-induced tumours in other organs (pancreas, mammary, stomach, testis, adrenal, thyroid), nor was there any

Table 44. Effects of isothiocyanates (ITCs) on carcinogen-induced tumours in mice

Organ site, strain (sex)	Age at start	No. of animals per group	Carcinogen, route, dose, duration	ITC, dose, route	Length and timing of ITC treatment	Preventive efficacy by tumour incidence (TI) or multiplicity (TM) (low to high dose)	Summarized effect	Reference
Forestomach								
A/J (F)	9 weeks	15	Benzo[a]pyrene, gavage, 2 mg, once every 2 weeks, three times	Benzyl-ITC, gavage, 1 and 2.5 mg, once every 2 weeks, 3 times	15 min before benzo[a]pyrene	At 26 weeks, TI reduced by 22% with 2.5 mg TM reduced by 67% with 2.5 mg Carcinoma TI reduced by 67% and 100% with 1 and 2.5 mg	Benzyl-ITC inhibited carcinoma and other neoplasms	Wattenberg (1987)
A/J (F)	9 weeks	20	Benzo[a]pyrene, gavage, 7.9 µmol each, once every 2 weeks, three times	Benzyl-ITC and phenethyl-ITC, gavage, 6.7 µmol, once every 2 weeks, three times	15 min before benzo[a]pyrene	At 26 weeks, TI not inhibited TM reduced by 48% with phenethyl-ITC	Phenethyl-ITC, but not benzyl-ITC, inhibited tumours	Lin et al. (1993)
ICR (F)	9–12 weeks	20	Benzo[a]pyrene, gavage, 120 mg/kg bw, once a week, 4 weeks	Sulforaphane, 2.5 mmol/kg, diet	6 weeks, 1 week before to 2 days after benzo[a]pyrene	TM reduced by 39%. No inhibition in mice lacking the nrf2 gene	Sulforaphane inhibited tumours in nrf2-competent but not in nrf2-null mice	Fahey et al. (2002)
Liver								
C3H/HeNCr1Br (M)	13–15 days	18–37	N-Nitroso-diethylamine, i.p., 4 mg/kg bw, once on day 15	Phenethyl-ITC i.p., 82 mg/kg bw on days 13, 14, 15 and 0.65 g/kg diet, days 21–161	3 days before N-nitrosodiethyl-amine and days 21–161 in diet	No. of foci per mouse reduced by 55% No. of adenomas per mouse reduced by 77%	Phenethyl-ITC given before and after N-nitrosodiethyl-amine inhibited liver lesions	Pereira (1995)
Lung								
ICR/Ha (F)	9 weeks	15–20	DMBA, 0.05 mg/g, diet	Benzyl-ITC, 5 mg/g, diet Phenethyl-ITC, 5.5 mg/g, diet	4 weeks	At 20 weeks, benzyl-ITC and phenethyl-ITC inhibited lung TM but no TI		Wattenberg (1977)

Table 44 (contd)

Organ site, strain (sex)	Age at start	No. of animals per group	Carcinogen, route, dose, duration	ITC, dose, route	Length and timing of ITC treatment	Preventive efficacy by tumour incidence (TI) or multiplicity (TM) (low to high dose)	Summarized effect	Reference
A/J (F)	6–7 weeks	20–30	NNK, i.p., 10 µmol	Phenethyl-ITC, 5 and 25 µmol; benzyl-ITC and phenyl-ITC, 5 µmol; gavage, once a day, 4 days	4 days before NNK	16 weeks after NNK, TI reduced by 70% at 25 µmol phenethyl-ITC TM reduced by 76%, 97% with phenethyl-ITC; by 29% with benzyl-ITC	Phenethyl-ITC at 5 and 25 µmol inhibited TM. Phenethyl-ITC at 25 µmol inhibited TI	Morse et al. (1989b)
A/J (F)	7 weeks	20	NNK, i.p., 10 µmol	Phenethyl-ITC, 5 µmol; 6-phenyl-hexyl-ITC, 0.2 µmol, once by gavage or once a day, 4 days	1 or 4 days before NNK	TI reduced by 33% and 65% with one and four doses of 6-phenylhexyl-ITC TM reduced by 62% and 79% with one and four doses of phenethyl-ITC and reduced by 83% and 96% with 6-phenylhexyl-ITC	6-Phenylhexyl-ITC more inhibitory than phenethyl-ITC One dose as effective on multiplicity as four with either compound	Morse et al. (1992)
A/J (M, F)	7–8 weeks	24	Benzo[a]-pyrene, i.p., 100 mg/kg bw, once	Phenethyl-ITC, 0.075, 0.25, 0.50, 1.25 µmol/g, gavage, once a day, 6 days	6 days, 4 days before and 2 days after benzo[a]pyrene	After 7 months, no significant difference between benzo[a]pyrene control and ITC-treated mice	Phenethyl-ITC did not inhibit lung tumours	Adam-Rodwell et al. (1993)
A/J (F)	9 weeks	20	Benzo[a]-pyrene, once every 2 weeks, three times	Benzyl-ITC or phenethyl-ITC, 6.7 µmol, gavage, once every 2 weeks, three times	3 days, 15 min before carcinogen	After 26 weeks, TI not significantly inhibited by either agent TM reduced by 46% by benzyl-ITC	Phenethyl-ITC did not inhibit lung tumours, but benzyl-ITC reduced no. of tumours per mouse	Lin et al. (1993)
A/J (F)	7–8 weeks	10–20	Benzo[a]-pyrene, 3 µmol; 5-methyl-chrysene, 2 µmol; dibenz[a,h]-anthracene, 1 µmol Once a week, 8 weeks, gavage	Benzyl-ITC, 13.4 and 6.7 µmol, gavage, once a week, 8 weeks	8 days, 15 min before benzo[a]-pyrene	19 weeks after final dose of carcinogen, TI reduced by 39% at 13.4 µmol, TM reduced by 64% and 81% with benzo[a]pyrene TM reduced by 73% and 77% with 5-methyl-chrysene TM reduced by 80% and 91% with dibenz[a,h]-anthracene	Dibenz[a,h]-anthracene most potent lung carcinogen. Only higher dose of benzyl-ITC inhibited TI	Hecht et al. (2002)

Table 44 (contd)

Organ site, strain (sex)	Age at start	No. of animals per group	Carcinogen, route, dose, duration	ITC, dose, route	Length and timing of ITC treatment	Preventive efficacy by tumour incidence (TI) or multiplicity (TM) (low to high dose)	Summarized effect	Reference
A/J (M)	10 weeks	25–32	ETS, 6 h/day, 5 days/week, 5 months	Phenethyl-ITC, 0.05%, diet	9 months, 1 week before and during ETS	TI and TM not reduced	ETS a weak carcinogen for mouse lung. Phenethyl-ITC did not reduce lung tumours	Witschi et al. (1998)
A/J (F)	7–8 weeks	15	NNK, i.p., 100 mg/kg bw, once	6-Methyl-thiohexyl-ITC, 5 µmol/day, gavage, once a day, 4 days	4 days, 2 h before NNK	After 16 weeks, TI not reduced. TM reduced by 38% (total tumours and tumours per mouse)	6-Methyl-thiohexyl-ITC inhibited tumours	Yano et al. (2000)
A/J (F)	7 weeks	10–24	NNK, i.p., 10 µmol, once	Phenethyl-ITC or benzyl-ITC, 1 or 3 µmol/g, diet	16 weeks, 1 week after NNK	TI and TM not reduced by phenethyl-ITC. TM reduced by 33% by 3 µmol of benzyl-ITC	Phenethyl-ITC and benzyl-ITC less effective when given post-initiation	Morse et al. (1990a)
A/J (F)	7 weeks	30–35	Benzo[a]-pyrene, gavage, 20 µmol, once	Benzyl-ITC–N-acetyl-cysteine and phenethyl-ITC–N-acetyl-cysteine, 15 µmol/g, diet	140 days, 2 days after benzo[a]-pyrene	TM reduced by 39% and 45% by benzyl-ITC–N-acetylcysteine and phenethyl-ITC–N-acetyl-cysteine	Both agents effective post-initiation	Yang et al. (2002)
A/J (F)	7 weeks	15–30	NNK, i.p., 10 µmol, once	Phenethyl-ITC, phenethyl-ITC–GSH, phenethyl-ITC–N-acetylcysteine, 6-phenylhexyl-ITC, 6-phenyl-hexyl-ITC–GSH, 6-phenylhexyl-ITC–N-acetyl-cysteine, gavage, 1–20 µmol	4 days, 2 h before NNK	After 16 weeks, TI reduced by 21% and 72% at 1 and 5 µmol 6-phenyl-hexyl-ITC–N-acetylcysteine. TM reduced by 28% (5 µmol phenethyl-ITC), 32% (8 µmol phenethyl-ITC–GSH and 5 µmol phenethyl-ITC–N-acetylcysteine). TM reduced by 70% and 97% by 1 and 5 µmol 6-phenylhexyl-ITC–N-acetyl-cysteine	Thiol conjugates of phenethyl-ITC and 6-phenyl-hexyl-ITC significantly inhibited TM. 6-Phenyl-hexyl-ITC–N-acetyl-cysteine inhibited TI	Jiao et al. (1997)

Table 44 (contd)

Organ site, strain (sex)	Age at start	No. of animals per group	Carcinogen, route, dose, duration	ITC, dose, route	Length and timing of ITC treatment	Preventive efficacy by tumour incidence (TI) or multiplicity (TM) (low to high dose)	Summarized effect	Reference
A/J (F)	6–8 weeks	20	NNK, i.p., 10 µmol, once	Phenethyl-ITC, 3-phenylpropyl-ITC, 4-phenyl-butyl-ITC, 5-phenylpentyl-ITC, 6-phenyl-hexyl-ITC, gavage, 0.2, 1.0, 5.0 µmol, once a day, 4 days	4 days, 2 h before NNK	After 16 weeks, TI reduced by 25% and 89% with 3-phenylpropyl-ITC, by 58% and 89% with 4-phenylbutyl-ITC, by 47% and 75% with 5-phenylpentyl-ITC, by 100% and 95% with 6-phenylhexyl-ITC (1 and 5 µmol) TM reduced by 18% and 48% (phenethyl-ITC), 85% and 97%, 90% and 97%, 89% and 96%, 100% and 99%, respectively	Phenethyl-ITC did not reduce TI. All agents reduced TM. Efficacy related to alkyl chain length	Stoner & Morse (1997)
A/J (F)	7 weeks	18–39	NNK, i.p., 10 µmol, once	Phenyl-ITC, benzyl-ITC, phenethyl-ITC, 3-phenylpropyl-ITC, 4-phenyl-butyl-ITC, 4-oxo-4-(3-pyridyl)butyl-ITC, gavage, 5 µmol per mouse, once a day, 4 days	4 days, 2 h before NNK	After 16 weeks, TI reduced by 0%, 0%, 7%, 63%, 68% and 4%, respectively. TM reduced by 64%, 96% and 96% with phenethyl-ITC, 3-phenylpropyl-ITC and 4-phenylbutyl-ITC, respectively	3-Phenyl-propyl-ITC and 4-phenyl-butyl-ITC inhibited TI. Phenethyl-ITC, 3-phenyl-propyl-ITC, and 4-phenyl-butyl-ITC reduced TM	Morse et al. (1989c)
A/J (F)	7 weeks	20	NNK, i.p., 10 mmol, once	Phenethyl-ITC, 3-phenyl-propyl-ITC, 4-phenyl-butyl-ITC, 5-phenyl-pentyl-ITC, 6-phenyl-hexyl-ITC and 4-(3-pyridyl)-butyl-ITC, gavage, 0.2, 1.0 and 5 µmol, once a day, 4 days	4 days, 2 h before NNK	After 16 weeks, TI reduced by 89%, 89%, 75%, 95% at 5 mmol by 3-phenyl-propyl-ITC, 4-phenylbutyl-ITC, 5-phenylpentyl-ITC, 6-phenylhexyl-ITC TM reduced by 59%, 95%, 95%, 90%, 92% at 5 mmol by phenethyl-ITC, 3-phenylpropyl-ITC, 4-phenyl-butyl-ITC, 5-phenylpentyl-ITC, 6-phenylhexyl-ITC	Phenethyl-ITC and 4-(3-pyridyl)butyl-ITC did not inhibit TM. TM reduction associated with chain length	Morse et al. (1991a)

Table 44 (contd)

Organ site, strain (sex)	Age at start	No. of animals per group	Carcinogen, route, dose, duration	ITC, dose, route	Length and timing of ITC treatment	Preventive efficacy by tumour incidence (TI) or multiplicity (TM) (low to high dose)	Summarized effect	Reference
A/J (F)	7 weeks	20	NNK, i.p., 10 μmol, once	Phenethyl-ITC, allyl-ITC, 1-hexyl-ITC, 2-hexyl-ITC, 1-dodecyl-ITC, 2,2-diphenethyl-ITC, 1,2-diphenethyl-ITC, gavage, 5, 1, 0.2, 0.1 or 0.04 μmol, once	2 h before NNK dosing	After 16 weeks, TI reduced by 25%, 70%, 75%, 55%, 55% by 1-hexyl-ITC, 2-hexyl-ITC, 1-dodecyl-ITC, 2,2-diphenethyl-ITC, 1,2-diphenethyl-ITC at 5 μmol. TM reduced by 87%, 97%, 97%, 95%, 95% by 1-hexyl-ITC, 2-hexyl-ITC, 1-dodecyl-ITC, 1,2-diphenethyl-ITC at 5 μmol	Inhibition of tumours depended on chain length	Jiao et al. (1994a)
A/J (F)	6–7 weeks	25	NNK, i.p., 10 μmol, once	Phenethyl-ITC, 0.008%, diet	17 weeks, 1 week before, during and after NNK	TI not inhibited. TM reduced by 54%	Inhibition of multiplicity	El-Bayoumy et al. (1996)
A/J (F)	7 weeks	20	Benzo[a]pyrene plus NNK, gavage, 3 μmol each, once a week, 8 weeks	Phenethyl-ITC and benzyl-ITC alone and combined, gavage, 6 μmol each	8 weeks, 2 h before carcinogens	After 16 weeks, TI and TM not inhibited	Neither agent nor the combination inhibited tumours	Hecht et al. (2000)
A/J (F)	7 weeks	20	Benzo[a]pyrene plus NNK, gavage, 3 μmol each, once a week, 8 weeks	Phenethyl-ITC and benzyl-ITC, 3 and 1 μmol each in diet	10 weeks, 1 week before to 1 week after carcinogen	At 27 weeks, TI not inhibited. TM reduced by 44% by phenethyl-ITC (3 μmol) and 33% by phenethyl-ITC plus benzyl-ITC (3 plus 1 μmol)	TI not inhibited. TM inhibited by phenethyl-ITC and combination at lower doses	Hecht et al. (2000)

DMBA, 7,12-dimethylbenz[a]anthracene; ETS, environmental tobacco smoke; GSH, glutathione; NNK, 4-(methylnitrosamino)-butanone; i.p., intraperitoneally; s.c., subcutaneously; F, female; M, male

ICR/Ha mice. Later, Wattenberg (1987) showed that benzyl-ITC given by gavage inhibited both forestomach and pulmonary tumours in A/J mice when administered 15 min before benzo[a]pyrene; however, it inhibited only forestomach and not lung tumour formation when N-nitrosodiethylamine was used as the carcinogen.

To study the effects of the synthetic phenyl-ITC, benzyl-ITC and phenethyl-ITC on tumorigenesis and O^6-methylguanine adduct formation in the lungs of A/J mice, Morse et al. (1989b) administered these compounds by gavage for four consecutive days at doses of 5 µmol/day (phenyl-ITC and benzyl-ITC) or 5 and 25 µmol/day (phenethyl-ITC). Two hours after the last dose of isothiocyanate, the mice were given a single intraperitoneal dose of 10 µmol of the tobacco-specific nitrosamine NNK. The incidence of pulmonary adenomas in NNK-treated mice after 16 weeks was 100%, and the multiplicity was 10.7 tumours per mouse. Neither phenyl-ITC nor benzyl-ITC affected tumour incidence or multiplicity, but phenethyl-ITC at 25 µmol/day inhibited tumour formation by 70% and multiplicity by 97% and at 5 µmol/day inhibited multiplicity by 76% but had little effect on incidence. Six hours after NNK treatment, phenethyl-ITC had inhibited O^6-methylguanine adduct formation by 87% when given at 5 µmol/day and by 100% when given at 25 µmol/day. Neither benzyl-ITC nor phenyl-ITC inhibited adduct formation. Morse et al. (1992) later showed that a single dose of 5 µmol of phenethyl-ITC or 0.2 µmol of 6-phenylhexyl-ITC was as effective as the four-dose regimen in inhibiting pulmonary adenoma multiplicity induced by NNK, suggesting that, in the four-dose schedule, the last dose was responsible for the observed inhibition. In contrast, doses of phenethyl-ITC ranging from 0.075 to 0.75 mmol/kg bw given over 6 days were completely ineffective in inhibiting lung tumours induced by benzo[a]pyrene given 4 days after the beginning of phenethyl-ITC treatment (Adam-Rodwell et al., 1993).

The apparent disparity with regard to inhibition of benzo[a]pyrene-induced lung tumours by isothiocyanates was addressed by Lin et al. (1993), who gave female A/J mice 6.7 µmol of benzyl-ITC or phenethyl-ITC three times by gavage once every 2 weeks, 15 min before giving 7.9 µmol of benzo[a]pyrene. Benzyl-ITC, but not phenethyl-ITC, inhibited lung tumour multiplicity by approximately 50% when evaluated at 26 weeks; neither compound decreased tumour incidence. The authors suggested that the differential inhibition of NNK- and benzo[a]pyrene-induced tumours by the isothiocyanates was due to selective inhibition of the cytochrome P450 enzymes involved in activation or detoxification of these carcinogens.

Hecht et al. (2002) examined the effect of benzyl-ITC on lung tumorigenesis induced in female A/J mice by benzo[a]pyrene and two other polycyclic hydrocarbons found in cigarette smoke, i.e., 5-methylchrysene and dibenz[a,h]anthracene. The mice were treated weekly for 8 weeks by gavage with 3 µmol of benzo[a]pyrene, 2 µmol of 5-methylchrysene or 1 µmol of dibenz[a,h]anthracene given 15 min after benzyl-ITC at 13.4 or 6.7 µmol by gavage. Nineteen weeks after the final dose, the lungs were fixed and examined for tumour formation. Benzyl-ITC at the higher but not at the lower dose significantly inhibited the development of pulmonary adenomas, resulting in a reduction in tumour incidence from 95% in controls given benzo[a]pyrene alone to 61%. Neither dose of benzyl-ITC inhibited the incidence of pulmonary tumours induced by 5-methylchrysene or dibenz[a,h]anthracene, but the higher and the lower doses reduced tumour multiplicity by 81% and 64% (benzo[a]pyrene), 77% and 73% (5-methylchrysene) and 91% and 80% (dibenz[a,h]anthracene), respectively. 5-Methylchrysene and dibenz[a,h]anthracene induced three to four times more tumours per mouse than benzo[a]pyrene.

In an extension of this study, Witschi et al. (1998) assayed the ability of phenethyl-ITC to inhibit lung tumours in male A/J mice exposed to mainstream cigarette smoke and environmental tobacco smoke (ETS) for 6 h/day, 5 days/week for 5 months. A diet containing 0.05% phenethyl-ITC for 9 months had no effect on the multiplicity of pulmonary tumours induced by ETS alone, which only slightly increased the number of tumours per lung, from 0.5–1.0 to 1.1–1.6. When NNK was used to induce lung tumours, phenethyl-ITC given by gavage or in the diet significantly inhibited tumour multiplicity by 85% and 87%, respectively. [A comprehensive discussion of the prevention of lung cancer induced by carcinogens in tobacco smoke was given by Hecht (1997), using inhibition of tumours induced by benzo[a]pyrene and NNK by various isothiocyanates as examples.]

Female A/J mice were given 5 µmol of 6-methylthiohexyl-ITC, one of the main components of wasabi (Wasabia japonica), by gavage for 4 consecutive days and, 2 h after the final gavage, a single intraperitoneal injection of NNK at 100 mg/kg bw (Yano et al., 2000). When the mice were killed at week 16, the tumour incidence was 100% in both NNK controls and those also receiving 6-methylthiohexyl-ITC; however, the total number of tumours was reduced from 165 to 102 and the number of tumours per animal from 11 to 6.8 (38% inhibition). In addition, when the lungs were harvested 4 h after NNK treatment, the level of O^6-methylguanine adducts was reduced by more than twofold, equivalent to that seen with phenethyl-ITC.

Table 45. Effects of isothiocyanates (ITCs) on tumours induced by N-nitrosobis(2-oxopropyl)-amine (BOP) given subcutaneously at 20 mg/kg bw once a week for 2 weeks to groups of 10–30 female hamsters aged 5 weeks at start

Organ, ITC, dose, route	Length and timing of ITC treatment	Preventive efficacy by tumour incidence (TI) or multiplicity (TM)	Summarized effect	Reference
Pancreas				
Phenethyl-ITC, 3-phenylpropyl-ITC, 10 or 100 µmol, gavage	2 h before each BOP treatment	After 52 weeks, phenethyl-ITC: 100 µmol: TI reduced by 50%; TM reduced by 88% 10 µmol: no effect on TI or TM 3-Phenylpropyl-ITC: 100 and 10 µmol: no effect on TI or TM	Phenethyl-ITC decreased TI and TM	Nishikawa et al. (1996a,b)
4-Phenylbutyl-ITC, 10 or 100 µmol, gavage	2 h before each BOP treatment	After 52 weeks, 100 µmol: TI reduced by 26%; TM, no effect 10 µmol: TI and TM, no effect Dysplasia reduced by about 60%	4-Phenylbutyl-ITC did not inhibit adenocarcinoma but reduced dysplastic lesions	Son et al. (2000)
Lung				
Phenethyl-ITC, 3-phenylpropyl-ITC, 10 or 100 µmol, gavage	2 h before BOP	After 52 weeks, phenethyl-ITC: 100 µmol: TI reduced by 100%; TM reduced by 100% 10 µmol: TI reduced by 83%; TM reduced by 87% 3-Phenylpropyl-ITC: 100 µmol: TI reduced by 94–100%; TM reduced by 97% 10 µmol: TI reduced by 57–100%; TM reduced by 80%	Phenethyl-ITC and 3-phenylpropyl-ITC inhibited TI and TM	Nishikawa et al. (1996a,b)
4-Phenylbutyl-ITC, 10 or 100 µmol, gavage	2 h before each BOP treatment	After 52 weeks, 100 µmol: TI reduced by 93–100%; TM reduced by 96–100% 10 µmol: TI not changed; TM reduced by 60%	4-Phenylbutyl-ITC at 100 µmol inhibited TI and TM; at 10 µmol, it decreased TM but not TI	Son et al. (2000)

cinomas was inhibited by 93% and 100%, while the multiplicity was decreased by 96% and 100%, showing that 4-phenylbutyl-ITC, like phenethyl-ITC and 3-phenylpropyl-ITC, is an exceptionally potent inhibitor of lung tumours in hamsters.

Indoles

Studies of natural indoles as cancer preventive chemicals were pioneered by Wattenberg and Loub (1978) in mice and by Bailey et al. (1982) in rainbow trout. Since then, a wealth of evidence has arisen to show that natural indoles (those most frequently tested

are indole-3-carbinol and 3,3´-diindolylmethane) can be remarkably effective in preventing a wide range of tumour phenotypes in various animal models. Several extensive reviews, appearing between 1997 and 2001, offer an exhaustive synopsis of the use of indoles as chemopreventives in mice, rats and rainbow trout (Verhoeven et al., 1997; Broadbent & Broadbent, 1998a,b; Bradlow et al., 1999; Brignall, 2001; Murillo & Mehta, 2001). A recent search of the Medline database revealed 347 publications related to indole-3-carbinol since 1978. The end-point of 20 of these was

tumour prevention; others focused on preneoplastic lesions or other indoles (primarily 3,3´-diindolylmethane). The great majority of the studies were of mechanisms and metabolism. This section summarizes studies of tumours and precursor lesions that illustrate that indoles are effective in multiple species, against a range of chemical and viral carcinogens, in many target organs and in both initiation (carcinogen treatment) and post-initiation periods (Table 46).

The protocols of dietary intervention studies with indole-3-carbinol and 3,3´-diindolylmethane involve giving the indole before, during and/or after the carcinogen over a wide range of doses. The end-points were usually tumours or precursor lesions such as hepatic GST+ foci and aberrant crypt foci in the colon.

Forestomach
Female ICR/Ha mice received a diet containing indole-3-carbinol at 0.03 mmol/g, 3,3′-diindolylmethane at 0.02 mmol/g or indole-3-acetonitrile at 0.03 mmol/g (Wattenberg & Loub, 1978). Eight days after beginning the indole diets, the animals were given benzo[a]pyrene at 0.3 or 1 mg, orally, twice a week for 4 weeks. Significant reductions in the multiplicity of fore-stomach tumours were seen with indole-3-carbinol (5.0 to 1.9 tumours per mouse), 3,3′-diindolylmethane (5.0 to 3.2) and indole-3-acetonitrile (5.9 to 1.6). Controls given the indoles alone had no tumours.

Colon
Several studies have indicated that protection by indole-3-carbinol in models of colon carcinogenesis is dependent on the protocol used. Dashwood and co-workers (Guo et al., 1995) treated male Fischer 344 rats with PhIP by gavage (50 mg/kg bw every other day during weeks 3 and 4) and provided a diet containing indole-3-carbinol at 1000 mg/kg either before and during PhIP treatment, after PhIP or continuously. Aberrant crypt foci in the colon were measured at week 16. All the indole-3-carbinol treatments significantly and strongly reduced the total number of aberrant crypts per rat, the number of aberrant crypt foci per rat, the ratio of aberrant crypts:aberrant crypt foci and the number of large aberrant crypt foci (containing three or four aberrant crypts).

In an experiment in which azoxymethane was used as the colon carcinogen, male Fischer 344 rats received a diet containing indole-3-carbinol at 0.875 or 1.75 g/kg for 5 weeks and received azoxymethane intraperitoneally at 15 mg/kg bw twice a week during weeks 2 and 3. The number of aberrant crypt foci per colon, determined at the end of the 5-week feeding period, was reduced to 54–63% of that in control animals by inclusion of indole-3-carbinol in the diet (Wargovich et al., 1996).

Kim et al. (2003) examined the effects of dietary indole-3-carbinol on spontaneous intestinal polyps in C57BL/6J-Apc$^{Min/+}$ mice. In heterozygous [Min/+] male mice that ate a diet containing indole-3-carbinol at 100 or 300 mg/kg for 10 weeks, the multiplicity of polyps in all portions of the small intestine and in the colon was not significantly affected, although the low dose reduced the multiplicity of polyps (from 1.40 to 0.85 polyps per colon). In mice treated with azoxymethane subcutaneously at 5 mg/kg bw once a week for 4 weeks before receiving dietary indole-3-carbinol for 32 weeks, both dietary concentrations of indole-3-carbinol decreased the number of aberrant crypt foci per colon (to 43–44% of control) and the total number of aberrant crypts per colon (to 38–40% of control).

Liver
Indole-3-carbinol inhibits numerous hepatocarcinogens in experimental animals. Evidence that indole-3-carbinol protects against liver carcinogenesis was derived initially from studies of the lower vertebrate, the rainbow trout (Bailey et al., 1982). When trout were fed diets containing indole-3-carbinol at 1000 mg/kg before and during initiation with aflatoxin B$_1$, the incidence of hepatocellular carcinoma was reduced by 40% relative to that in trout not given the indole. It was found later, however, that feeding of indole-3-carbinol after initiation by aflatoxin B$_1$ strongly promoted liver tumour incidence in trout (Bailey et al., 1987;

Dashwood et al., 1991; Oganesian et al., 1999). The studies showing promotion of hepatocarcinogenesis in rodents and fish by administration of indole-3-carbinol post-initiation are reviewed in section 6.

Manson et al. (1998) examined the effects on hepatocarcinogenesis in male Fischer 344 rats treated with aflatoxin B$_1$ for 24 weeks, either alone or with a high concentration of indole-3-carbinol (5000 mg/kg) added to the diet in weeks 6–24. A second protocol involved feeding the diet containing indole-3-carbinol for weeks 1–24 and adding aflatoxin B$_1$ during weeks 3–24. All groups were reared on control diet for an additional 19 weeks. The animals were assessed for three hepatic biomarkers, GST-P+ and GGT foci; cytokeratin 18 at weeks 13 and 43; and tumours at week 43. Although only four to six animals were examined for tumour development, treatment with indole-3-carbinol in either protocol reduced the tumour response, from 4/4 tumour-bearing animals and 6.5 tumours per liver in controls receiving only aflatoxin B$_1$ to 0/5 tumour-bearing animals in each group given indole-3-carbinol. Hepatic biomarkers were also reduced in rats given indole-3-carbinol at week 43. Interestingly, at week 13, administration of indole-3-carbinol after aflatoxin B$_1$ did not reduce the numbers of GST-P+ or GGT foci, but, rather, the numbers of foci per amount of staining were greater than in the livers of rats receiving aflatoxin B$_1$ alone. These results indicate that administration of a high dose of indole-3-carbinol can reduce hepatocarcinogenesis induced in rats by prolonged treatment with aflatoxin B$_1$, even if the indole-3-carbinol is delayed for 6 weeks. Nevertheless, two of three early biomarkers (GST-P+ and γ-glutamyl transferase foci) predicted the ultimate effects of indole-3-carbinol on tumour outcome when given after aflatoxin B$_1$.

Table 46. Selected studies of chemoprevention by indoles in experimental animals

Species, strain (sex)	Age at start	No. of animals per group	Carcinogen, dose, route, duration	Indole, dose, route	Timing of treatment	Preventive efficacy by tumour incidence (TI) or multiplicity (TM)[a]	Summarized effect	Reference
Forestomach								
Mouse, ICR/Ha (F)	9 weeks	18–39	Benzo[a]-pyrene, 1 mg, orally, twice per week, 4 weeks	Indole-3-carbinol, 0.03 mmol/g, diet; 3,3′-diindolyl-methane, 0.02 mmol/g, diet	5 weeks, 8 days before and during carcinogen	No inhibition of TI. TM decreased by 62% by indole-3-carbinol and by 36% by 3,3′-diindolylmethane	Both compounds inhibited multiplicity	Wattenberg & Loub (1978)
Colon								
Rat, Fischer 344 (M)	Wean-ling	9 or more	PhIP, 50 mg/kg bw gavage, every other day, weeks 3–4 of study or single gavage at week 3 in adduct study	Indole-3-carbinol, 1000 mg/kg, diet	4 weeks, before and with PhIP, 12 weeks after PhIP or 16 weeks, before, during and after PhIP	Indole-3-carbinol before or with PhIP blocked no. of aberrant crypt foci per rat (3.3 to 0.1), after PhIP (3.3 to 1.6) or for entire period (3.3 to 0.3)	Indole-3-carbinol can block or suppress PhIP initiation of aberrant crypt foci	Guo et al. (1995)
Rat, Fischer 344 (M)	Wean-ling	15	IQ, weeks 3–4 of study, 50 mg/kg bw orally	Indole-3-carbinol, 1000 mg/kg, diet, weeks 1–8	Before, during and/or after IQ	Significant reduction in mean no. of aberrant crypts per colon compared with rats given IQ alone (11.5 to 4.2)	Indole-3-carbinol for 8 weeks inhibited aberrant crypt foci induced by IQ in weeks 3–4. Initiation effects	Xu et al. (1996)
Rat, Fischer 344 (M)	7 weeks	10	Azoxy-methane, twice a week, weeks 2–3, i.p., 15 mg/kg bw	Indole-3-carbinol, 5 weeks, 0.875 or 1.75 g/kg, diet	1 week before to 3 weeks after azoxymethane	Significant reduction in no. of aberrant crypt foci per colon (63% and 54% versus 100% in controls)	Indole-3-carbinol inhibited colon aberrant crypt foci. Pre- and post-initiation effects not distinguished	Wargovich et al. (1996)

Table 46 (contd)

Species, strain (sex)	Age at start	No. of animals per group	Carcinogen, dose, route, duration	Indole, dose, route	Timing of treatment	Preventive efficacy by tumour incidence (TI) or multiplicity (TM)[a]	Summarized effect	Reference
Mouse, C57Bl/6J-*Min/+ Apc* (M)	6 weeks	10–25	Azoxymethane, once a week for 4 weeks before indole-3-carbinol, 5 mg/kg bw	Indole-3-carbinol, 10 or 32 weeks, 100 or 300 mg/kg, diet	After azoxymethane, 32 weeks, or no azoxymethane, 10 weeks	100 mg/kg indole-3-carbinol reduced spontaneous polyp multiplicity (1.40 to 0.83) Significant reduction in no. of aberrant crypt foci per colon induced by azoxymethane (44% and 43% versus 100% in controls)	Indole-3-carbinol had no significant effect on intestinal polyps in control Min^+ mice but inhibited aberrant crypt foci after azoxymethane	Kim *et al.* (2003)
Rat, Sprague-Dawley (M)	5 months	5–7	Azoxymethane on days 2 and 9 of indole-3-carbinol treatment, 19 mg/kg bw, i.p.	Indole-3-carbinol, 50, 100, 150 mg/kg bw orally, daily for 7 weeks	Before, during and after azoxymethane	No effect on no. or multiplicity of aberrant crypt foci	Indole-3-carbinol did not inhibit aberrant crypt foci	Exon *et al.* (2001)
Liver Trout, Shasta-derived rainbow	Finger-ling	200	Aflatoxin B_1, 20 µg/kg, diet, 4 weeks	Indole-3-carbinol, 1000 mg/kg, diet	2 weeks before and 4 weeks with aflatoxin B_1	40% reduction in hepatocellular carcinoma TI	Indole-3-carbinol effectively blocked aflatoxin B_1-induced tumour initiation	Bailey *et al.* (1982)
Trout, Shasta-derived rainbow	Finger-ling	200	Aflatoxin B_1, 20 µg/kg, diet, 2 weeks	Indole-3-carbinol, 1000 mg/kg, diet	8 weeks before, 2 weeks with, 6 weeks after aflatoxin B_1	Reduction in hepatocellular carcinoma TI from 36% in positive controls to 4% with indole-3-carbinol	Indole-3-carbinol inhibited aflatoxin B_1-induced liver tumours; initiation and post-initiation not distinguished	Nixon *et al.* (1984)
Rat, ACI/N (M)	7 weeks	8–12	N-Nitroso-diethylamine, 40 mg/l, drinking-water, 5 weeks	Indole-3-carbinol, 1000 mg/kg, diet, 7 weeks	1 week before, 5 weeks with, 1 week after carcinogen	Reduction in liver iron-altered foci (48.3/cm² to 17.6/cm²), TI (100% to 75%), TM (9.5 to 02.4)	Indole-3-carbinol blocked nitrosamine-initiated liver tumours	Tanaka *et al.* (1990)

Table 46 (contd)

Species, strain (sex)	Age at start	No. of animals per group	Carcinogen, dose, route, duration	Indole, dose, route	Timing of treatment	Preventive efficacy by tumour incidence (TI) or multiplicity (TM)[a]	Summarized effect	Reference
Rat, Fischer 344 (M)	19 weeks	4–6	Aflatoxin B_1, diet, 22–24 weeks	Indole-3-carbinol, 5000 mg/kg, diet	2 weeks before and 22 weeks with aflatoxin B_1 or during weeks 7–24 of a 26-week exposure to aflatoxin B_1	After 43 weeks, TI (100%) and TM (6.5 per animal) reduced to 0 by both indole-3-carbinol protocols. Cytokeratin biomarker reduced at weeks 13 and 43 by indole-3-carbinol. GGT and GST-P^+ foci reduced at week 43 but not at week 13 in group given indole-3-carbinol after aflatoxin B_1	Indole-3-carbinol inhibited liver tumours by prolonged co-exposure or if started 6 weeks after aflatoxin B_1. Post-initiation not distinguished	Manson et al. (1998)
Mouse, C57/Bl/6J (M)	15 days	9–12	N-Nitroso-diethylamine, 2 or 5 mg/kg bw, i.p.	Indole-3-carbinol, 1500 mg/kg, diet, 5.5 or 7.5 months	After carcinogen	After high dose of carcinogen, indole-3-carbinol reduced liver TM at 6 months (16.1 to 9.7) and 8 months (35.4 to 12.5)	Indole-3-carbinol suppressed nitrosamine-induced hepatocarcino-genesis	Oganesian et al. (1997)
Lung Mouse, A/J (F)	6–7 weeks	25	NNK, 10 µmol, i.p.	Indole-3-carbinol, 1800 mg/kg, diet	1 week before until 16 weeks after single NNK injection	TI not inhibited TM reduced from 8.1 to 4.9 tumours per mouse	Indole-3-carbinol inhibited NNK-induced lung tumour multi-plicity. Initiation and post-initiation not distinguished	El-Bayoumy et al. (1996)

Cancer preventive effects

Table 46 (contd)

Mammary gland

Species, strain (sex)	Age at start	No. of animals per group	Carcinogen, dose, route, duration	Indole, dose, route	Timing of treatment	Preventive efficacy by tumour incidence (TI) or multiplicity (TM)[a]	Summarized effect	Reference
Rat, Sprague-Dawley (F)	7 weeks	10–16	DMBA, 12 mg once, orally	Indole-3-carbinol, 0.10 mmol orally 20 h before; 0.014 mmol/g diet, for 8 days before 3,3'-Diindolyl-methane, 0.05 mmol orally 20 h before	Before carcinogen	At 28 weeks of age, 77% reduction in mammary TI by indole-3-carbinol orally; 73% by dietary indole-3-carbinol. 40–70% reduction by 3,3'-diindolylmethane orally	Blocking effects with one application of indole before carcinogen; indole-3-carbinol inhibited tumours when fed in diet 8 days before DMBA	Wattenberg & Loub (1978)
Mouse, C3H/OuJ (F)	21–28 days	30	Spontaneous	Indole-3-carbinol, 500 or 2000 mg/kg diet up to age 250 days	Not applicable	Inhibition of mammary TI and TM over time by ~50% at low dose and 75% at high dose	Inhibition of 'spontaneous' tumours	Bradlow et al. (1991)
Rat, Sprague-Dawley (F)	43 days	10–20	DMBA, 12 mg orally at age 50 days N-Methyl-N-nitrosourea, 50 mg/kg bw i.v. at age 50 days	Indole-3-carbinol, 50–100 mg/day, 5 times per week to 100 days after carcinogen	During and after carcinogen	$\geq$ 51% reduction in mammary TM at day 100; > 90% delay in time to tumour	Reduction of TM with both carcinogens. Design does not distinguish blocking from suppression.	Grubbs et al. (1995)
Mouse, BALB/cfC 3H, (F)	0 days	10–21	Spontaneous, driven by murine mammary tumour virus	Indole-3-carbinol, 2000 mg/kg in diet, up to 52 weeks	Not applicable	69% reduction in TI and increase in latency at age 36 weeks TI reduced from 50% to 20% in oncomouse at week 54	Reduction of spontaneous tumorigenesis	Malloy et al. (1997)
Rat, Sprague-Dawley (F)	55 days	8–10	DMBA, 20 mg, orally, single dose	3,3'-Diindolyl-methane, 0.5, 1.0 and 5 mg/kg bw, 10 doses over 20 days, gavage	After tumours reached 100–200 mm^3	Highest dose of indole significantly inhibited further tumour growth relative to controls; no effect at lower doses	Mammary tumour suppression by 3,3'-diindolyl-methane after DMBA. Anti-estrogenic effects seen	Chen, I. et al. (1998)

Table 46 (contd)

Species, strain (sex)	Age at start	No. of animals per group	Carcinogen, dose, route, duration	Indole, dose, route	Timing of treatment	Preventive efficacy by tumour incidence (TI) or multiplicity (TM)[a]	Summarized effect	Reference
Cervix Mouse, K14-HPV16 transgenic (F)	4–5 weeks	25	17β-estradiol, 0.125 or 0.250 mg/kg, 60-day release pellet, chronically	Indole-3-carbinol, 2000 mg/kg, diet, 6 months	Long-term	Decreased dysplasia and hyperplasia relative to mice fed estrogen alone TI decreased from 76% to 58%	Dietary indole-3-carbinol reduced tumours of cervix in mice bearing HPV-16	Jin et al. (1999)
Endometrium Rat, Donryu (F)	6 weeks	32–35	Spontaneous	Indole-3-carbinol, 200, 500, 1000 mg/kg, diet, for duration of study (660 days)	Not applicable	At 1000 mg/kg reduced endometrial adenocarcinoma (12/32 to 5/35) and uterine adeno-carcinoma TI	Indole-3-carbinol inhibited spontaneous endometrial cancer	Kojima et al. (1994)
Skin Mouse, Swiss albino (M, F)	12–15 g	20 M, 20 F	DMBA, 52 µg, once topically; TPA, 5 µg, twice a week, 28 weeks	Indole-3-carbinol, 250 µg, topically, twice a week, 28 weeks	1 week after DMBA 1 h before each TPA treatment	Final TI reduced from 100% to 56% (M) and 71% (F) Delay in tumour induction time	Topical indole-3-carbinol suppressed skin tumours in two-stage model	Srivastava & Shukla (1998)
Mouse, CD-1 (M)	5–6 weeks	20	DMBA, 50 µg topically, once TPA, 2.5 ng twice a week, 12 weeks	Brassinin, 1 or 2 µg twice a week, 12 weeks	After DMBA, 1 h before each TPA treatment	Incidence reduced from 95% to 50% at 2 µg No. of tumours per mouse reduced from 17.5 to 7.8 (1 µg) and 5.4 (2 µg)	Anti-promotion in two-stage model	Mehta et al. (1995)
Multiple organs Rat, Fischer 344 (M)	6 weeks	16–20	N-Nitroso-diethylamine, N-methyl-N-nitrosourea, N,N-nitroso-dibutylamine	Indole-3-carbinol, 5000 mg/kg, diet, for 36 weeks	After carcinogens	Reduction in liver hyperplastic nodules; no significant effect on lung, thyroid, kidney or bladder carcino-genesis	High dose of indole-3-carbinol inhibited liver hyperplastic nodules and GST-P[+] foci	Jang et al. (1991)

Species, strain (sex)	Age at start	No. of animals per group	Carcinogen, dose, route, duration	Indole, dose, route	Timing of treatment	Preventive efficacy by tumour incidence (TI) or multiplicity (TM)[a]	Summarized effect	Reference
Rat, Sprague-Dawley (F)	54 days	20	DMBA, aflatoxin B$_1$, azoxymethane	Indole-3-carbinol, 2000 mg/kg, diet, 25 weeks, weeks 5-30	After last carcinogen treatment on day 29	Colon: aberrant crypt foci decreased from 285 to 170 per colon Mammary: 3-4-week delay in time to first mammary tumour and significant reduction in kinetics of mammary tumour appearance No reduction in final mammary TI, TM or size	Post-initiation indole-3-carbinol suppressed colon aberrant crypt foci, delayed mammary tumour onset, but strongly promoted GST-P$^+$ foci. Also increased foci by 69-fold in unitated group	Stoner et al. (2002)

Table 46 (contd)

[a] All effects listed statistically significant at $p \leq 0.05$

DMBA, 7,12-dimethylbenz[a]anthracene; GGT, γ-glutamyl transferase; GST-P$^+$, glutathione S-transferase placental form; IQ, 2-amino-3-methyl-imidazo[4,5-f]quinoline; NNK, 4-(methylnitrosamino)-1-(3-pyridyl)-1-butanone; PhIP, 2-amino-1-methyl-6-phenylimidazo[4,5-b]pyridine; TPA, 12-O-tetradecanoylphorbol 13-acetate; i.p., intraperitoneally; i.v., intravenously; F, female ; M, male

Cytokeratin 18 was the best marker for tumour outcome.

Mammary gland

Wattenberg and Loub (1978) provided the classic demonstration of the chemo-prevention of mammary tumours by indoles in rodents. Female Sprague-Dawley rats were initiated with DMBA (12 mg, orally) at 7 weeks of age and then received either standard chow or diets containing indole-3-carbinol at 0.014 mmol/g 8 days before DMBA. Additional groups received a single oral dose of indole-3-carbinol at 0.10 mmol, 3,3′-diindolylmethane at 0.05 mmol or indole-3-acetonitrile at 0.1 mmol 20 h before DMBA. Mammary tumour development was assessed at 28 weeks of age. After a single treatment, indole-3-carbinol significantly reduced the mammary tumour incidence in each of three experiments (e.g. from 91% to 21%) and the tumour multiplicity (e.g. from 1.45 to 0.29 tumours per rat). Diindolylmethane provided a similar degree of protection (e.g. reduction in incidence from 91% to 27%) when administered at half the dose of indole-3-carbinol. Indole-3-acetonitrile did not provide significant protection. Protracted dietary indole-3-carbinol also reduced the incidence (73% to 20%) and multiplicity (1.20 to 0.33 tumours per rat) of mammary tumours.

In a more recent study (Mehta et al., 1995), cultured BALB/c mouse mammary organ explants were incubated for 10 days with synthesized brassinin (10^{-9} to 10^{-5} mol/l of medium), and DMBA was added at 2 µg/ml to the medium on days 3 and 4 to generate mammary lesions ex vivo. Mammary lesions were detected in 10/15 glands with DMBA alone, and this incidence was reduced significantly with brassinin (2/15, 80% inhibition) and cyclobrassinin (1/15, 91% inhibition) but not with 2-methyl-brassinin (11/15).

Cervix

Indole-3-carbinol and 3,3′-diindolyl-methane can negatively regulate estrogen activity (Auborn et al., 2003). For instance, Jin et al. (1999) studied the effects of these indoles in the K14-HPV16 mouse, which expresses oncogenes from HPV 16 and develops cervical cancer in response to long-term exposure to estrogens. In positive control mice receiving estradiol at 0.125 mg/day, 19 of 25 developed cervical–vaginal cancer within 6 months, and the remaining animals had hyperplasia. In mice that also received a diet containing indole-3-carbinol at 2000 mg/kg, only two of 24 developed cancer, and the remainder had dysplasia and hyperplasia. This result was taken to suggest that indole-3-carbinol negatively affected the proliferative effects of estrogen by restoring tissue homeostasis. In support of this, the authors showed that the increased expression of proliferating cell nuclear antigen (PCNA) in the cervical epithelium after estrogen treatment is reduced by dietary indole-3-carbinol (Jin et al., 1999), and that indole-3-carbinol and 3,3′-diindolylmethane induce apoptosis in the cervical epithelium of estrogen-treated mice (Chen, D.Z. et al., 2001).

Skin

The anti-tumour promoting potential of indole-3-carbinol was examined in a mouse skin cancer model (Srivastava & Shukla, 1998). Swiss albino mice were initiated with a single topical dose (52 μg) of DMBA, and 1 week later were given 250 μg of indole-3-carbinol topically with 5 μg of 12-O-tetradecanoylphorbol 13-acetate (TPA) twice a week for 28 weeks. At the end of the experiment, the indole-3-carbinol-supplemented animals had a significantly reduced incidence (from 33/34 to 21/34) and cumulative number of tumours (from 267 to 155). The multiplicity was reduced in males but not in females, and tumour induction time

was significantly delayed by indole-3-carbinol.

Mehta et al. (1995) initiated 5–6-week-old CD-1 mice with DMBA (50 μg, painted once) and promoted them with TPA (2.5 mg, twice weekly, 12 weeks). In the group that received brassinin (1 or 2 μg in 0.2 ml acetone) 1 h before each TPA treatment, the tumour incidence at termination and the multiplicity were reduced, with a dose–response relationship.

Multiple organs

Stoner et al. (2002) examined the effects of post-initiation administration of dietary indole-3-carbinol at 2000 mg/kg in a multi-organ model, with azoxymethane to initiate colon carcinogenesis. Indole-3-carbinol given for 25 weeks after carcinogen treatment significantly reduced the number of aberrant crypt foci, from 285 to 170 crypts per colon. The number of aberrant crypt foci containing more than four crypts was also reduced, from 167 to 113 per colon, but this result was not significant.

Intermediary biomarkers
Cruciferous vegetables

The xenobiotic-metabolizing enzymes are among the most important of the defence systems that modulate the access of chemical carcinogens to DNA in target tissues. The regulation of this complex enzyme system by dietary constituents is thought to be the principle mechanism underlying the ability of certain food components to block the induction of tumours by chemical carcinogens, in animal models of carcinogenesis (Wattenberg, 1990). Induction of phase I metabolism enhances detoxification but also often activates procarcinogens, and can either enhance or suppress carcinogenesis. In contrast, induction of phase II metabolism usually reduces the biological activity of carcinogenic intermediates and accelerates their excretion.

Phase I enzymes

Whitty and Bjeldanes (1987) explored the effect of a diet containing freeze-dried cabbage on phase I enzymes and on the binding of aflatoxin B_1 to hepatic DNA in vivo. Rats received a diet supplemented with 25% freeze-dried cabbage for 21 days. Radio-labelled aflatoxin was administered intraperitoneally, and hepatic DNA was isolated for analysis. The treated group had an 87% reduction in aflatoxin binding when compared with the control group, which was associated with increases in the activity of hepatic (2.6-fold) and intestinal (1.4-fold) epoxide hydrolases and of intestinal Ah hydroxylase (2.3-fold) and ethoxycoumarin O-deethylase (2.5-fold). No increases in the hepatic activities of the latter enzymes were observed. The authors discussed the possible roles of various phase I and II enzymes as modulators of aflatoxin B_1 metabolism and concluded that induction of either epoxide hydrolase or GST (2.1- and 2.3-fold increases in the liver and intestine, respectively) might have accounted for the striking reduction in aflatoxin binding observed in their study.

Phase II enzymes

Godlewski et al. (1985) studied the effects of Brussels sprouts and of glucosinolate-rich and glucosinolate-free sprout extracts on the induction of hepatic GST activity and on aflatoxin-induced hepatic foci in weanling rats. All three dietary treatments increased hepatic GST activity, but only Brussels sprouts and the glucosinolate-rich fractions inhibited hepatic focus formation. This important observation suggests that glucosinolates and their breakdown products are anticarcinogenic through mechanisms other than by induction of hepatic GST.

Kassie et al. (2003a) studied the effects of Brussels sprouts and red cabbage juices on the IQ-induced activity of the hepatic phase II enzymes. The activities of UDP-glu-curonosyl transferase (UGT)-2 and CYP1A2 were increased by both vegetables. The induction of UGT-2 activity by Brussels sprouts (and inhibition of IQ-induced aberrant crypt foci) was more marked than that by red cabbage cultivars, suggesting that greater glucuronidation of IQ may account for reductions in preneoplastic lesions. The authors suggested that Brussels sprouts are more effective because they have a higher glucosinolate content than red cabbage. Interestingly, cooking the vegetables had no influence on their protective effect. Therefore, the effect was probably due to intact glucosinolates, which were presumably metabolized to breakdown products in the intestinal lumen. The effects could not, however, be attributed to any particular glucosinolate.

DNA adducts

The relationship between carcinogen–DNA adduct formation and the induction of tumours in animals is well established, and it is generally considered that DNA adduct formation is a prerequisite for a mutational event which, in turn, may trigger the carcinogenic process (see reviews by Hemminki, 1993; Schut & Snyderwine, 1999). For instance, the main genotoxic metabolite of the polycyclic aromatic hydrocarbon benzo[a]pyrene forms adducts in the same codon of the p53 gene in which characteristic mutations are formed in the lungs of smokers (Denissenko et al., 1996). Furthermore, in lung tumours induced by polycyclic aromatic hydrocarbons in mice, a correlation was found between DNA adducts and the induction of ras mutations (Nesnow et al., 1998). If DNA adduct formation is a prerequisite for tumour formation, it follows that inhibition of DNA adduct formation should lead to inhibition of carcinogenesis. The correlation between inhibition of carcinogen–DNA adduct formation

and inhibition of carcinogen-induced tumour formation has indeed been established in several experimental systems (Dashwood et al., 1989b; Morse et al., 1989a; Liu et al., 1991; Singletary & Nelshoppen, 1991; Liu et al., 1992). Thus, inhibition of carcinogen–DNA adduct formation by, e.g. dietary components can be an excellent measure of its chemopreventive properties.

As mentioned previously, Whitty and Bjeldanes (1987) studied the effects of dietary cabbage (25% w/w) on the binding of aflatoxin B_1 to hepatic DNA, and on hepatic phase I and II enzymes in weanling male Fischer 344 rats. An increase in liver weight, upregulation of hepatic enzymes and an 87% reduction in the binding of aflatoxin B_1 to hepatic DNA were found in animals receiving cabbage, 2 h after treatment with the carcinogen. Tan et al. (1999), used a similar approach to explore the protective effects of Chinese cabbage against tumour initiation by the food-borne carcinogen PhIP, which induces colon and mammary gland tumours in rats and has been implicated as a cause of colorectal cancer. Rats were fed a diet containing freeze-dried Chinese cabbage (20% w/w) for 10 days before oral administration of a single dose of PhIP (10 mg/kg bw). The levels of DNA adducts in the colon, heart, lung and liver were determined with a ^{32}P-postlabelling technique, and the activity of hepatic CYP1A1 and CYP1A2 and cytosolic GSTs were also measured. There were substantial reductions (50–80%) in the levels of adduct formation in target organs, significant upregulation of both CYP1A1 and CYP1A2 and up-regulation of hepatic GST. The results are therefore consistent with the proposed protective effects of Chinese cabbage, although in this, as in many such studies, the amount of the vegetable administered was very high.

Markers of oxidative damage

In only a few of the published studies on Brassica vegetables were biochemical indices of oxidative damage used as biomarkers of effect. Deng et al. (1998) used purified glucosinolates, crude extracts of raw and cooked Brussels sprouts and a standardized aqueous extract of Brussels sprouts to explore the effects of a complex mixture of Brassica vegetable constituents in an animal model. The standardized extract, used by this group in several other studies, was produced by homogenizing the raw sprouts, collecting the juice and the residues and cooking them in a microwave oven. Soluble material was then leached out of the residues and mixed with the juice extract, and the liquid was freeze-dried and re-suspended in distilled water for use. It is probable that the material contained a complex mixture of non-volatile glucosinolate breakdown products, but its composition was not well defined by the authors. The effects on spontaneous oxidative damage were studied in male Wistar rats, and modulation of induced damage was studied in animals treated with 2-nitropropane (at 100 mg/kg bw). The end-point measured was the DNA oxidation product 8-oxo-7,8-dihydro-2-deoxyguanosine (8-oxodG). Oral administration of cooked Brussels sprouts homogenate (3 g) for 4 days reduced spontaneous urinary excretion of 8-oxodG by 31%, whereas raw sprouts, isolated indole glucosinolates or their breakdown products had no effect. The standardized aqueous extract of sprouts also substantially decreased both the spontaneous and the induced level of 8-oxodG excretion. Pretreatment with the aqueous sprout extract also reduced the levels of DNA oxidation induced by 2-nitropropane in several target tissues (kidney, liver and bone marrow), but the spontaneous levels of 8-oxodG were reduced only in the kidney. The authors drew attention to the parallels between their own results and the findings of one of the few human interventions in this area, which showed that oral administration of Brussels sprouts reduced oxidative DNA damage in healthy volunteers (Verhagen et al., 1995, 1997).

The protective effects of the sprout extract (Deng et al., 1998), which appeared to be due to antioxidant effects in the target tissues, were observed only when the sprouts were cooked. This is somewhat surprising because the bioavailability of glucosinolate breakdown products in animals and humans is known to be reduced by cooking, as a consequence of the inactivation of myrosinase (see sections 2 and 3). Cooking has, however, been shown by other groups to enhance the antioxidant effects of many types of non-cruciferous vegetable, so that the effects may be unrelated to glucosinolates or their breakdown products (Maeda et al., 1992).

To resolve some of these issues, the same group subsequently explored the antioxidant effects of their sprout extract in vitro, using calf thymus DNA in which oxidative damage was induced with Fenton reagents and ultraviolet light (Zhu et al., 2000). The aqueous extract and several sub-fractions derived by HPLC had a consistently protective effect against the production of 8-oxodG, at levels that the authors interpreted as consistent with those achievable in humans eating modest amounts of Brussels sprouts. The antioxidant factors in the extract were not convincingly identified, but the authors noted that the glucosinolate sinigrin co-eluted with the most effective HPLC fraction derived from the extract. It has been reported that a substantial proportion of intact sinigrin is absorbed from the small intestine of rats, but its metabolic fate and biological effects are unknown (Elfoul et al., 2001).

In their most recent study on this topic (Sorensen et al., 2001), the same group treated rats with the aqueous Brussels sprout extract for periods of between 3 and 7 days and studied a range of end-points, including phase I enzymes (CYP1A2, CYP2B1/2 and CYP2E1) and two phase II enzymes, NADPH:quinone reductase and GST π7. They also explored the effects on antioxidant enzymes and on 8-oxodG and malondialdehyde excretion, as before. In agreement with many previous studies, induction of both GST and quinone reductase was observed, but there was no effect on phase I enzymes. Unexpectedly, a statistically significant increase in oxidative DNA damage was found in the liver (8-oxodG), with no effect on antioxidant enzyme activity or malondialdehyde excretion. The authors commented that Brussels sprouts appeared to have both adverse and beneficial effects, depending on the conditions of the experiment and the target organs observed, and they speculated that advising the public to eat large quantities of Brassica vegetables might not be entirely justified. [The Working Group considered that the levels of the biomarkers were probably overestimated.]

Apoptosis

Suppression of apoptosis is thought to occur at every stage of cancer progression, from normal tissue to fully established invasive carcinoma. Conversely, high levels of apoptosis were shown in a large human cohort to protect against colorectal adenoma (Martin et al., 2002). There is a substantial body of evidence that isothiocyanates induce apoptosis in vitro, and several groups using animal models to study the blocking effects of isothiocyanates have acknowledged that induction of apoptosis in vivo may also play a role in the anticarcinogenic effects of Brassica vegetables. At present, however, there are few studies on the ability of intact

glucosinolates or Brassica vegetables to induce apoptosis in vivo.

Smith et al. (1998) studied the effects of purified sinigrin on apoptosis in an animal model, in which dimethylhydrazine was used to induce apoptosis in colonic crypts at 48 h and aberrant crypt foci after 16 weeks. Sinigrin had no effect on apoptosis in crypt cells in untreated animals, but amplification of the apoptotic response to dimethylhydrazine was seen after 48 h, which was associated with a reduction in aberrant crypt foci at the later time. It was shown subsequently that supplementation with raw sprout extract in the form of freshly prepared juice slowed mitosis and amplified apoptosis by about threefold in dimethylhydrazine-treated animals but had no effect on controls (Smith et al., 2003). A freeze-dried whole-sprout supplement had a similar, although slightly less marked, effect, but cooked sprouts were ineffective. These results indicate that large quantities of Brassica vegetable tissue exert a pro-apoptotic effect in the colonic mucosa of rats in which the epithelial cells have previously been challenged with a mutagenic carcinogen.

Isothiocyanates
Phase I enzymes

Guo et al. (1992) studied the effects of a single acute oral dose (1 mmol/kg bw) of phenethyl-ITC on phase I and phase II enzymes in the liver, lung and nasal tissues of Fischer 344 rats. Their main observation was a prompt and complex change in the pattern of activities of hepatic phase I enzymes. For example, the activity of N-nitrosodimethylamine demethylase, which is primarily a function of CYP2E1, was reduced by 80% 2 h after administration of phenethyl-ITC and was still 40% below baseline levels at 48 h. The activity of CYP1A2 and CYP3A was decreased to a somewhat lesser degree, but that of hepatic PROD, which is a marker for CYP2B1, was increased by 10-fold after 24 h. The last effect was associated with a sevenfold increase in CYP2B1 protein. The rates of oxidation of NNK were substantially reduced in liver, lung and nasal tissue microsomes 2 h and 24 h after treatment. Administration of phenethyl-ITC resulted in a reduction in the metabolic activation of the oesophageal carcinogen *N*-nitrosomethylamylamine and a reduction in the formation of methylated DNA in rat oesophagus (Huang *et al.*, 1993).

Studies with radioactively labelled phenethyl-ITC indicate that the compound, or a metabolite, is distributed to the liver, lung and other target tissues within a few hours (Eklind *et al.*, 1990) and that it combines both covalently and non-covalently with cellular proteins. Phenethyl-ITC is also a competitive inhibitor of NNK oxidation in lung microsomes (Smith *et al.*, 1990), and it seems probable that the overall effect of the compound or its metabolites is a combination of covalent inactivation and competitive inhibition of microsomal enzymes (Guo *et al.*, 1992). The last authors speculated that competitive inhibition is more important early on, while longer-term reductions in enzyme activity are due primarily to covalent inactivation.

Using a similar protocol, Guo *et al.* (1993) examined the effects of phenethyl-ITC, benzyl-ITC and two synthetic compounds, 4-phenylbutyl-ITC and 6-phenylhexyl-ITC, on NNK oxidation and on phase I and II enzymes. In general, a single dose of 0.25 or 1.0 mmol/kg bw of these compounds given 6 or 24 h before death resulted in significant reductions in NNK oxidation by lung, liver and nasopharyngeal microsomes. Phenethyl-ITC was generally a more potent inhibitor than benzyl-ITC, but both were less effective than the synthetic compounds. The effects and the relative potencies of the different isothio-

cyanates correlated reasonably well with their relative effectiveness as inhibitors of carcinogenesis in vivo (Morse *et al.*, 1989b, 1991).

The chemistry of tobacco smoke is extremely complex, as is the sequence of carcinogenic events leading ultimately to lung cancer. Sticha *et al.* (2000) explored the hypothesis that benzyl-ITC inhibits the formation of DNA adducts induced by benzo[*a*]pyrene by blocking production of the highly reactive metabolite 7,8-dihydroxy-9,10-epoxy-7,8,9,10-tetrahydrobenzo[*a*]pyrene (BPDE). The metabolism of benzo[*a*]pyrene by mouse lung and liver microsomes 6 or 24 h after treatment with benzyl-ITC or phenethyl-ITC was used as an intermediate end-point of anticarcinogenic activity. Both benzyl-ITC and phenethyl-ITC inhibited the formation of benzo[*a*]pyrene metabolites and BPDE–DNA adducts. This finding was interpreted as support for the hypothesis for the mechanism of action of benzyl-ITC. Although there were some differences in the activities of the two isothiocyanates, they did not entirely explain the inefficacy of phenethyl-ITC against lung tumours in this model. The authors speculated that other mechanisms, such as suppression of tumorigenesis by benzyl-ITC by induction of apoptosis, might explain the different effects of the two isothiocyanates.

One unresolved issue is the relative importance of native isothiocyanates and their conjugates as inhibitors of phase I enzyme activity. The main route of isothiocyanate metabolism in humans is conjugation with GSH, followed by urinary excretion as *N*-acetyl-L-cysteine conjugates (Brüsewitz *et al.*, 1977). The target tissues are therefore exposed primarily to GSH conjugates of isothiocyanates rather than the native compounds. Conaway *et al.* (1996) studied the structure–activity relationships of isothiocyanates and their conjugates with

regard to inhibition of CYP1A1, CYP1A2 and CYP2B1, using hepatic microsomes from 3-methylcholanthrene- or phenobarbital-treated rats as an assay system. In general, the parent isothiocyanates were more potent inhibitors than the conjugates. The same group compared phenethyl-ITC–GSH and 6-phenylhexyl-ITC–GSH conjugates in the assay system and showed that the 6-phenylhexyl-ITC–GSH conjugates were several times more potent than those of phenethyl-ITC; however both conjugated species showed anticarcinogenic activity against NNK in the A/J mouse pulmonary carcinogenesis model (Jiao *et al.*, 1997). Studies on the decomposition of isothiocyanate–GSH conjugates in vitro (Conaway *et al.*, 2001) suggested that, in solution, an equilibrium is established between free isothiocyanate and its conjugate, and that it is the free species (Moreno *et al.*, 1999) or another metabolite (Goosen *et al.*, 2001) that inhibits enzyme activity by covalently modifying the protein.

Phase II enzymes

GST activity is abundant throughout the mammalian alimentary tract and in the liver, and in both locations it is highly responsive to diet. In mice, a diet of unrefined rodent chow led to greater activity of small intestinal and hepatic GST than semi-synthetic diets. *Brassica* vegetables, as well as other foods, including coffee and tea, all induce GSTs in the alimentary tract, as do benzyl-ITC, indole-3-carbinol and indole-3-acetonitrile (Sparnins *et al.*, 1982a,b), but induction of phase II enzymes has not been used as an intermediate biomarker of carcinogenesis.

Guo *et al.* (1992) studied the effects of a single oral dose of 1 mmol/kg bw of phenethyl-ITC on phase I and phase II enzymes in the liver, lung and nasal tissues of Fischer

344 rats. The activities of the phase II enzymes NQO1 and GST were increased in the liver, but a more variable pattern of effects was observed in other target tissues.

To explore the dose–response relationship of the effects of isothiocyanates on the induction of phase II enzymes, Kore et al. (1993) administered iberin [1-isothiocyanato-3-(methylsulfinyl)propane] over a concentration range of 1–100 µmol/kg bw per day. Intestinal GST and NQO1 activities were significantly enhanced by treatment, but only at the highest dose. The authors estimated that the human population is exposed to about 1 mmol/kg bw per day of iberin, and they concluded that a conventional diet was unlikely to have a significant effect on phase II enzyme activity.

Haemoglobin adducts

Prolonged administration of 6-phenyl-hexyl-ITC and phenethyl-ITC strongly inhibited lung carcinogenesis induced by NNK in rats (see above). In one study, under conditions in which the induction of tumours by NNK was reduced from around 70% in control groups to less than 30% in treated groups, the latter showed reduced blood-borne biomarkers of DNA adduct formation [4-hydroxy-1-(3-pyridyl)-1-butanone-releasing haemoglobin adducts], together with increased NNK detoxification and urinary excretion (Hecht et al., 1996b).

DNA adducts

If modulation of phase I and/or II enzyme activity is effective in blocking mutagenesis, then the reduction in carcinogen activation should be accompanied by a reduction in the level of DNA adducts induced by model carcinogens, and this should be detectable in target tissues. Chung et al. (1985) explored the effects of phenyl-ITC, phenethyl-ITC and the glucosinolate sinigrin on the α-hydroxy-

lation of N-nitrosodimethylamine and NNK by liver microsomes in vitro, and observed that the isothiocyanates inhibited demethylation of the nitrosamines. Pretreatment of rats with the isothiocyanates or with sinigrin inhibited the formation of 7-methylguanine and O^6-methylguanine in rat hepatic DNA. The authors concluded that this was the probable mechanism for the anticarcinogenic effects of the isothiocyanates towards these carcinogens.

Certain isothiocyanates have been shown to exert significant anticarcinogenic effects in rat models of oesophageal carcinogenesis, and these effects appeared to be well correlated with inhibition of adduct formation. Stoner et al. (1991) showed that administration of phenethyl-ITC before and during treatment of Fischer 344 rats with N-nitrosobenzylmethylamine suppressed oesophageal tumours and preneoplastic lesions by as much as 99–100%. In cultured explants of rat oesophageal tissue, phenethyl-ITC reduced N-nitrosobenzylmethylamine metabolism, reduced the formation of DNA adducts by 53–97% and inhibited DNA methylation at the 7 and O^6 positions of guanine. A similar inhibitory effect of phenethyl-ITC on the metabolism of N-nitrosomethyl-amylamine and methylation of DNA in rat oesophagus was described later (Huang et al., 1993).

Phenethyl-ITC and a number of synthetic isothiocyanates inhibited lung carcinogenesis and DNA methylation induced by NNK in mouse models (Morse et al.,1989b, 1991). Staretz et al. (1997a) investigated the effects of phenethyl-ITC on the induction of pyridyloxobutyl DNA adducts in the NNK model of rat lung tumorigenesis. Having established that there was a significant relationship between the extent of tumour induction and the level of adducts in the appropriate target cells in lung tissue, they demonstrated a 50% reduction in pyridyloxobutyl DNA adducts in target cells,

which was consistent with the 50% reduction in NNK-induced lung tumours by phenethyl-ITC.

Wattenberg (1987) showed that benzyl-ITC inhibited lung neoplasia induced by benzo[a]pyrene in a mouse model. This was confirmed by Lin et al. (1993) but, as others have observed (Adam-Rodwell et al., 1993), phenethyl-ITC was not effective under the same conditions. Sticha et al. (2000) tested the hypothesis that inhibition by benzyl-ITC of benzo[a]pyrene-induced lung carcinogenesis in the murine model is due directly to suppression of DNA adduct formation. They found a significant reduction in the formation of BPDE–DNA adducts in lung and hepatic DNA from A/J mice treated with benzyl-ITC and phenethyl-ITC, 2–120 h after treatment with the carcinogen. Phenethyl-ITC was a somewhat less effective inhibitor of adduct formation than benzyl-ITC, but the differences were not considered great enough to explain the marked differences in the anticarcinogenic activity of the two isothiocyanates. In a more complex model, Sticha et al. (2002) studied the effects of phenethyl-ITC and a mixture of phenethyl-ITC and benzyl-ITC on the formation of DNA adducts after treatment with a mixture of benzo[a]pyrene and NNK. The adducts quantified were BPDE–N^2-deoxyguanosine from benzo[a]pyrene, O^6-methylguanine and 4-hydroxy-1-(3-pyridyl)-1-butanone-releasing adducts from NNK. Both phenethyl-ITC and the mixture with benzyl-ITC inhibited the formation of the adducts from NNK, but they had no effect on BPDE–N^2-deoxyguanosine or O^6-methylguanine.

Administration of phenethyl-ITC resulted in a reduction in the metabolic activation of the oesophageal carcinogen N-nitrosomethylamylamine and a reduction in the formation of methylated DNA adducts in rat oesophagus (Huang et al., 1993).

Apoptosis

Samaha *et al.* (1997) studied the effects of various candidate chemopreventive agents on the level of apoptosis in colorectal tumours of rats treated with azoxymethane and observed a correlation between the induction of apoptosis and the effectiveness of the treatment. Sulindac and curcumin both increased apoptosis and suppressed tumorigenesis; however, the synthetic 6-phenylhexyl-ITC, which is highly protective against pulmonary tumorigenesis (Morse *et al.*, 1991) but enhances both oesophageal (Stoner *et al.*, 1995) and colonic tumorigenesis (Rao *et al.*, 1995), suppressed the rate of apoptosis. This finding provides circumstantial evidence for a role of apoptosis in tumour suppression and shows that isothiocyanates can have adverse as well as beneficial effects.

Yang *et al.* (2002) investigated the anticarcinogenic effects of *N*-acetylcysteine conjugates of benzyl-ITC and phenethyl-ITC against lung tumorigenesis induced by benzo[*a*]pyrene in A/J mice. Both conjugates reduced tumour multiplicity, and the reductions were associated with increased apoptosis in lung tissue, together with biochemical evidence for activation of apoptosis-related signalling pathways.

D'Agostini *et al.* (2001) reported that phenethyl-ITC amplified cigarette smoke-induced apoptosis in rat bronchial and bronchiolar epithelium.

Srivastava *et al.* (2003) reported that a bolus intraperitoneal injection of allyl-ITC (10 µmol) given to mice three times a week after implantation of human prostate cancer (PC-3) xenografts significantly inhibited tumour growth by reducing mitotic activity and inducing apoptosis. This effect may be similar to that observed by Smith *et al.* (1998) in dimethylhydrazine-treated rats fed sinigrin, which is the parent glucosinolate of allyl-ITC.

Indoles

Effects on enzymes

Studies on the induction and inhibition of enzymes by indole-3-carbinol are reviewed in section 3. In this section, only those effects observed in protocols for chemical carcinogenesis or effects that are clearly related to chemoprevention are summarized. Studies on the effects of indole-3-carbinol on the metabolism of carcinogens in vivo, as measured by quantification of their metabolites, are not included. The relevant studies are described below and those in rats are summarized in Table 47.

After 2 weeks of feeding male Fischer 344 rats with an indole-3-carbinol-containing diet (30 µmol/g), the activity of O^6-methylguanine–DNA transmethylase, an enzyme that removes O^6 methyl groups from guanine bases in DNA, was quantified in liver, lung and nasal mucosa. The indole-3-carbinol-containing diet had no effect on this enzyme (Morse *et al.*, 1988).

In a study of mammary tumours induced by DMBA or MNU in female Sprague-Dawley rats, Grubbs *et al.* (1995) measured induction of various alkoxyresorufin-*O*-dealkylases by a hepatic microsomal preparation (9000 x *g* supernatant) after prolonged oral dosing (by gavage) with indole-3-carbinol (50 or 100 mg/day for 100 days). In parallel experiments, these doses were shown to be effective in preventing mammary tumour induction when given either during or both during and after carcinogen administration. The activities of methoxyresorufin-*O*-dealkylase (MROD, specific for CYP1A2), EROD (specific for CYP1A1) and benzyloxyresorufin-*O*-dealkylase (BROD, specific for CYP2B1) were increased in relation to dose of indole-3-carbinol (up to 121-fold for CYP2B1). The induction was parallelled by induction of the respective mRNAs; mRNA analysis also showed induction of hepatic GST sub-

family α (GST Ya/Yc) and epoxide hydrolase.

The induction of hepatic alkoxyresorufin-*O*-dealkylases (MROD, EROD, BROD and pentoxyresorufin-*O*-dealkylase [PROD]) in female Sprague-Dawley rats was confirmed by Malejka-Giganti *et al.* (2000), in animals that received indole-3-carbinol at a dose of 250 mg/kg bw three times a week for 12 weeks. In contrast to the results of Grubbs *et al.* (1995), this regimen failed to result in inhibition of DMBA-induced mammary tumours when DMBA was given as a single dose three weeks before the start of indole-3-carbinol treatment.

The induction by 0.1% dietary indole-3-carbinol of hepatic microsomal MROD and EROD activities was also confirmed in male Fischer 344 rats (Xu *et al.*, 1996) in a protocol whereby the animals received a dose of IQ that was sufficient to induce colonic aberrant crypt foci. Xu *et al.* (1997) also examined the dose–response relationship of single oral doses of indole-3-carbinol in male Fischer 344 rats. At doses equal to or higher than the equivalent of 100 mg/kg of diet, the activities of both EROD and MROD were induced (EROD twofold more than MROD) in hepatic and colonic microsomes. The induction was parallelled by decreased formation of colonic IQ–DNA adducts and by mutagenic activation of IQ catalysed by hepatic microsomes in vitro. In contrast, at doses of indole-3-carbinol less than the equivalent of 50 mg/kg of diet, hepatic EROD and MROD were both inhibited, accompanied by an increase in colonic IQ–DNA adducts and by an increase in IQ mutagenicity catalysed by hepatic microsomes from animals receiving these low doses. The authors considered it possible that the different effects of indole-3-carbinol at lower and higher doses might be related to the profile of acid condensation products formed

Table 47. Modulation by indole-3-carbinol of enzymes relevant to carcinogenesis in rats

Strain (sex); organ(s) analysed	Dose and schedule of indole-3-carbinol	Dose and schedule of carcinogen	Enzyme(s) measured	Summary of results	Reference
Fischer 344 (M); liver, lung, nasal mucosa	30 µmol/g of diet for 2 weeks	None	O^6-Methylguanine DNA methyltransferase	No effect	Morse et al. (1988)
Sprague-Dawley (F); liver	50 or 100 mg/day orally for 100 days	None	MROD, EROD, BROD, GST-YaYc, epoxide hydrolase	Increase in all	Grubbs et al. (1995)
Sprague-Dawley (F); liver	250 mg/kg bw orally 3 times per week for 12 weeks, 3 weeks after DMBA	DMBA, 20 mg/rat, orally, single dose	MROD, EROD, BROD, pentoxy-ROD	Increase in all	Malejka-Giganti et al. (2000)
Fischer 344 (M); liver	0.1% in diet for 8 weeks	IQ, 50 mg/kg bw, orally, every other day, weeks 3 and 4	MROD, EROD	Increase in both	Xu et al. (1996)
Fischer 344 (M); liver, colon	Single oral dose, equivalent to 0–1000 mg/kg of diet	None	MROD, EROD (activities), CYP1A1, CYP1A2 (by western blot)	Dose-related increase in all; decrease in hepatic MROD, EROD at low (0–50 mg/kg) concentrations	Xu et al. (1997)
Fischer 344 (M); liver	0.5% in diet for up to 13 weeks	Aflatoxin B_1, 2 mg/kg of diet for 13 weeks	CYP1A1, CYP1A2, CYP3A, CYP2B1/2, GST-Yc2, GST-P, AFAR (all by western blot)	Increase in all	Manson et al. (1998)

DMBA, 7,12-dimethylbenz[a]anthracene; IQ, 2-amino-3-methylimidazo[4,5-f]quinoline; MROD, methyl resorufin-O-dealkylase; EROD, ethoxy-; ROD, BROD, benzyloxy ROD-; CYP, cytochrome P450; GST, glutathione S-transferase; AFAR, aflatoxin B; aldehyde reductase ; M, male, F, female from this compound in the stomach, which differs with high and low doses. At low doses, these products, which act as agonists for the *Ah* receptor, are less likely to bind to this receptor.

In a protocol of aflatoxin B_1 and hepatocarcinogenesis, Manson *et al.* (1998) examined a number of hepatic enzymes relevant for carcinogenesis. Male Fischer 344 rats were given diets containing aflatoxin B_1 (2 mg/kg) or aflatoxin B_1 (2 mg/kg) plus indole-3-carbinol (5000 mg/kg, w/w). After 13 weeks, western blot analysis showed induction of the phase I enzymes, CYP1A1, CYP1A2, CYP3A and CYP2B1/2 and of the phase II enzymes aflatoxin B_1 aldehyde reductase (AFAR), GST-Yc2 and GST-P (the latter only in a group receiving aflatoxin B_1 or aflatoxin B_1 before indole-3-carbinol). Immunohistochemistry of liver sections showed a protective effect of indole-3-carbinol against GGT and GST-P+ foci, but only when indole-3-carbinol was given in the diet for 2 weeks before dietary aflatoxin B_1. The numbers of foci positive for aflatoxin B_1 aldehyde reductase and particularly cytokeratin 18 were decreased when indole-3-carbinol was provided in the diet either before or after aflatoxin B_1, but most prominently when given before. The activities of ornithine decarboxylase and tyrosine kinase were also decreased, when measured in liver extracts after exposure to indole-3-carbinol with or without aflatoxin B_1.

The effect of dietary indole-3-carbinol on liver enzymes possibly involved in aflatoxin B_1 activation and deactivation has also been studied in rainbow trout. Liver microsomal 7-ethoxycoumarin deethylase and EROD activities were not induced significantly in fish fed diets containing indole-3-carbinol at 500–2000 mg/kg for 8 days, concentrations that are effective in lowering hepatic aflatoxin B_1–DNA adduct formation. Similarly, the indole-3-carbinol diets did not affect liver CYP-LM$_2$ or CYP-LM$_{4b}$ isozymes (both specific for trout), nor did they affect liver microsomal UDPG-transferase or cytosolic GST activity (Fong *et al.*, 1990). In trout embryos, however, microinjection of an 'acid reaction mixture' (indole-3-carbinol treated with hydrochloric acid and partially purified before administration), 3,3′-diindolylmethane or a symmetrical cyclic trimer, 5,6,11,12,17,18-hexahydrocyclononal[1,2-*b*:4,5-*b*′:7,8-*b*″]triindole (CT) resulted in induction of total embryonic CYP1A. The same effect could be demonstrated in the livers of fingerlings (3 months old) injected intraperitoneally with these three derivatives. Indole-3-carbinol itself was a weak and only transient inducer of CYP1A. In the livers of fingerlings exposed to dietary indole-3-carbinol (2000 mg/kg for 21 days), weak but transient induction of EROD was found (Takahashi *et al.*, 1995a). After 7 days of feeding fingerlings a diet containing indole-3-carbinol at 500–4000 mg/kg, a dose-related increase in liver EROD activity was found at 2000–4000 mg/kg; at 500–1000 mg/kg, liver EROD activity was slightly inhibited. The induction of EROD activity at higher concentrations of indole-3-carbinol (2000–4000 mg/kg) was negatively correlated with hepatic [^{3}H]aflatoxin B_1–DNA binding, determined after administration of [^{3}H]aflatoxin B_1 in vivo (Takahashi *et al.*, 1995b).

DNA adducts

Rats: In male Sprague-Dawley rats pretreated intraperitoneally or orally with indole-3-carbinol or with the acid reaction mixture described above, total binding of [^{3}H]benzo[*a*]pyrene to hepatic DNA was reduced by 30–50% as compared with that in untreated controls. In contrast, inhibition of binding to pulmonary DNA was effective (50–70% decrease) only after oral administration of indole-3-carbinol or the acid reaction mixture, and not after intraperitoneal pretreatment with these compounds (Park & Bjeldanes, 1992) (Table 48). These results are consistent with rapid clearance of [^{3}H]benzo[*a*]pyrene in the intestine, aided by induction of benzo[a]pyrene-metabolizing enzymes such as CYP1A1, by indole-3-carbinol and the acid reaction mixture in this organ.

Indole-3-carbinol in the diet of male Fischer 344 rats increased the formation of hepatic 7-methylguanine after subcutaneous administration of the tobacco-specific carcinogen NNK but decreased this adduct in the lung and nasal cavity. In this experiment, indole-3-carbinol had no effect on the activity of O^6-methylguanine–DNA methyltransferase, an enzyme that catalyses the repair of O^6-methylguanine (Morse *et al.*, 1988).

In the only study on the effects of indole-3-carbinol on aflatoxin B_1–DNA binding in rats in vivo, dietary indole-3-carbinol inhibited the total binding of [^{3}H]aflatoxin B_1 to liver DNA in male Fischer 344 rats (Stresser *et al.*, 1994b).

Inhibition of the formation of DNA adducts with heterocyclic amines (food mutagens) by indole-3-carbinol has been studied in rats under a variety of experimental conditions. Male Fischer 344 rats pretreated for 4 weeks with a diet containing 0.1% (w/w) indole-3-carbinol and a single oral dose of IQ showed an initial (8 h after the last dose of IQ) increase in hepatic IQ–DNA adducts but significant decreases at later times (24–48 h) (Xu *et al.*, 1996). Inhibition of colonic IQ–DNA adducts in male Fischer 344 rats was shown to depend on the dietary concentration (10–1000 mg/kg) of indole-3-carbinol (Xu *et al.*, 1997).

Both the liver and colon are target organs for IQ in male Fischer 344 rats (reviewed by Schut & Snyderwine, 1999). When female Sprague-Dawley rats were maintained on a diet containing 0.02% (w/w) or 0.1% indole-3-

Table 48. Modulation by indole-3-carbinol and derivatives of carcinogen–DNA adduct formation in vivo

Species, strain (sex); organ(s) analysed	Indole-3-carbinol (I3C) or derivative, dose and schedule[a]	Carcinogen, dose and schedule	Method of DNA adduct analysis	Summary of effects[b]	Reference
Rat					
Sprague-Dawley (M); liver, lungs	I3C or RXM, 500 μmol/kg bw, single dose, i.p. or oral	[³H]Benzo[a]pyrene, 0.2 μmol/animal, oral	TBRM	Decrease (except in lungs after i.p.)	Park & Bjeldanes (1992)
Fischer 344 (M); liver, lung, nasal mucosa	I3C, 30 μmol/g diet for 2 weeks	[³H]NNK, 0.6 mg/kg bw, subcutaneous, 4 doses	HPLC (7-methylguanine only)	Increase (liver), decrease (lung, nasal mucosa)	Morse et al. (1988)
Fischer 344 (M); liver	I3C 0.2% in diet for 7 days	[³H]Aflatoxin B₁, 0.5 mg/kg bw, i.p., single dose	TBRM	Decrease	Stresser et al. (1994b)
Fischer 344 (M); liver	I3C, 0.1% in diet for 8 weeks	IQ, 50 mg/kg bw, oral, single dose	³²P-Postlabelling	Increase 8 h after IQ; decrease 24–48 h after IQ	Xu et al. (1996)
Fischer 344 (M); colon	I3C, single oral dose equivalent to 0–1000 mg/kg of diet	IQ, 5 mg/kg bw, loral single dose	³²P-Postlabelling	Decrease at doses > 25 mg/kg and increase at 10 mg/kg	Xu et al. (1997)
Sprague-Dawley (F); multiple organs	I3C, 0.02% or 0.1% of diet for 42 days	IQ, 0.01% of diet, days 15–42	³²P-Postlabelling	Decrease (in almost all of 14 organs)	He & Schut (1999a)
Fischer 344 (M); colon	I3C, 0.1% of diet for 10 days	PhIP, 50 mg/kg bw, oral single dose	³²P-Postlabelling	Decrease	Huber et al. (1997)
Fischer 344 (M); multiple organs	I3C, 0.1% of diet for 4 weeks	PhIP, 50 mg/kg bw, oral single dose	³²P-Postlabelling	Increase in some organs 6 h after PhIP; decrease in all organs 24 h to 6 days after PhIP	Guo et al. (1995)
Fischer 344 (F); liver, colon, mammary epithelial cells	I3C, 0.1% of diet for 4 weeks	PhIP, 0.01% of diet	³²P-Postlabelling	Decrease	Schut & Dashwood (1995)

Table 48 (contd)

Species, strain (sex); organ(s) analysed	Indole-3-carbinol (I3C) or derivative, dose and schedule[a]	Carcinogen, dose and schedule	Method of DNA adduct analysis	Summary of effects[b]	Reference
Fischer 344 (F); liver, colon, mammary epithelial cells, leukocytes	I3C, 0.02% or 0.1% of diet for 58 days	PhIP, 0.04% of diet, days 15–42	^{32}P-Postlabelling	Decrease only with 0.1% I3C	He et al. (1997)
Fischer 344 (F); multiple organs	I3C, 0.1% of diet for 29 days	PhIP, 10 or 50 mg/kg bw, single oral dose on day 13	^{32}P-Postlabelling	Decrease	He & Schut (1999)
Fischer 344 (F); multiple organs	I3C, 0.02% or 0.1% of diet for 3 weeks	PhIP, 1 mg/kg bw per day, oral, for 3 weeks	^{32}P-Postlabelling	Decrease in almost all organs and cells	He et al. (2000)
Sprague-Dawley (F); lungs, trachea, bladder, heart	I3C, 1.36 or 3.40 mmol/kg bw per day for 5 weeks	Cigarette smoke, 6 h/day, 7 days/week for 4 weeks	^{32}P-Postlabelling	Decrease	Arif et al. (2000)
Mouse					
ICR Swiss (M); liver	I3C, 167 mg/kg bw, single oral dose	[^{14}C]Benzo[a]pyrene, 5 µCi per mouse, oral	TBRM	Decrease	Shertzer (1983)
ICR Swiss (M); liver	I3C, 167 mg/kg bw, single oral dose	[^{14}C]Benzo[a]pyrene, 5 µCi per mouse, oral	TBRM	Decrease	Shertzer (1984)
ICR Swiss (M); liver	167 mg I3C/kg bw, single oral dose	[^{14}C]NDMA, 5 µCi per mouse, oral	TBRM	Decrease	Shertzer (1984)
A/J (F); liver, lungs	25 or 125 µmol I3C per mouse per day for 4 days, gavage	[^{3}H]NNK, 10 µmol per mouse, i.p.	HPLC (O^6-methylguanine and 7-methylguanine)	Decrease in lung O^6-methylguanine; increase in liver O^6-methylguanine and 7-methylguanine	Morse et al. (1990b)
Trout					
Rainbow; liver	2000 mg/kg of diet for 1 week	NDEA, 250 mg/kg of diet for 24 h	HPLC (O^6-ethylguanine and 7-ethylguanine)	Decrease in both O^6-ethylguanine and 7-ethylguanine	Fong et al. (1988)
Rainbow; liver	1000 mg/kg of diet for 12 weeks	[^{3}H]Aflatoxin B$_1$, 0.44 µCi per fish, i.p.	TBRM	Decrease	Nixon et al. (1984)
Rainbow; liver	2000 mg/kg of diet for 8 days	[^{3}H]Aflatoxin B$_1$, 2.6 nmol/kg bw, i.p.	TBRM	Decrease	Fong et al. (1990)

Table 48 (contd)

Species, strain (sex); organ(s) analysed	Indole-3-carbinol (I3C) or derivative, dose and schedule[a]	Carcinogen, dose and schedule	Method of DNA adduct analysis	Summary of effects[b]	Reference
Rainbow; liver	I3C, 1000–4000 mg/kg of diet for 7 days	[³H]Aflatoxin B_1, 30 µCi/10 µg/kg bw), i.p.	TBRM	Decrease	Takahashi et al. (1995b)
Rainbow; liver	I3C, 0–4000 mg/kg of diet for 6 weeks	[³H]Aflatoxin B_1, 10–320 µg/kg of diet, weeks 5 and 6	TBRM	Decrease	Dashwood et al. (1988)
Rainbow; whole embryo	I3C, 5 µg/egg; DIM, 8.6 µg/egg; CT, 13.5 µg/egg; RXM, 13.5 µg/egg	[³H]Aflatoxin B_1, 0.17 mCi per egg or 10 ng per egg	TBRM	Decrease with DIM, CT and RXM, but not with I3C	Dashwood et al. (1994)

I3C, indole-3-carbinol; DIM, 3,3´-diindolylmethane; RXM, acid reaction mixture of I3C; CT, 5,6,11,12,17,18-hexahydrocyclononal[1,2-b:4,5-b´:7,8-b´´]-triindole; DMBA, 7,12-dimethylbenz[a]anthracene; NNK, 4-(methylnitrosoamino)-1-(3-pyridyl)-1-butanone; IQ, 2-amino-3-methylimidazo[4,5-f]quinoline; PhIP, 2-amino-1-methyl-6-phenylimidazo[4,5-b]pyridine; NDEA, N-nitrosodiethylamine; NDMA, N-nitrosodimethylamine; TBRM, total binding of radioactive material; HPLC, high-performance liquid chromatography; i.p., intraperitoneally; M, male ; F, female

[a] I3C and derivatives were given before and/or during administration of the carcinogen.
[b] Only results statistically different from those for control animals not treated with indole-3-carbinol are listed; see text for percentage changes

carbinol for 7 weeks, followed by 2 weeks of control diet, and received 0.01% (w/w) IQ in their diet during weeks 3–6, IQ–DNA adduct formation was inhibited in almost all of the 14 organs examined, including the mammary gland and the liver, the target organs of IQ in female Sprague-Dawley rats. In most organs, the extent of inhibition was related to the dietary concentration of indole-3-carbinol. Dietary indole-3-carbinol did not, however, affect the rate of adduct removal, measured at the end of weeks 7 and 9 (He & Schut, 1999).

Indole-3-carbinol has also been studied as a potential inhibitor of carcinogenesis induced by another heterocyclic amine, PhIP. This compound is a mammary carcinogen as well as a weak colon carcinogen in female Fischer 344 rats and a colon and prostate carcinogen in male Fischer 344 rats (reviewed by Schut & Snyderwine, 1999). Maintaining male Fischer 344 rats on a diet containing 0.1% (w/w) indole-3-carbinol for 10 days, followed by a single oral dose of PhIP (50 mg/kg bw) resulted in significant inhibition (64% of control) in PhIP–DNA adduct formation in the colon (Huber et al., 1997). Incorporating 0.1% (w/w) indole-3-carbinol into the diet of male Fischer 344 rats for 4 weeks inhibited DNA adduct formation with PhIP in a number of tissues, including the colon, 1 or 7 days after a bolus oral dose of PhIP given at the end of week 3. PhIP–DNA adducts were increased 6 h after dosing with PhIP, however, in the colon, heart, caecum and spleen of indole-3-carbinol-treated animals (Guo et al., 1995). In a virtually identical protocol, except that PhIP was given in the diet (0.01% w/w) during week 3, 0.1% (w/w) indole-3-carbinol inhibited PhIP–DNA adduct formation in the colon, liver and epithelial cells isolated from the mammary glands of female Fischer 344 rats (Schut & Dashwood,

1995). This finding was confirmed in a study of similar design, in which a higher dietary concentration of PhIP (0.04%, w/w) and two concentrations of indole-3-carbinol (0.02% and 0.1%, w/w) were used. Only the highest concentration of indole-3-carbinol inhibited PhIP–DNA adducts in mammary epithelial cells, leukocytes, colon and liver (by 67–92%) of female Fischer 344 rats (He et al., 1997). In another experiment, female Fischer 344 rats were maintained on a diet containing 0.1% (w/w) indole-3-carbinol for 29 days and received an oral dose of PhIP at 10 or 50 mg/kg bw on day 13. PhIP–DNA adducts were determined on days 14, 15, 19 and 29 in a number of organs. Indole-3-carbinol inhibited PhIP–DNA adduct formation in virtually all organs, including the mammary gland and colon, by 33–100% at the four times. As before, dietary indole-3-carbinol did not affect the rate of adduct removal during the 14–29 days (He & Schut, 1999). In a similar protocol, but with repeated oral administration (daily for 3 weeks) of much lower doses of PhIP that were closer to human intake (1 mg/kg bw per day), diets containing 0.02% or 0.1% (w/w) indole-3-carbinol inhibited PhIP–DNA adducts (by 35–95%) in 12 organs, including the colon, but not in the mammary gland, of female Fischer 344 rats (He et al., 2000).

Only one study addressed the effect of indole-3-carbinol on cigarette smoke-induced DNA adducts in rats. Female Sprague-Dawley rats were exposed to cigarette smoke (6 h/day, 7 days per week) for 4 weeks while receiving indole-3-carbinol daily by gavage (1.36 or 3.40 mmol/kg) during this period as well as during the week preceding exposure to smoke. The main smoke-related adducts, some of which were also detectable (albeit in much smaller amounts) in animals receiving only indole-3-carbinol or no treatment, were inhibited (by 40–65%)

in the lungs, trachea, bladder and heart (Arif et al., 2000).

Mice: Total covalent binding of ^{14}C to hepatic DNA in ICR Swiss mice pre-treated with indole-3-carbinol (167 mg/kg bw) and then given a single dose of [^{14}C]benzo[a]pyrene by gavage was inhibited by up to 63% within 2–24 h (Shertzer, 1983, 1984). A single oral dose of indole-3-carbinol (167 mg/kg bw) administered to male ICR Swiss mice 1 h before a single oral dose of [^{14}C]N-nitrosodimethylamine inhibited binding of ^{14}C to hepatic DNA by 69% 1 h after dosing with the nitrosamine (Shertzer, 1984). In a study of the effects of indole-3-carbinol on DNA methylation of the tobacco-specific nitrosamine NNK, A/J mice received the indole by gavage for 4 days at a dose of 25 or 125 mmol/mouse per day. The last dose was followed 2 h later by an intraperitoneal injection of [^3H]NNK (10 mmol/mouse). Liver and lung DNA was analysed for O^6-methylguanine and 7-methylguanine after 2 and 6 h. Both doses of indole-3-carbinol inhibited pulmonary O^6-methylguanine by at least 50% but enhanced both O^6-methylguanine and 7-methylguanine in the liver at both times. The decrease in O^6-methylguanine in the lungs corresponded to a similar decrease in lung tumour multiplicity in mice receiving the same doses of NNK and indole-3-carbinol (Morse et al., 1990b).

Rainbow trout: The only other species in which the chemopreventive effects of indole-3-carbinol have been studied is the rainbow trout. Aflatoxin B_1 was used as the liver carcinogen in all except one study, in which N-nitrosodiethylamine was used (Fong et al., 1988). Fingerling trout were given diets containing N-nitrosodiethylamine at 250 mg/kg for 24 h, and liver DNA was then analysed for O^6-ethylguanine and

7-ethylguanine. Addition of indole-3-carbinol at 2000 mg/kg of diet for 1 week before exposure to N-nitrosodiethylamine resulted in 41% inhibition of both O^6-ethylguanine and 7-ethylguanine.

In an early study on the chemopreventive effects of indole-3-carbinol against the carcinogenicity of aflatoxin B_1 (Nixon et al., 1984), trout were fed diets containing indole-3-carbinol at 1000 mg/kg for 12 weeks and then injected with [^3H]aflatoxin B_1. When their liver DNA was analysed for total binding of ^3H 24 h later, indole-3-carbinol was found to have reduced the binding to 55% of that in control fish. Using a slightly different protocol (diet containing indole-3-carbinol at 2000 mg/kg for 8 days), Fong et al. (1990) found 58% inhibition of total binding of ^3H in trout liver DNA. Similarly, Takahashi et al. (1995b) showed dose-dependent inhibition of total hepatic binding of [^3H]aflatoxin B_1 to DNA in trout given diets containing indole-3-carbinol at 1000–4000 mg/kg for 7 days. In a detailed study of the dose–response relationship, Dashwood et al. (1988) gave trout diets containing a range of concentrations of indole-3-carbinol (0–4000 mg/kg) for 6 weeks. During the last 2 weeks, the fish also received aflatoxin B_1 (10–320 µg/kg) and a trace of [^3H]aflatoxin B_1. Liver DNA was analysed for total ^3H binding on days 7 and 14 after the start of feeding aflatoxin B_1. Binding depended linearly on both dose of aflatoxin and time of concomitant treatment. Indole-3-carbinol at all concentrations $\leq$ 2000 mg/kg linearly inhibited binding of aflatoxin B_1. At the highest concentration of indole-3-carbinol (4000 mg/kg), aflatoxin B_1 binding was suppressed by almost 95%. The linear inhibition observed with low doses of indole-3-carbinol indicates that there may be no significant threshold for protection against aflatoxin B_1–DNA binding. In a concurrent study with a similar

Table 51. Phenotypic changes effected by isothiocyanates (ITCs) relevant to gene regulation

Cell line	Change	Reference
Hepa-1c1c7	Buthionine-(R,S)-sulfoximine increased the potency of NQO1 induction by allyl-ITC, benzyl-ITC and phenethyl-ITC, but not sulforaphane	Zhang & Talalay (1998)
RL-34	Marked increase in intracellular level of reactive oxygen species after treatment with benzyl-ITC	Nakamura et al. (2000b)
Hepa-1c1c7	Sulforaphane and benzyl-ITC accumulated in cells as glutathione conjugate, causing decrease in glutathione	Zhang (2000)
Primary hepatocytes	Induction of MRP-2 by sulforaphane associated with generation of reactive oxygen species	Payen et al. (2001)
Various	Sulforaphane exported from cells by MRP-1 or P-glycoprotein-1	Zhang & Callaway (2002)
Hepa-1c1c7	Antioxidant response element in 5' upstream region of NQO1 defined as 5'-TcACaGTgAGtCggCA-3'	Nioi et al. (2003)
RL-34	Stabilization and nuclear translocation of Nrf2 stimulated by sulforaphane	McMahon et al. (2003)

NQO1, NADP(H):quinone reductase; MRP, multidrug resistance protein; Nrf2, nuclear factor–erythroid 2 p45-related factor 2

2002; Scharf et al., 2003; Zhang et al., 2003). As shown in Table 52, the proteins or mRNAs that are induced include the antioxidant and detoxication proteins aldo-keto reductase 1C1, γ-glutamalcysteine synthetase heavy subunit and γ-glutamalcysteine synthetase light chain, GSTA1, GSTP1, NQO1, thioredoxin reductase and UGT1A1. The efflux pump MRP-2 was also induced (Payen et al., 2001), as were the regulators of cell proliferation cyclin A and cyclin B_1 (Gamet-Payrastre et al., 2000). In mammary MCF-10F cells and colon LS-174 cells, induction of gene expression by sulforaphane provided protection against the genotoxic effects of benzo-[a]pyrene (Singletary & MacDonald, 2000; Bonnesen et al., 2001).

Many of the genes regulated by cancer chemopreventive agents contain an antioxidant response element in their 5' upstream promoter regions (Hayes & McMahon, 2001). This cis-acting element was originally defined by Rushmore et al. (1991) as 5'-RGTGACnnnGC-3', although the consensus sequence was subsequently further refined by Wasserman and Fahl (1997) as 5'-TMAnn-RTGAYnnnGCR-wwww-3'. The antioxidant response element in the 5' upstream region of the mouse NQO1 gene that is functionally required for its induction by sulforaphane is 5'-gagTcACaGTgA-GtCggCAaaatt-3' (non-essential resi-dues in lower case) (Nioi et al., 2003). Antioxidant response elements in different genes appear to be influenced to varying degrees by their surrounding sequence context. Thus, care should be taken in interpreting the results obtained from transfection experiments. Various groups have used antioxidant response element-driven reporter constructs to show that isothiocyanates can transcriptionally activate gene expression through the antioxidant response element (Table 53) (Prestera et al., 1993; Bonnesen et al., 2001). In the case of NQO1, the dose of isothiocyanate required to stimulate antioxidant response element-driven reporter gene expression was similar to the dose required to induce the endogenous gene in Hepa-1c1c7 or RL-34 cells (Prestera et al., 1993; Nioi et al., 2003).

Induction of antioxidant response element-driven genes is mediated by the cap 'n' collar basic region leucine zipper (bZIP) transcription factor, nuclear factor–erythroid 2 p45-related factor 2 (Nrf2), which binds to the enhancer as a heterodimer with small Maf proteins (Itoh et al., 1997). Experiments in nrf2−/− mice have shown that this transcription factor controls both basal and inducible expression of antioxidant and detoxication genes (McMahon et al., 2001; Chanas et al., 2002; Thimmulappa et al., 2002; Jowsey et al., 2003; Kwak et

Table 52. Induction of genes by isothiocyanates (ITCs) in human cells cultured in vitro

Cell type	ITC	Concentration (µmol/l)	mRNA or protein induced	Remarks	Reference
Hep-G2 (liver)	Sulforaphane	30	UGT1A1, GSTA1	GSH conjugate also induced	Basten et al. (2002)
Hep-G2 (liver)	Benzyl-ITC	5	GCS	Only enzyme activity measured	Scharf et al. (2003)
Hep-G2 (liver)	Sulforaphane	12	Thioredoxin reductase	Selenium acted synergistically	Zhang et al. (2003)
Primary human hepatocytes	Sulforaphane	50	MRP-2		Payen et al. (2001)
CaCo-2 (colon)	Sulforaphane	5	NQO1, AKR1C1, GCS$_h$	NQO1 mRNA, not protein, induced	Bonnesen et al. (2001)
CaCo-2 (colon)	Benzyl-ITC	5	NQO1, AKR1C1, GCS$_h$	NQO1 mRNA, not protein, induced	Bonnesen et al. (2001)
CaCo-2 (colon)	Phenethyl-ITC	5	NQO1, AKR1C1, GCS$_h$	NQO1 mRNA, not protein, induced	Bonnesen et al. (2001)
CaCo-2 (colon)	Sulforaphane	25	GSTA1	Induction only in subconfluent cells	Rouimi et al. (2001)
HT-29 (colon)	Benzyl-ITC	25	NQO1	Also an increase in GST activity	Kirlin et al. (1999a)
HT-29 (colon)	Sulforaphane	15	Cyclin A, cyclin B1	Caused growth arrest and apoptosis	Gamet-Payrastre et al. (2000)
HT-29 (colon)	Sulforaphane	30	UGT1A1	GSH conjugate also induced	Basten et al. (2002)
HT-29 (colon)	Sulforaphane	25	AKR	Only enzyme activity measured	Jiang et al. (2003)
LS-174 (colon)	Sulforaphane	5	NQO1, AKR1C1, GCS$_h$	Induction protected against hydrogen peroxide- and benzo[a]pyrene-stimulated single-strand DNA breaks	Bonnesen et al. (2001)
LS-174 (colon)	Benzyl-ITC	5	NQO1, AKR1C1, GCS$_h$		Bonnesen et al. (2001)
LS-174 (colon)	Phenethyl-ITC	5	NQO1, AKR1C1, GCS$_h$		Bonnesen et al. (2001)
MCF-10F (breast)	Sulforaphane	2	NQO1, GSTP1	Induction protected against formation of benzo[a]pyrene–DNA adducts	Singletary & MacDonald (2000)
MDA PCa 2a (prostate)	Sulforaphane	10	NQO1		Brooks et al. (2001)
PC3 (prostate)	Sulforaphane	10	NQO1		Brooks et al. (2001)
LNCaP (prostate)	Sulforaphane	10	NQO1, GCS$_l$	Addition of N-acetylcysteine blocked NQO1 induction	Brooks et al. (2001)
LNCaP (prostate)	Sulforaphane	25	NQO1, GST, AKR	Only enzyme activity measured	Jiang et al. (2003)

UGT, UDP-glucuronosyl transferase; GST, glutathione S-transferase; GCS, γ-glutamylcysteine synthetase; GSH, glutathione; MRP, multidrug-resistant protein; NQO1, NAD(P)H:quinone oxidoreductase 1; AKR, aldo-keto reductase; GCLC, glutamate cysteine ligase catalytic; GCS$_h$, γ-glutamylcysteine synthetase heavy subunit; GCS$_l$, γ-glutamylcysteine synthetase light chain al., 2003; Lee et al., 2003). In embryonic fibroblasts from nrf2⁻/⁻ mice, the absence of the cap 'n' collar bZIP factor results in loss of basal NQO1 expression and failure of induction of NQO1 by sulforaphane (Nioi et al., 2003). Nrf2 is itself regulated negatively by an actin-binding protein called Keap1 (Itoh et al., 1999; Wakabayashi et al., 2003). This negative regulation entails proteasomal degradation of Nrf2 (McMahon et al., 2003; Nguyen et al., 2003). Sulforaphane treatment antagonizes the negative regulation of Nrf2, resulting in stabilization of the bZIP transcription factor and its nuclear translocation (McMahon et al., 2003).

The levels of endogenous Nrf2 protein appear to vary significantly in different cells, being essentially undetectable in untransformed rat liver RL-34 cells (McMahon et al., 2003) but readily detectable in human hepatocarcinoma Hep-G2 cells (Nguyen et al., 2003).

The fact that isothiocyanates are selective inhibitors of cytochrome P450 enzymes involved in carcinogen metabolism may be particularly important in their inhibitory effects on nitrosamine carcinogenicity (Conaway et al., 1996, 2001). The covalent binding of isothiocyanates to the cytochrome P450 apoprotein can result in structural modification and loss of

activity. Inactivation may also occur due to release of atomic sulfur produced through oxidative desulfuration (conversion to isocyanates). Isothiocyanates can also bind reversibly to cytochrome P450 active sites, thus acting as competitive inhibitors.

Isothiocyanates inhibited CYP1A2. For example, phenethyl-ITC was a competitive inhibitor of cytochrome P450-catalysed NNK activation, with an apparent K_i value of 180 nmol/l (Smith et al., 1996). It also decreased the activity of MROD, with a median inhibitory concentration of 340 nmol/l. Other isothiocyanates decreased the activities of MROD and EROD, CYP1A-linked activities, in rodent hepatocytes and liver microsomes (Hamilton & Teel, 1996; Mahéo et al., 1997; Goosen et al., 2001). Various isothiocyanates were effective inhibitors of CYP2B1. They decreased PROD activity (due to CYP2B) in liver microsomes of rats treated with phenobarbital and in rat hepatocytes (Hamilton & Teel, 1996; Mahéo et al., 1997) and also inhibited CYP2E1 (Conaway et al., 1996; Moreno et al., 1999; Conaway et al., 2001).

Nakajima et al. (2001) studied the inhibition and inactivation of human cytochrome P450 enzymes by phenethyl-ITC using microsomes from insect cells expressing specific human

enzymes. Phenethyl-ITC competitively inhibited CYP1A2 and, to a lesser extent, CYP2A6. This compound was a strong, non-competitive inhibitor of CYP2B6, a non-competitive inhibitor of CYP2C9 and a mechanism-based inactivator of CYP2E1. These results are generally consistent with those described above.

Hollenberg and coworkers studied the effects of benzyl-ITC on rat and human cytochrome P450 enzymes (Goosen et al., 2000, 2001). This isothiocyanate was a potent mechanism-based inactivator of rat CYP2B1, primarily through protein modification. It was also a mechanism-based inactivator of rat CYP1A1, CYP1A2 and CYP2E1 and human CYP2B6 and CYP2D6. It was most effective in inactivating CYP2B1, CYP2B6, CYP1A1 and CYP2E1. Benzylamine was the major benzyl-ITC metabolite in the CYP2B1 reactions, suggesting conversion of benzyl-ITC to benzyl isocyanate, which modified the cytochrome P450 apoprotein or was hydrolysed to benzylamine. Phenethyl-ITC was shown to be a competitive and suicide inhibitor of CYP2E1 (Ishizaki et al., 1990); the inhibition by benzyl-ITC was irreversible (Moreno et al., 1999). These results indicate differences in the mechanisms by which phenethyl-ITC and benzyl-ITC interact with CYP2E1.

Conaway et al. (2001) investigated the inhibition of cytochrome P450-mediated reactions by thiol conjugates of benzyl-ITC and phenethyl-ITC. Inhibition of PROD, for CYP2B1, and EROD, for CYP1A1, roughly paralleled the extent of decomposition of the conjugates to the corresponding isothiocyanates, suggesting that the parent compounds were responsible for the observed inhibition.

Effects on glutathione metabolism
Isothiocyanates react with protein and non-protein thiols. These reactions are rapid and reversible, and isothio-

Table 53. Potency of isothiocyanates (ITCs) to stimulate antioxidant response element-driven gene expression

Isothiocyanate	Cell line	Concentration (µmol/l) required to double reporter gene expression	Reference
Sulforaphane	Hep-G2	0.4	Prestera et al. (1993)
Sulforaphane	Caco-2	1.3	Bonnesen et al. (2001)
Benzyl-ITC	Hep-G2	0.7	Prestera et al. (1993)
Phenethyl-ITC	Caco-2	1.7	Bonnesen et al. (2001)

cyanates and their cysteine conjugates both induced a decrease in the cellular concentrations of GSH and reduced GSH (GSSG) during the initial 2–3 h of incubation with tumour cells in vitro. During the first hour, there was rapid formation of the GSH conjugate inside cells, catalysed by GST, which was then exported from the cells by a GSH conjugate transporter (Zhang, 2000; Xu & Thornalley, 2001a; Zhang, 2001). The GSH conjugate was unstable in the extracellular medium, even when γ-glutamyl transferase had been inhibited, suggesting that spontaneous fragmentation to isothiocyanate and GSH occurred. Isothiocyanate–GSH conjugates are unstable under physiological conditions (Table 54 and Figure 25). In the extracellular medium, GSH was oxidized and formed GSSG and GSH–protein mixed disulfides. Extra-cellular GSH and GSSG degraded to cysteine and cystine, which re-entered the cells and stimulated GSH synthesis. The cellular concentration of GSH had thereby recovered to normal levels after 12 h. After incubation for 24 h, however, the concentration of GSH decreased again as apoptosis developed (Xu & Thornalley, 2001a; Zhang & Callaway, 2002).

The formation and cellular efflux of isothiocyanate–GSH conjugates decreased the cellular concentration of both GSH and GSSG during the initial 2 h of incubation, perhaps due to GSH–GSSG thiol–disulfide exchange reactions and activation of GSH reductase as the ratio of GSSG:GSH concentrations increased (Kirlin et al., 1999b; Xu & Thornalley, 2001a). The cellular concentration of GSSG increased over 2–6 h, perhaps due to increased oxidative stress associated with the decrease in total GSH. High concentrations of isothiocyanates (0.5–2 mmol/l), 100- to 1000-fold higher than the median growth inhibiting concentrations, formed low concentrations of superoxide (3–40 μmol/l) and induced oxidative damage to DNA in HL60 cells: the cellular concentration of the DNA oxidative marker 8-hydroxy-deoxyguanosine was increased by 18% in cells treated with the median growth inhibiting concentration of allyl-ITC. The order of potency for inducing DNA oxidative damage in a cell-free system was: allyl-ITC >> benzyl-ITC > phenethyl-ITC (Murata et al., 2000), which is the reverse of the potency order for decreases in GSH in HL60 cells by isothiocyanates (Xu & Thornalley, 2001a). This suggests that export of GSH from cells, rather than the spontaneous degradation of isothiocyanates, is important in the induc-tion of oxidative stress associated with isothiocyanate-induced apoptosis.

Expulsion of the GSH conjugate from cells was a critical feature for activation of isothiocyanate-induced cellular responses (Xu & Thornalley, 2001a; Zhang & Callaway, 2002). Indeed, expulsion of the GSH conjugate, extra-cellular fragmentation of the conjugate and re-entry of isothiocyanate into cells for further GSH conjugation could be considered an 'engine' for depletion of cellular GSH, only running out of 'fuel' when the isothiocyanate was hydrolysed (Figure 26). GSH depletion is not the only critical determinant of the potency of induction of apoptosis by an isothiocyanate. There was no strong correlation between the ability to decrease cellular GSH and potency of inhibition of tumour cell growth in vitro (Xu & Thornalley, 2000a). While GSH depletion is important for the pharmacological activity of isothiocyanates, other activities—effect on protein folding and protein membrane translocation when thiocarbamoylated—are probably also influential.

Expulsion of GSH conjugates is mediated by the MRPs. Indeed, sulforaphane induced the expression of MRP-2 (Payen et al., 2001). The expression of these proteins is increased in some tumours and particularly in relapsed tumours with

Table 54. Stability of isothiocyanates (ITCs) and their cysteinyl conjugates at pH 7.4 and 37 °C

Isothiocyanate	Half-life (min)			
	Parent compound	Cysteine conjugate	Glutathione conjugate	N-Acetylcysteine conjugate
Benzyl-ITC	Not determined	12	67	157
Phenethyl-ITC	141	13, 16	44,58	100
Sulforaphane	Not determined	14	58	173

From Conaway et al. (2001); Xu & Thornalley (2000a, 2001a)

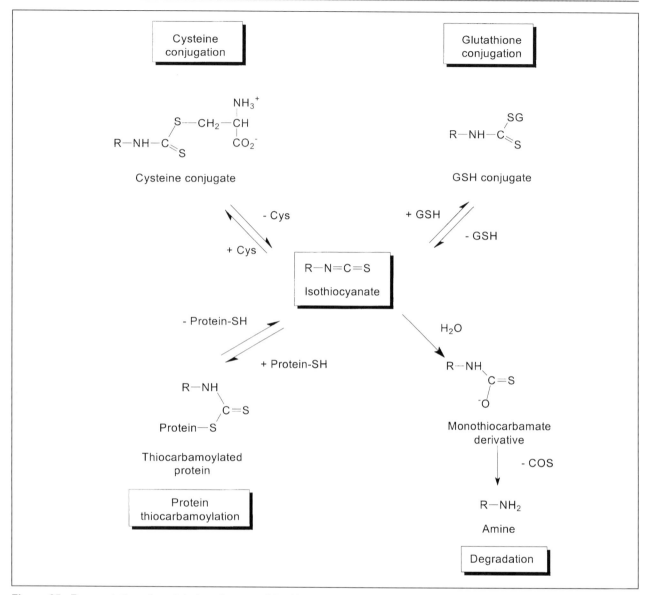

Figure 25 Fragmentation of cysteinyl conjugates of isothiocyanates and degradation of isothiothiocyanates under physiological conditions

GSH, glutathione

multidrug resistance (Borst *et al.*, 1999). GSH conjugates of isothiocyanates have high affinity for these proteins and may block antitumour drug expulsion. This suggests that isothiocyanates may be active against multidrug-resistant cells. Indeed, isoth- iocyanates inhibited the export of anti- tumour drugs from P-glycoprotein- and MRP-1-mediated resistant human can- cer cell lines (Tseng *et al.*, 2002). Strong expression of these proteins can also be expected to result in rapid expulsion of the GSH conjugate from cells. This may increase the effect, since depletion of GSH is critical to activating cellular responses.

Allyl-ITC, benzyl-ITC and sul- foraphane (at 5 µmol/l) induced one- to fourfold increases in the GSH concen- tration of human breast carcinoma

MCF-7 cells, murine hepatoma Hepa 1c1c7 cells and murine skin papilloma cells after 24 h of exposure (Ye & Zhang, 2001). This was accompanied by induction of GST and quinone reductase activity and may have been due to increased expression of γ-gluta-mylcysteine synthetase activity via the *Nrf2*-regulated response (Thimmulappa *et al.,* 2002). The increase in GSH occurred probably during the rebound of synthesis after the decrease in GSH concentration during the initial 3–6 h (Xu & Thornalley, 2001a). In the study showing increased cellular GSH concentration, no measurements were made before 12 h of exposure (Ye & Zhang, 2001).

Induction of apoptosis

Isothiocyanates inhibited growth and induced apoptosis of human tumour cells in vitro (Table 55). The median growth inhibitory concentrations were 0.7–55 µmol/l. At higher concentrations, isothiocyanates induced necrotic cell death (Fimognari *et al.*, 2002a,b; Nakamura *et al.*, 2002). Cysteine conjugates and cysteinyl conjugates in the mercapturic acid pathway also inhibited tumour cell growth; this was attributed to fragmentation of the conjugate to the corresponding isothiocyanate. The fragmentation of cysteine and GSH conjugates is relatively rapid under physiological conditions (Figure 25 and Table 54). The thiocarbamoyl group may also be transferred from

one cysteinyl thiol residue to another in an exchange reaction (Bruggeman *et al.*, 1986).

Isothiocyanates are also toxic to non-malignant cells in vitro. They have relatively little toxicity in colon, prostate, bronchus and oral mucosal epithelial cells but significant toxicity in keratinocytes and renal tubular, cervical and mammary epithelial cells (Table 56). Sulforaphane inhibited the growth of proliferating human lymphocytes, inducing growth arrest in G_1 phase through a decrease in cyclin D3. It also induced *p53*-mediated apoptosis (Fimognari *et al.*, 2002b), indicating that isothiocyanates may have tissue-specific toxicity (Elmore *et al.*, 2001). The cysteine conjugates were signifi-

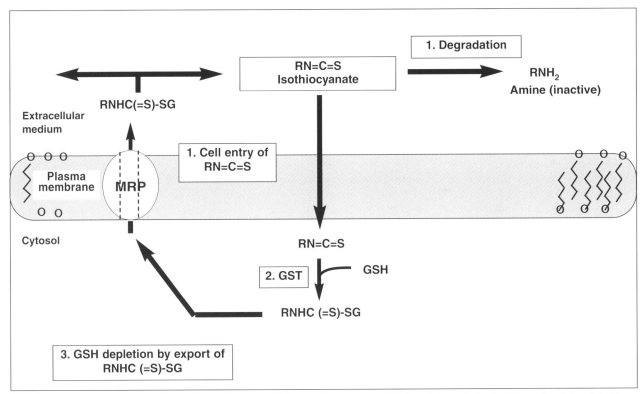

Figure 26 Isothiocyanate–glutathione *S*-transferase–multidrug-resistance-associated protein cycle for depletion of cellular glutathione
GSH, glutathione; MRP, multidrug-resistance-associated protein; GST, glutathione *S*-transferase

cantly less toxic to non-malignant cells than the corresponding isothio-cyanates (Bruggeman et al., 1986; Xu & Thornalley, 2000a). The toxicity to differentiated human colorectal tumour HT29 cells was less than that to undif-ferentiated control cells (Musk & Johnson, 1993).

Tumour cell growth was arrested in G_2 or M, and apoptosis was associ-ated with activation of caspase-8, c-Jun N-terminal kinase-1 and tyrosine phosphorylation (Hasegawa et al., 1993; Adesida et al., 1996; Yu et al., 1996; Chen Y.R. et al., 1998; Gamet-Payrastre et al., 2000; Xu & Thornalley, 2000a; Lund et al., 2001; Xu & Thornalley, 2001a,b; Fimognari et al., 2002a,b). Apoptosis can be p53-dependent (Huang et al., 1998; Fimognari et al., 2002b) or p53-inde-pendent (Xu & Thornalley, 2000a). The cytotoxicity of isothiocyanates was selective for tumour cells in vitro, but the basis for this selectivity is unknown.

c-Jun N-terminal kinase-1 was acti-vated during phenethyl-ITC-induced apoptosis of HeLa cells (Yu et al., 1996) and Jurkat cells in vitro (Chen, Y.R. et al., 1998), and this was associ-ated with activation of mitogen-acti-vated protein kinase/extracellular sig-nal-regulated kinase 1 (Chen & Tan, 1998, 2000). Overexpression of Bcl-2 and Bcl-x$_L$ suppressed both phenethyl-ITC-induced activation of c-Jun N-ter-minal kinase-1 and apoptosis, sug-gesting that Bcl-2 and Bcl-x$_L$ could intervene upstream of c-Jun N-termi-nal kinase-1 activation in phenethyl-ITC-induced apoptosis (Chen, Y.R. et al., 1998). Curcumin, an inhibitor of c-Jun N-terminal kinase signalling upstream of mitogen-activated pro-teinkinase/-extracellular signal-regu-lated kinase 1 (Chen & Tan, 1998), delayed the induction of apoptosis by phenethyl-ITC (Xu & Thornalley, 2001b). Exogenous GSH (15 mmol/l) prevented this activation but simply by binding to phenethyl-ITC, thereby inter-

cepting it before it entered the cell and decreasing the effective dose that did enter the tumour cells (Xu & Thornalley, 2001a,b). Similar effects were found with mercaptoethanol and N-acetylcysteine (Chen, Y.R. et al., 1998). The general caspase inhibitor Z-VAD-fmk prevented apoptosis but not c-Jun N-terminal kinase activation, thus excluding a role for caspases in this context, whereas curcumin pre-vented c-Jun N-terminal kinase activa-tion but only delayed apoptosis. Total protein tyrosine phosphatase activity was unchanged (Xu & Thornalley, 2001b). As genotoxic-sensitive and -resistant prostate cancer cells were similarly sensitive to phenethyl-ITC-induced apoptosis and c-Jun N-termi-nal kinase activation, isothiocyanate-induced apoptosis probably does not involve direct DNA damage (Chen et al., 2002). The M-associated protein (MAP) kinases MKK4 and MKK7 acti-vate c-Jun N-terminal kinase (Chen & Tan, 2000), but they were not activated in phenethyl-ITC-induced apoptosis. Rather, inhibition of the c-Jun N-terminal kinase phosphatase M3/6 was impli-cated in activation of the kinase in phenethyl-ITC-induced apoptosis. c-Jun N-terminal kinase phosphatase M3/6 protein was decreased in phenethyl-ITC-induced apoptosis by proteasomal degradation (Chen et al., 2002).

Other MAP kinases such as P38 protein kinase were activated in human prostate carcinoma P-3 cells, but c-Jun N-terminal kinase was not (Xiao & Singh, 2002). This is surpris-ing, since c-Jun N-terminal kinase phosphatase M3/6 also deactivates and inhibits p38 protein kinase (Muda et al., 1996), and inhibition of this phosphatase may also be involved in phenethyl-ITC-induced activation of P38 MAP kinase in apoptosis. P38 pro-tein kinase is thought to down-regulate the induction of NQO1 and phase II enzyme activities controlled by the antioxidant response element (Yu et

al., 2000). Hence, isothiocyanates that activate P38 protein kinase may have characteristic apoptotic activity and diminished phase II enzyme induction.

Phenethyl-ITC-induced apoptosis in PC-3 cells was associated with acti-vation of extracellular signal-regulated kinases, and a specific inhibitor of kinases 1/2 blocked phenethyl-ITC-induced apoptosis (Xiao & Singh, 2002). It is possible that isothio-cyanates also inhibit the phosphatase that inactivates extracellular signal-regulated kinases 1/2 MAP kinase phosphatase-3 (Muda et al., 1996). Activation of extracellular signal regu-lated kinase 2 by sulforaphane was associated with induction of phase II enzymes regulated by the antioxidant response element (Yu et al., 1999).

When HL60 cells were incubated with phenethyl-ITC in vitro, caspase-8 and caspase-3 were activated (Xu & Thornalley, 2000a). These caspases cleaved BID protein into three frag-ments, p15, p13 and p11 (Xu & Thornalley, 2001b). An inhibitor of caspase-1 blocked phenethyl-ITC-induced apoptosis in Jurkat cells (Chen, Y.R. et al., 1998). In HeLa cells, however, phenethyl-ITC increased the activity of caspase-3, and a caspase-3 inhibitor but not a caspase-1 inhibitor attenuated phenethyl-ITC-induced apop-tosis (Yu et al., 1998). Caspase-3 activ-ity was activated by benzyl-ITC at 25 µmol/l in human colonic adenocarci-noma HT29 cells in vitro (Kirlin et al., 1999a). This suggests that activation of caspases is important in the mecha-nism of phenethyl-ITC-induced apoptosis but that the role of individual caspases may vary with cell type.

The p15 fragment of BID formed by the action of caspase-8 and caspase-3 interacted with Bcl-x$_L$ in mitochondria, leading to release of cytochrome c and loss of mitochondrial membrane poten-tial (Li et al., 1998). Over-expression of Bcl-2 and Bcl-x$_L$ suppressed phen-ethyl-ITC-induced apoptosis (Chen,

Table 55. Inhibition of human tumour cell growth and induction of cytotoxicity in vitro by dietary isothiocyanates

Isothiocyanate (ITC)	Cell line	GC$_{50}$ (μmol/l)	TC$_{50}$ (μmol/l)	Reference
3-Methylsulfonylpropyl-ITC	K562	6.0	–	Nastruzzi et al. (2000)
Sulforaphane	HT29	15	–	Gamet-Payrastre et al. (1998)
	K562	15	–	Nastruzzi et al. (2000)
	LS-174	40	–	Bonnesen et al. (2001)
	Caco-2	55	–	Bonnesen et al. (2001)
	Jurkat	~ 15	–	Fimognari et al. (2002a)
	P-3	20	–	Frydoonfar et al. (2003)
Allyl-ITC	HeLa	15		Hasegawa et al. (1993)
	HL60	2.6	11	Xu & Thornalley (2000a)
	ML-1	2.6	7.7	Xu & Thornalley (2000a)
2-Hydroxybut-3-enyl-ITC	K562	32	–	Nastruzzi et al. (2000)
Benzyl-ITC	HeLa	1.9	–	Hasegawa et al. (1993)
	K562	1.5	–	Nastruzzi et al. (2000)
	LS-174	15	–	Bonnesen et al. (2001)
	Caco-2	2	–	Bonnesen et al. (2001)
Phenethyl-ITC	HeLa	2.5		Hasegawa et al. (1993)
	HL60	1.5		Chen, Y.R. et al. (1998)
	Jurkat	3	5	Adesida et al. (1996)
	HL60	1.5	5.0	Xu & Thornalley (2000a)
	ML-1	2.7	3.3	Xu & Thornalley (2000a)
	LS-174	20	–	Bonnesen et al. (2001)
	Caco-2	12	–	Bonnesen et al. (2001)
	PC-3	~ 6		Xiao & Singh (2002)
S-(N-Allylthiocarbamoyl)cysteine	HL60	3.2	12	Xu & Thornalley (2000a)
	ML-1	3.2	11	Xu & Thornalley (2000a)
S-(N-Benzylthiocarbamoyl)cysteine	HL60	0.7	2.3	Adesida et al. (1996)
S-(N-Phenethylthiocarbamoyl)cysteine	HL60	2.5	4.8	Xu & Thornalley (2000a)
	ML-1	2.4	3.6	Xu & Thornalley (2000a)
S-(N-Phenethylthiocarbamoyl)glutathione	HL60	5.5	15	Adesida et al. (1996)

Cell lines: CaCo-2, human colonic adenocarcinoma; HCEC, SV40 T-antigen immortalized human colonic epithelial cells; HeLa, human cervical carcinoma; HL60, human acute myeloblastic leukaemia; HT29, human colonic adenocarcinoma; Jurkat, human T-cell leukaemia; K562, human erythroleukaemia; LS-174, human colorectal adenocarcinoma; ML-1, human myeloblastic leukaemia; PC-3, human prostate cancer
GC$_{50}$, median growth inhibitory concentration; TC$_{50}$, median toxic inhibitory concentration

Y.R. et al., 1998). Sulforaphane-induced apoptosis in Jurkat cells in vitro was associated with a marked induction of bax (Fimognari et al., 2002a). Bax binds to mitochondria in apoptosis and facilitates cytochrome c release (Scorrano & Korsmeyer, 2003). Benzyl-ITC induced activation of caspase-9 and changes in mitochondrial membrane potential in rat liver epithelial RL34 cells in vitro, with inhibition of respiration, mitochondrial swelling and cytochrome c release (Nakamura et al., 2002).

Other cellular effects
The anti-inflammatory properties of some isothiocyanates have been investigated. Phenethyl-ITC inhibited phorbol ester-activated production of superoxide radicals by HL-60-derived neutrophils (Gerhäuser et al., 2003), at a median inhibitory concentration of 3.5 μmol/l. Phenethyl-ITC also scavenged alkylperoxy radicals and hydroxyl radicals, at median inhibitory concentrations of 0.4 and 2.5 μmol/l in a free radical-generating test system.

Table 56. Toxicity of dietary isothiocyanates to non-malignant cells in vitro

Compound	Species origin	Cell type	TC$_{50}$ (µmol/l)			Reference
			Cell growth	PCNA	Mitochon-drial function	
Sulforaphane	Human	Lymphocytes	~ 33	–	–	Fimognari et al. (2002a)
	Human	Colon epithelial	95	–	–	Bonnesen et al. (2001)
Allyl-ITC	Rat	RL-4 liver epithelial	~ 175			Bruggeman et al. (1986)
Benzyl-ITC	Human	Colon epithelial	22	–	–	Bonnesen et al. (2001)
	Rat	RL-4 liver epithelial	~ 25	–	–	Bruggeman et al. (1986)
Phenethyl-ITC	Human	Liver epithelial (Chang)	~ 20	–	–	Bruggeman et al. (1988)
	Human	Lymphocytes	53	–	–	Xu & Thornalley (2000a)
	Human	Colon epithelial	20	–	–	Bonnesen et al. (2001)
	Human	Keratinocytes	0.5	6.2	38	Elmore et al. (2001)
	Human	Renal tubular epithelial	4.5	6.7	> 61	Elmore et al. (2001)
	Human	Mammary epithelial	1.3	30	11	Elmore et al. (2001)
	Human	Cervical epithelial	3.2	7.4	9.3	Elmore et al. (2001)
	Human	Prostate epithelial	12	> 61	> 61	Elmore et al. (2001)
	Human	Bronchial epithelial	15	> 61	18	Elmore et al. (2001)
	Human	Oral mucosal epithelial	19	9.6	5.5	Elmore et al. (2001)
	Human	Hepatocytes	–	20	29	Elmore et al. (2001)
Allylthiocyanate–cysteine	Rat	RL-4 liver epithelial	200	–	–	Bruggeman et al. (1986)
Allylthiocyanate–glutathione	Rat	RL-4 liver epithelial	250	–	–	Bruggeman et al. (1986)
Benzylthio-cyanate–cysteine	Rat	RL-4 liver epithelial	150	–	–	Bruggeman et al. (1986)
Benzylthio-cyanate–glutathione	Rat	RL-4 liver epithelial	80	–	–	Bruggeman et al. (1986)
Phenethylthio-cyanate–cysteine	Human	Lymphocytes	91	–	–	Xu & Thornalley (2000a)

TC$_{50}$, median toxic inhibitory concentration; PCNA, proliferating cell nuclear antigen

Isothiocyanates inhibited lipopolysaccharide-induced formation of nitric oxide in a murine macrophage line, at median inhibitory concentrations of: sulforaphane, 0.7 µmol/l; allyl-ITC, 1.6 µmol/l; benzyl-ITC, 2.7 µmol/l; and phenethyl-ITC, 5 µmol/l (Ippoushi et al., 2002; Gerhäuser et al., 2003). This was associated with inhibition of inducible nitric oxide synthase expression (Gerhäuser et al., 2003). Some isothiocyanates (allyl-ITC and benzyl-ITC; 1 and 10 µmol/l) increased lipopolysaccharide-stimulated secretion of tumour necrosis factor-α (Ippoushi et al., 2002), but sulforaphane inhibited its secretion at a median inhibitory concentration of 7.8

μmol/l (Heiss *et al.*, 2001). Sulforaphane also inhibited the lipopolysaccharide-induced expression of COX-2 and associated formation of prostaglandin E_2; the median inhibitory concentration was 1.4 μmol/l (Heiss *et al.*, 2001). Sulforaphane and phenethyl-ITC (20 μmol/l) inhibited activation of NF-κB (Heiss *et al.*, 2001; Gerhäuser *et al.*, 2003), perhaps mediated by thiocarbamoylation of the NF-κB protein complex. Sulforaphane induced the expression of thioredoxin reductase-1. In the presence of selenium supplementation, but not alone, sulforaphane prevented chemically induced oxidative stress (Zhang *et al.*, 2003).

Sulforaphane at a median minimal inhibitory concentration of 2 μg/ml was bacteriostatic against *Helicobacter pylori* and eliminated *H. pylori* infections in human epithelial Hep-G2 cells in culture (Fahey *et al.*, 2002).

Isothiocyanates afforded some protection against damage to DNA in cultured cells induced by hydrogen peroxide (Bonnesen *et al.*, 2001). Sulforaphane was a potent inducer of haem oxygenase-1 (Prestera *et al.*, 1995), which is thought to confer resistance to oxidative stress (Lee *et al.*, 1996).

Indoles
Effect on antioxidant and drug-metabolizing enzymes
Indole-3-carbinol and derived chemicals are effective inducers of CYP1A1 (Table 57), which displays high EROD activity. In many studies, therefore, an increase in cellular EROD activity has been used as a marker of induction of CYP1A1. Table 57 shows that EROD activity or CYP1A1 can be induced in a wide range of rodent and human cell lines. CYP1A1 is induced through the xenobiotic response element, mediated by the Ah receptor (Hankinson, 1995).

Indoles can induce other cytochrome P450 enzymes, such as CYP1B1 and CYP19 (Sanderson *et al.*, 2001), as well as the drug-metabolizing enzymes aldo–keto reductase, GSTT1, sulfotransferase and UGT1 (Li *et al.*, 2003)

Indolo[3,2-*b*]carbazole is a much more potent inducing agent than 3,3′-diindolylmethane, indole-3-carbinol or ascorbigen (Table 58). Binding of indoles to the Ah receptor in vitro showed a similar trend, indolo[3,2-*b*]carbazol having a much lower dissociation constant for the receptor than either 3,3′-diindolylmethane or indole-3-carbinol (Bjeldanes *et al.*, 1991). CT had weaker binding activity to the Ah receptor in MCF-7 breast cancer cell lines, as shown by EROD induction, than indolo[3,2-*b*]carbazole (Riby *et al.*, 2000a).

Protection against mutagenicity in bacteria and mammalian cells
Several studies addressed the ability of indoles to prevent mutagenicity in the Ames test for reverse mutation or to block carcinogen-induced DNA damage, with various end-points.

The mutagenicity of MNU, MNNG, benzo[*a*]pyrene and 2-aminoanthracene was not reduced by indole-3-carbinol (Birt *et al.*, 1986). This compound was also ineffective in inhibiting genotoxicity in *Salmonella* tester strains and Chinese hamster ovary cells after treatment with 1-nitropyrene or 1,6-dinitropyrene (Kuo *et al.*, 1992).

Jongen *et al.* (1989) found that the effects of indole-3-carbinol and indole-3-acetonitrile on induction of sister chromatid exchange depended on the type of mutagen. Pretreatment of primary chick embryo hepatocytes with indole-3-carbinol (at 25 μg/ml) resulted in a 30–45% decrease in the number of sister chromatid exchanges induced by benzo[*a*]pyrene and *N*-nitrosodimethylamine in co-cultured V79 cells, but had no effect on sister chromatid exchanges induced by 2-aminoanthracene or ethylmethanesulfonate. It increased the frequency of sister chromatid exchange induced by dibromoethane. Indole-3-acetonitrile (at 35 μg/ml) decreased the frequency of benzo[*a*]pyrene-induced sister chromatid exchanges by 20–40%.

The ability of indole-3-carbinol, two of its oligomers and an acid reaction mixture (formed by mixing indole-3-carbinol under conditions that mimic the conditions in the stomach) to inhibit mutagenesis and aflatoxin B_1–DNA binding was investigated (Takahashi *et al.*, 1995c). Using a trout post-mitochondrial activation system in the reverse mutation test, they found that indole-3-carbinol (at concentrations up to 35 μmol/l) was not protective. At concentrations as low as 3.5 μmol/l, 3,3′-diindolylmethane, the cyclic trimer CT and the acid reaction mixture caused about 80% inhibition when compared with the control. 3,3′-Diindolylmethane also inhibited microsome-catalysed aflatoxin B_1–DNA binding. In a previous study of the ability of the acid reaction mixture to inhibit the production of covalent DNA adducts in the presence of aflatoxin B_1-8,9-Cl_2, a surrogate for aflatoxin B_1-epoxide, the same group observed no protective effect (Fong *et al.*, 1990).

Pretreatment of LS-174 human colon cells for 24 h with indolo[3,2-*b*]carbazole (1 μmol/l) plus sulforaphane (5 μmol/l), followed by continued exposure to these agents in the presence of benzo[*a*]pyrene (25 μmol/l) reduced the number of DNA single-strand breaks induced by the carcinogen by > 80% (Bonnesen *et al.*, 2001). Indolo[3,2-*b*]carbazole on its own was much less effective. No such protection was afforded when indolo[3,2-*b*]carbazole or sulforaphane was given 24 h after the carcinogens. Similar results were obtained with hydrogen peroxide (100 μmol/l) as the genotoxic agent.

The induction of *his*[+] revertant colonies in the reverse mutation assay in *S. typhimurium* by benzo[*a*]pyrene

Table 57. Indoles that induce metabolizing enzymes, drug metabolizing enzymes, transcription factors or cell cycle proteins in cell culture models

Indole	Dose	Biochemical end-point	Cell line	Reference
Ascorbigen	700 µmol/l	EROD, CYP1A1	Hepa-1c1c7	Stephensen et al. (1999)
Ascorbigen	700 µmol/l	EROD, CYP1A1	CaCo-2	Bonnesen et al. (2001)
Ascorbigen	700 µmol/l	EROD, CYP1A1	LS-174	Bonnesen et al. (2001)
2,3-Bis(3-indolylmethyl)-indole	5 µmol/l	EROD	Primary rat hepatocytes	Wortelboer et al. (1992c)
3,3'-Diindolylmethane	36 nmol/l	EROD	Primary rat hepatocytes	Wortelboer et al. (1992b)
3,3'-Diindolylmethane	50 µmol/l	CYP1A1	MCF-7	Chen, I. et al. (1998)
3,3'-Diindolylmethane	25 µmol/l	EROD, CYP1A1	CaCo-2	Bonnesen et al. (2001)
3,3'-Diindolylmethane	25 µmol/l	EROD, CYP1A1	LS-174	Bonnesen et al. (2001)
3,3'-Diindolylmethane	3 µmol/l	EROD, CYP1A1, CYP1B1, CYP19	H295R	Sanderson et al. (2001)
3,3'-Diindolylmethane	100 µmol/l	GADD153, ATF3, c-Jun, NF-IL6	C33A, HaCat	Carter et al. (2002)
3,3'-Diindolylmethane	40 µmol/l	AKR, CYP1A1, GSTT1, sulfotransferase, UGT1, phospholipase A_2	PC3	Li et al. (2003)
3,3'-Diindolylmethane	100 µmol/l	GADD34, GADD45α, GADD153	MCF-7	Auborn et al. (2003)
5,6,11,12,17,18-Hexahydrocyclonona[1,2-b:4,5-b':7,8-b'']tri-indole	5 µmol/l	EROD	Primary rat hepatocytes	Wortelboer et al. (1992c)
Indole-3-carbinol	68 nmol/l	EROD	Primary rat hepatocytes	Wortelboer et al. (1992b)
Indole-3-carbinol	125 µmol/l	CYP1A1	T47D	Chen, I. et al. (1996)
Indole-3-carbinol	100 µmol/l	p21	MCF-7	Cover et al. (1999)
Indole-3-carbinol	100 µmol/l	EROD, CYP1A1	CaCo-2	Bonnesen et al. (2001)
Indole-3-carbinol	100 µmol/l	EROD, CYP1A1	LS-174	Bonnesen et al. (2001)
Indole-3-carbinol	60 µmol/l	AKR, CYP1A1, GSTT1	PC3	Li et al. (2003)
Indolo[3,2-b]carbazole	0.1 µmol/l	EROD	Hepa-1c1c7	Bjeldanes et al. (1991)
Indolo[3,2-b]carbazole	0.1 µmol/l	EROD	MCF-7	Liu et al. (1994)
Indolo[3,2-b]carbazole	0.05 µmol/l	CYP1A1	HaCaT	Wei et al. (1998)
Indolo[3,2-b]carbazole	1 µmol/l	EROD, CYP1A1	CaCo-2	Bonnesen et al. (2001)
Indolo[3,2-b]carbazole	1 µmol/l	EROD, CYP1A1	LS-174	Bonnesen et al. (2001)
2-(Indol-3-ylmethyl)-3,3-diindolylmethane	1 µmol/l	EROD	MCF-7	Chang et al. (1999)
N-Methoxyindole-3-carbinol	50 µmol/l	EROD, CYP1A1	Hepa-1c1c7	Stephensen et al. (2000)

CYP, cytochrome P450 isozyme; NF-IL6, nuclear factor–interleukin 6; GADD, growth arrest in response to DNA damage; ATF, activating transcription factor; AKR, aldo-keto reductase; GST, glutathione S-transferase; UGT, UDP glucuronsyl transferase; EROD, othoxyresorufin-O-dealkylase

Table 58. Potency of indoles to bind to the aryl hydrocarbon (Ah) receptor or stimulate xenobiotic response element-driven gene expression

Indole	Cell line	Binding to Ah receptor (Kd, nmol/l)	Concentration required to double reporter gene expression (nmol/l)	Reference
Ascorbigen	CaCo2	–	3.7×10^4	Bonnesen et al. (2001)
3,3′-Diindolylmethane	None	90	–	Bjeldanes et al. (1991)
3,3′-Diindolylmethane	CaCo2	–	1.0×10^4	Bonnesen et al. (2001)
Indole-3-carbinol	None	2.7×10^4	–	Bjeldanes et al. (1991)
Indole-3-carbinol	CaCo2	–	6×10^4	Bonnesen et al. (2001)
Indolo[3,2-b]carbazole	None	0.19	–	Bjeldanes et al. (1991)
Indolo[3,2-b]carbazole	CaCo2	–	5	Bonnesen et al. (2001)

(20 µg/plate) and cyclophosphamide (10 mg/plate) was prevented by indole-3-carbinol (inhibition: 25%, 41% and 65% with 30, 60 and 120 µg/plate) (Shukla et al., 2003). In Chinese hamster ovary cells, indole-3-carbinol was protective against the cytotoxicity of 1-nitropyrene and 1,6-dinitropyrene, but did not reduce the frequency of sister chromatid exchange induced by these agents (Kuo et al., 1992).

Effects on cell proliferation and apoptosis

Some of the main biological responses to indoles are summarized in Table 59.

Inhibition of cell proliferation

Many reports indicate that indoles inhibit proliferation in a wide range of mammalian cell types, tumour cells often showing greater sensitivity than non-transformed cells.

In mouse mammary epithelial cells stably transfected with ras or myc oncogenes to induce transformation, indole-3-carbinol (50 µmol/l) inhibited proliferation by 98% and 83%, respectively, but was not particularly effective in inhibiting Ras p21-GTP binding in the ras-transfected cells (Telang et al., 1997b). Exposure to indole-3-carbinol

for 2 days resulted in 54–61% inhibition of anchorage-independent growth in three mammary cell lines (Telang et al., 1997c). The results with MDA-MB-231 cells in this study appeared to contradict those of an earlier study (Tiwari et al., 1994), which suggested no effect of indole-3-carbinol on growth.

The effects of indole-3-carbinol, indole-3-acetic acid, indole-3-carboxylic acid and 3,3′-diindolylmethane on the growth of two colon cell lines, HT29 (undifferentiated) and CaCo2 (which undergo post-confluence differentiation) were examined (Gamet-Payrastre et al., 1998). Indole-3-carboxylic acid and indole-3-acetic acid had no effect on the viability of HT29 cells after treatment at 100 µmol/l for 24 or 48 h. The same dose of indole-3-carbinol decreased viability by nearly 70% after 48 h, but no effect was seen after 24 h and lower doses were not effective. 3,3′-Diindolylmethane was the most potent compound, leading to an 80% decrease only 24 h after treatment with 100 mmol/l, with a median inhibitory concentration of 10 µmol/l after 48 h. The effect of 3,3′-diindolylmethane at 10 µmol/l on HT29 cells was reversible only if it was removed from the medium within 12 h. When the

cultures were serum-starved, causing a high percentage of cells to accumulate in G_0 and G_1, 3,3′-diindolylmethane inhibited the re-initiation of serum-induced DNA synthesis. This effect was not reversible. The median inhibitory concentration of 3,3′-diindolylmethane for inhibiting the growth of undifferentiated CaCo2 cells was 20 µmol/l, but it was ineffective at doses up to 100 µmol/l in differentiated cells.

After treatment with benzo[a]pyrene (39 µmol/l, 24 h) of human mammary epithelial 184-B5 cells, a 50% decrease in the ratio of quiescent (G_0) to proliferative (S + M) cells was observed (Katdare et al., 1998), which was reversed by simultaneous treatment with indole-3-carbinol at 10 µmol/l (equivalent to the median inhibitory concentration).

Growth of MCF7 (median inhibitory concentration, 50 µmol/l) and T47D (median inhibitory concentration, 180 µmol/l) breast cells was inhibited by indole-3-carbinol (Ge et al., 1999). The median inhibitory concentration was 120 µmol/l for HBL100 non-tumorigenic cells and only 30 µmol/l for the MDA-MB-468 carcinoma cell line, both being estrogen

Table 59. Main biological responses to indole-3-carbinol and indoles in vitro

Indole	Effect	Cell line
Indole-3-carbinol	Inhibition of cell proliferation	Mouse mammary epithelial cell (+ Ras, + Myc) Breast: 184-B5 (+ B[a]P, + HER2), MDA-MB-231, MCF7, T47D, HBL100, MDA-MB-468, MDA-MB-435 (± HER2), ZR-75-1 Colon: HT29, HCEC, SW480 Prostate: LNCaP, DU145, PC-3
	Decreased ODC activity	Breast: HBL100, MCF7, MDA-MB-468 Colon: HCEC, SW480, HT29
	Decreased EGFR expression and phosphorylation	Prostate: PC-3
	Increased ODC activity	Colon: HT-29
	G_0/G_1 growth arrest	Breast: 184-B5 (+ B[a]P, + HER2), MDA-MB-231, MCF7 Prostate: PC-3
	Decreased CDK6 expression	Breast: MCF7, MDA-MB-231 Prostate: PC-3
	Decreased CDK2 activity	Breast: MCF7
	Decreased Rb phosphorylation	Breast: MCF7 Prostate: PC-3
	Decreased cyclin activity	Prostate: PC-3
	Increased *p21*, *p27* expression	Breast: MCF7 Prostate: PC-3
	Increased *p16* expression	Breast: 184-B5 (+ B[a]P)
	Increased *p53* expression	Breast: 184-B5
	Induction of apoptosis	Breast: 184-B5 (+ B[a]P + HER2), MDA-MB-231, MCF7, MDA-MB-435 (± HER2), MDA-MB-468 Colon: LS-174, CaCo2 Cervix: C33A, C33AE6, CaSki Prostate: LNCaP, PC-3
	Increased *Bax* expression	Breast: MDA-MB-435 (± HER2), MCF10A, MCF10CA1a Prostate: PC-3
	Decreased *Bcl2* expression	Breast: MDA-MB-435 (± HER2) Prostate: PC-3 Cervix: C33A, C33AE6, CaSki
	Decreased *Bcl-x$_l$* expression	Breast: MCF10CA1a Prostate: PC-3
	Decreased *BAD* expression	Prostate: PC-3
	Release of cyt C from mitochondria	Breast: MCF10CA1a
	Induction of TRAIL receptors DR4 and DR5	Prostate: LNCaP

Table 59 (contd)

Indole	Effect	Cell line
	Decreased NF-κB-DNA binding	Breast: MDA-MB-468 Prostate: PC-3
	Decreased Akt phosphorylation	Breast: MDA-MB-468 Prostate: PC-3, LNCaP
	Decreased PI3K phosphorylation	Prostate: PC-3
	Induction of E-cadherin, catenins, BRCA1	Breast: MCF7, T47D
	Induction of PTEN	Breast: T47D
	Inhibition of ER signalling	Breast: MCF7, T47D, ZR75-1, 184-B5, MDA-MB-231 Keratinocyes: HPV immortalized Cervix: CaSKi, C33A, SiHa
3,3′-Diindolyl-ethane	Inhibition of cell proliferation	Breast: MCF7, MDA-MB-231, T47D Colon: HT29, CaCo2 (undifferentiated) Prostate: LNCaP, PC-3, DU145 Osteosarcoma: Saos2 Ishikawa endometrial cancer cells
	Inhibition of ligand binding to p-glycoprotein G_0/G_1 growth arrest	Melanoma: B16 (+ MDR-1) Breast: MCF7, MDA-MB-231
	Up-regulation of GADD proteins Decreased CDK2 activity Increased p21 activity Induction of apoptosis	Breast: MCF7 Breast: MCF7, MDA-MB-231 MCF7, MDA-MB-231 Breast: MCF7, T47D, MDA-MB-468, MDA-MB-231 Colon: LS-174, CaCo2 Prostate: LNCaP, PC-3, DU145 Cervix: C33A, C33AE6, CaSki Osteosarcoma: Saos2 Ishikawa endometrial cancer cells
	Decreased Bcl2/Increased Bax	Breast: MCF7, MDA-MB-231
	Inhibition of ER signalling	Breast: MCF7
	Induction of TGFα mRNA	Ishikawa endometrial cancer cells
	Inhibition of androgen-induced proliferation	Prostate: LNCaP
	Decreased PSA expression	Prostate: LNCaP
Indolo[3,2-b]carbazole	Inhibition of signalling through ER	Breast: MCF7
LTr1	Inhibition of proliferation	Breast: MDA-MB-231
	Inhibition of signalling through ER	Breast: MCF7
CTr	Increased cell proliferation (ER agonist)	Breast: MCF7
	Inhibition of ligand binding to p-glycoprotein	Melanoma: B16 (+ MDR1)

Cell lines shown in parentheses are transfected cells. Unless otherwise indicated, cells are of human origin.
 B[a]P, benzo[a]pyrene; ER, estrogen receptor; ODC, ornithine decarboxylase; EGFR, epidermal growth factor; CDK, cyclin-dependent kinase; Rb, retinoblastoma gene; TRAIL, tumour necrosis factor-related apoptosis-inducing ligand; Akt, serine–threonine protein kinase; PI3K, phosphatidylinositol 3′-kinase; PTEN, phosphatase and tensin homologue deleted in chromosome 10; GADD, growth arrest in response to DNA damage; TGF, transforming growth factor; PSA, prostate-specific antigen; LTr1, 2-(indol-3-ylmethyl)-3,3′-diindolymethane; CTr, 5,6,11,12,17,18-hexahydrocyclononal[1,2-b:4,5-b′,7,8-b′′]triindol

receptor-α-negative (Howells et al., 2002).

Indole-3-carbinol at 30 or 60 µmol/l slightly stimulated the growth of LNCaP cells over 2 days, while 90 µmol/l slightly suppressed growth from the second day of treatment (Jeon et al., 2003). After treatment with indole-3-carbinol for 5 h, median inhibitory concentrations of 22 µmol/l and 48 µmol/l were estimated for the LNCaP and DU145 prostate cell lines, respectively (Howells et al., 2002). The growth of PC-3 prostate cancer cells was inhibited by indole-3-carbinol (0.2 mmol/l for 72 h) (Frydoonfar et al., 2003).

At concentrations above 10 µmol/l, 3,3′-diindolylmethane inhibited DNA synthesis and proliferation of MCF-7 and MDA-MB-231 cells (Hong et al., 2002a).

Ornithine decarboxylase is the rate-limiting enzyme in the biosynthesis of polyamines and, as such, is critical for cell proliferation. It is often overexpressed in tumour cells and is a target for chemoprevention. Indole-3-carbinol inhibited cell growth in a range of breast and colon cell lines (HBL100, MDA-MB-468, MCF-7, HCEC, HT29, SW480), in a time- and dose-dependent manner in all lines. The MDA-MB-468 line was the most sensitive, showing complete inhibition at 100 µmol/l, the lowest concentration tested. The other lines were inhibited by 250 µmol/l. Indole-3-carbinol caused significant inhibition of basal ornithine decarboxylase activity after 5 h in normal colon-derived HCEC and HBL100 breast cells at concentrations above 250 µmol/l and in MDA-MB-468 cells above 500 µmol/l. SW480 and MCF-7 cells were inhibited to a lesser extent, while in the HT29 cells ornithine decarboxylase activity appeared to be stimulated at lower concentrations. The effect of indole-3-carbinol on ornithine decarboxylase activity at 5 h did not always correlate with the final growth inhibition (Hudson et al., 1998).

The involvement of ornithine decarboxylase in chemoprevention by indole-3-carbinol was investigated further in colon cells (Hudson et al., 2003). The median inhibitory concentrations (after 168 h) in SW480, HT29 and HCEC cells were 123, 127 and 164 µmol/l, respectively. The basal levels of ornithine decarboxylase activity of 171, 1079 and 156 pmol CO_2 produced per hour per milligram of protein in these cells were decreased by indole-3-carbinol after 24 h of treatment. The HCEC line showed the greatest inhibiton of ornithine decarboxylase activity but the least growth inhibition at this time. The SW480 cells showed the least inhibition of ornithine decarboxylase activity. While administration of exogenous putrescine reversed the growth inhibitory effects of a direct inhibitor of ornithine decarboxylase, difluoromethylornithine, it did not reverse inhibition by indole-3-carbinol and, in the SW480 cells, even enhanced the effect. Putrescine in combination with indole-3-carbinol did not, however, predispose the cells to apoptosis. The results obtained in this study suggested that inhibition of ornithine decarboxylase is unlikely to be a major mechanism for inhibition of growth by indole-3-carbinol.

Induction of cell cycle arrest

In the few studies in which growth arrest in a specific phase of the cell cycle has been reported in response to treatment with indoles, the phase has usually been G_0 or G_1. Treatment with indole-3-carbinol (50 µmol/l) of reduction mammoplasty-derived 184-B5 cells initiated with benzo[a]pyrene or the oncogene HER, and of MDA-MB231 cells, resulted in a 137–210% increase in the quiescent:proliferative ratio, i.e. G_0/G_1 arrest (Telang et al., 1997c).

Treatment of MCF-7 breast cells with indole-3-carbinol (30–100 µmol/l)

reversibly suppressed incorporation of tritiated thymidine, without affecting viability or estrogen receptor responsiveness (Cover et al., 1998). Arrest of cells in the G_1 phase of the cycle was associated with specific inhibition of the expression of the cyclin-dependent kinase CDK6 (also observed in MDA-MB-231 cells), which resulted in inhibition of phosphorylation of the retinoblastoma tumour suppressor gene Rb. No effect was observed on CDK2, CDK4, cyclin D1 or cyclin E expression, although indole-3-carbinol and 3,3′-diindolylmethane apparently affected CDK2 activity (Firestone & Bjeldanes, 2003). After maximal growth arrest, the levels of the CDK inhibitors p21 and p27 were increased by 50% (Cover et al., 1998). A combination of indole-3-carbinol and tamoxifen was found to inhibit the growth of MCF-7 cells more stringently than either agent alone. Taken together, the results suggest that indole-3-carbinol can suppress the growth of breast cancer cells in an estrogen receptor-independent manner. The combination of tamoxifen and indole-3-carbinol was explored further (Cover et al., 1999), and was found to cause a more pronounced decrease in CDK2 activity than either compound on its own. Protein expression of CDK2 was not affected. The combination also completely prevented phosphorylation of the Rb protein, whereas either compound on its own was only partially effective.

In exploring the mechanism by which indole-3-carbinol down-regulates CDK6, Cram et al. (2001) showed that the indole could inhibit the activity of the CDK6 promoter contained in a luciferase reporter construct. By deletion analysis, they identified an Sp1 and an Ets-like binding site, both of which were required for indole-3-carbinol responsiveness. With electrophoretic mobility-shift analysis (EMSA) and an antibody against Sp1, it appeared that the Sp1 binding site in the *CDK6* promoter leads to a specific indole-3-carbinol-responsive DNA–protein complex that contains the Sp1 transcription factor. Thus, indole-3-carbinol appeared to down-regulate *CDK6* transcription by targeting Sp1 at a composite site in the promoter of this gene.

A synthetic stable tetrameric derivative of indole-3-carbinol, prepared by oxidation, suppressed the growth of MCF7, 734B and BT474 (estrogen receptor-positive) and BT20, MDA-MB-231 and BT539 (estrogen receptor-negative) breast tumour cells, inducing G_1 arrest, without evidence of apoptosis (Brandi *et al.*, 2003). It was about five times more active than indole-3-carbinol in this respect. The tetramer inhibited *CDK6* expression and activity, increased p27 and reduced Rb protein expression. No change was observed in *CDK4*.

Indole-3-carbinol (30 µmol/l) inhibited the growth of PC-3 prostate cancer cells by inducing G_1 arrest, leading to apoptosis (Chinni *et al.,* 2001). This was accompanied by significant induction of *p21* and *p27* CDK inhibitors. The induction of *p21* appeared to be independent of *p53*, but deletion of an Sp1 site reduced promoter activity. Induced expression of the CDK inhibitors led to decreased kinase activity of the cyclin D1 and E complexes. Exposure to indole-3-carbinol also led to a dose-dependent decrease in *CDK6* expression, apparent from 24 h with a dose of 50 or 100 µmol/l. *CDK6* activity was decreased by as much as 70% in the presence of 100 µmol/l indole-3-carbinol for 48 h. Indole-3-carbinol treatment also resulted in progressive inhibition of Rb phosphorylation, which was pronounced after 48 h of treatment with 60–100 µmol/l. These results in a prostate cell line are similar to those described above for a breast cell line (Cover *et al.*, 1998, 1999).

3,3′-Diindolylmethane induced arrest in the G_1 phase of the cycle in both MCF-7 and MDA-MB-231 breast cells (Hong *et al.*, 2002b). This was accompanied by a decrease in the activity of *CDK2* and increase in $p21^{Waf1/Cip1}$ mRNA (six- to sevenfold) and protein in both cell lines, suggesting that the latter was independent of estrogen receptor signalling and *p53*. Transient transfection with a series of deletion constructs suggested that 3,3′-diindolylmethane responsiveness is dependent on a segment of the $p21^{Waf1/cip1}$ promoter containing six Sp1 elements. This conclusion was reinforced by electrophoretic mobility shift assays that showed that 3,3′-diindolylmethane induced binding of Sp1 and Sp3 to the consensus Sp1 responsive element. In a comparison of the effects of indole-3-carbinol and 3,3′-diindolylmethane on cell cycle arrest (Firestone & Bjeldanes, 2003), a fraction of indole-3-carbinol was found to be converted intracellularly to 3,3′-diindolylmethane, which accumulated in the nucleus. In contrast, 3,3′-diindolylmethane had no effect on the *CDK6* promoter. These results indicate that the control of cell cycle gene expression is mediated by a combination of the specific effects of indole-3-carbinol and 3,3′-diindolylmethane.

Proteins of the growth arrest and DNA damage (GADD) family, GADD153, 45α, β and γ and 34, induce growth arrest and apoptosis by various pathways. Microarray analysis suggested that 3,3′-diindolylmethane up-regulates genes of the GADD family (Carter *et al.*, 2002). BRCA1, which was induced by indole-3-carbinol and 3,3′-diindolylmethane (Meng *et al.,* 2000a), induced expression of *GADD45* but also inhibited signalling by estrogen through estrogen receptor-α. Auborn *et al.* (2003) investigated the ability of 3,3′-diindolylmethane to up-regulate *GADD* genes as a mechanism for overcoming estrogen induction of tumour growth. They showed in MCF7 breast cells that 3,3′-diindolylmethane (50 or 100 µmol/l, 6 h) increased expression of *GADD34*, *153* and *45*. Significant loss of cell viability was also found at these concentrations. 3,3′-Diindolylmethane at 25 µmol/l was not effective, but when it was combined with genistein (5 µmol/l), even greater induction of *GADD* genes was observed, with significant induction of apoptosis at 48 h.

Induction of apoptosis
A number of studies have been reported on the efficacy of indoles in inducing apoptosis. In some cases, tumour cells were more sensitive than non-transformed cells, and often the condensation products of indole-3-carbinol were more effective than the parent compound.

In a study with reduction mammoplasty-derived 184-B5 cells initiated with benzo[*a*]pyrene or the oncogene *HER*, and with MDA-MB-231 cells, treatment with indole-3-carbinol at 50 µmol/l resulted in a twofold increase in apoptosis, as measured by the sub-G_1 fraction after 24 h (Telang *et al.*, 1997c).

Treatment of human mammary epithelial 184-B5 cells with benzo[*a*]pyrene reduced the sub-G_1 population by more than 85%; this effect was partially reversed (reduced to 41% of control) by indole-3-carbinol at 10 µmol/l (Katdare *et al.*, 1998). The reversal was accompanied by a twofold or greater increase in p53 immunoreactivity. Treatment with indole-3-carbinol in combination with benzo[*a*]pyrene doubled the immunoreactivity for the CDK inhibitor p16[INK4C] compared with treatment with benzo[*a*]pyrene alone.

Induction of apoptosis, as determined by DNA fragmentation and nuclear condensation, was observed in MCF-7 cells after 24 h of treatment with indole-3-carbinol at 250 μmol/l or 72 h of treatment at 50 μmol/l (Fares et al., 1998; Ge et al., 1999). No change was observed in the level of wild-type p53 in MCF-7 cells up to 8 h after treatment with indole-3-carbinol or 3,3′-diindolylmethane at 250 μmol/l. Additionally, no change was observed in Bax levels in MCF-7 (estrogen receptor-positive) or T47D (estrogen receptor-negative) cell lines. The authors observed some conversion of indole-3-carbinol to 3,3′-diindolylmethane in the culture medium (up to 30% after 72 h).

Working with parental MDA-MB-435 breast cancer cells and a line transfected with Her-2/Neu, Rahman et al. (2000) found that indole-3-carbinol (30–100 μmol/l) inhibited the growth of both lines and induced apoptosis, as measured by poly(ADP–ribose)polymerase cleavage and caspase-3 activation. Up-regulation of *Bax*, in combination with down-regulation of *Bcl-2*, led to an increased *Bax:Bcl-2* ratio, favouring apoptosis. Indole-3-carbinol caused relocation of Bax from the cytoplasm to the mitochondria, which would be predicted to cause mitochondrial depolarization, release of cytochrome c and activation of caspases. In a subsequent study (Rahman et al., 2003; Sarkar et al., 2003) with MCF10A (non-tumorigenic) and MCF10CA1a (tumorigenic) cell lines, indole-3-carbinol (30–100 μmol/l) induced translocation of *Bax* to the mitochondria in both cell lines but resulted in a loss of mitochondrial membrane potential and release of cytochrome c only in the tumour cells, which were much more sensitive to growth inhibition and induction of apoptosis. Indole-3-carbinol up-regulated the *Bax:Bcl2* ratio and down-regulated *Bcl-x$_L$* expression only in CA1a tumour cells.

In a study of the effects of indole-3-carbinol and 3,3′-diindolylmethane on three human cervical cancer cell lines, C33A, C33AE6 and CaSki, Chen, D.Z. et al. (2001) found that both agents induced apoptosis, while 3,3′-diindolylmethane was more potent (50–60 μmol/l versus 200 μmol/l) and faster acting than indole-3-carbinol in C33A cells. Indole-3-carbinol reduced Bcl-2 protein levels in total cell lysates in a time- and dose-dependent manner, but had no effect on total Bax levels. Neither compound caused apoptosis in normal human keratinocytes.

Apoptosis was observed in PC-3 cells after treatment with indole-3-carbinol at 100 μmol/l for 48 h, as measured by DNA laddering and poly(ADP-ribose)polymerase cleavage (Chinni et al., 2001). The levels of Bcl2 were down-regulated (by 80%) after 24–72 h of treatment, while Bax protein expression was up-regulated (1.9-fold). Indole-3-carbinol (60 μmol/l) was also found to inhibit tumour necrosis factor-α-stimulated NF-κB (p65/p50)–DNA binding after treatment for 48 h. In a subsequent study (Chinni & Sarkar, 2002), indole-3-carbinol (at doses from 30 μmol/l) affected another survival pathway by inhibiting the phosphorylation of Akt/protein kinase B in unstimulated and epithelial growth factor (EGF)-stimulated cells. Western blot analysis revealed down-regulation of both EGF receptor levels and autophosphory-lation of EGF receptor. This was accompanied by inhibition of EGF-induced phosphorylation of phosphatidylinositol 3′-kinase. Downstream of *Akt*, *Bcl-x$_L$* and *BAD* showed decreased expression after indole-3-carbinol treatment.

In a comparative study of the effects of indole-3-carbinol in two breast cell lines, HBL100 derived from normal tissue and MDA-MB-468 from a carcinoma, Howells et al. (2002) found that the tumour line underwent apoptosis after treatment with 10–100 μmol/l, while the HBL100 line was resistant. At higher doses (> 250 μmol/l), however, the HBL100 cells underwent increasing necrosis. Indole-3-carbinol inhibited phosphorylation of Akt in the MDA-MB-468 line, which lacks the tumour suppressor phosphatase and tensin homologue deleted on chromosome 10 (PTEN), but not in the HBL100 cells which are positive for PTEN. Indole-3-carbinol also reduced NF-κB–DNA binding, independently of an effect on IκB kinase, but only in the tumour cell line. Phospho-PKB levels were also decreased and apoptosis induced by indole-3-carbinol at doses > 250 μmol/l in the prostate cell line LNCaP, which expresses very low levels of PTEN, but not to the same extent in PTEN-positive DU145 cells. Indole-3-carbinol had no effect on PTEN levels in either the breast or the prostate cell lines.

In one study, indole-3-carbinol caused no significant change in the level of Akt or in its phosphorylation in LNCaP cells over 48 h (Jeon et al., 2003). [The Working Group noted that the corresponding data were not presented. Doses of 30–90 μmol/l were used in other parts of the study, which would explain the absence of an effect and would be in agreement with the results of Howells et al. (2002).]

A range of cell lines with different p53 status were used to examine the chemopreventive potential of 3,3′-diindolylmethane (Ge et al., 1996). Dose-dependent growth inhibition (at 1–100 μmol/l) was found in MCF-7 (wild type *p53*), T47D (mutant *p53*) breast and Saos-2 (*p53*-deficient) osteosarcoma lines. Apoptosis (affecting 12–14% of cells) was induced after 48 h of treatment with 3,3′-diindolylmethane at 50 μmol/l, as determined by altered morphology and DNA laddering. In MCF-7 cells, the lowest dose to induce apoptosis was 10 μmol/l after 72 h of treatment, while 24 h of treatment at 100 μmol/l resulted in 19% apoptotic cells, as estimated by FACScan analysis. Induction of apoptosis appeared to be independent of p53 status.

In a later study, concentrations of 3,3´-diindolylmethane > 10 μmol/l, were found to induce apoptosis in MCF-7 and MDA-MB-231 cells, as evidenced by externalization of phosphatidyl serine, chromatin condensation and DNA fragmentation (assessed in the TUNEL assay). The protein levels of Bcl2 were decreased in both cell lines (by 90% in MCF-7 and 60% in MDA-MB-231). The mRNA levels of Bcl2 were also decreased by 70% after treatment of MCF-7 cells with 3,3´-diindolylmethane at 100 μmol/l, as was the amount of Bcl2 bound to Bax. The levels of the latter were increased by 3,3´-diindolylmethane treatment, by up to fourfold in MCF-7 and by sixfold in MDA-MB-231 cells, with a maximum effect after 48 h of treatment (Hong et al., 2002a). After co-immunoprecipitation of Bcl2–Bax complexes, 3,3´-diindolylmethane caused a time- and concentration-dependent decrease in the amount of Bcl2 associated with Bax in both cell lines (80% after exposure to 100 μmol/l for 24 h). Ectopic expression of Bcl2 in MCF-7 cells blocked the apoptotic effect of 3,3´-diindolylmethane (by 50% after 24 h).

3,3´-Diindolylmethane and indolo-[3,2-b]carbazole induced apoptosis in the human colon LS-174 and CaCo2 adenocarcinoma cell lines (Bonnesen et al., 2001), but no apoptosis was observed in the SV40-T antigen immortalized normal colon-derived cell line HCEC.

The ability of indole-3-carbinol (10–400 μmol/l) and 3,3´-diindolylmethane (10–100 μmol/l) to affect proliferation and apoptosis was examined in three prostate cell lines with different p53 status (LNCaP, wild-type; PC-3, deficient; and DU145, mutant). The results after 48 h of treatment suggested the following median inhibitory concentrations for inhibition of prolifer-ation: indole-3-carbinol, 150 μmol/l for LNCaP, 160 μmol/l for DU145 and 285 μmol/l for PC-3; 3,3´-diindolylmethane, 40 μmol/l for LNCaP and PC-3 and 20 μmol/l for DU145. Both compounds induced apoptosis in all cell lines in a p53-independent manner (LNCaP, 24 h with 200 μmol/l indole-3-carbinol or 75 μmol/l 3,3´-diindolylmethane; DU145, 72 h with 200 μmol/l indole-3-carbinol, 48 h with 75 μmol/l 3,3´-diindolylmethane; PC-3, 72 h with 400 μmol/l indole-3-carbinol or 75 μmol/l 3,3´-diindolylmethane) (Nachshon-Kedmi et al., 2003). No effect were observed on the levels of Bcl-2, Bax or fas$_L$. The results suggest that the well-differentiated LNCaP cells were more sensitive to inhibition of apoptosis by 3,3´-diindolylmethane and indole-3-carbinol than the moderately (DU145) and poorly (PC-3) differentiated cells.

After treatment for 24 h with indole-3-carbinol (30 or 90 μmol/l), the LNCaP cell line was sensitized to tumour necrosis factor-related apoptosis-inducing ligand (TRAIL)-mediated (100 ng/ml) apoptosis. Treatment with indole-3-carbinol (90 μmol/l) induced two TRAIL death receptors (DR4 and DR5) at both the transcriptional and translational level, without affecting the expression of two decoy receptors (Jeon et al., 2003). Treatment with indole-3-carbinol (90 μmol/l) alone for 24 h did not induce apoptosis, although viability was affected (see above).

Effects on invasion and metastasis
Limited evidence from one laboratory indicates that indoles can inhibit the invasive capacity or metastasis of breast cells. Nevertheless, a study with rat hepatocytes suggested the opposite effect.

Indole-3-carbinol (50 or 100 μmol/l) inhibited the adhesion, migration and invasive properties of both MCF-7 and MDA-MB-468 breast tumour cells in vitro and also inhibited their ability to metastasize to the lung when injected into the tail vein of mice. Indole-3-carbinol could also suppress 17β-estradiol-induced migration and invasion of MCF-7 cells (Meng et al., 2000a). It induced the expression of several genes, including E-cadherin, α-, β-, and γ-catenin and BRCA1, whose functions include suppression of invasion. Disruption of the E-cadherin–catenin complex has been shown to correlate with progression of breast cancer by increasing proliferation, invasion and metastasis, while restoration of E-cadherin function reduces invasiveness dramatically.

Up-regulation of the tumour suppressor PTEN and the cell adhesion molecule E-cadherin in T47D cells in response to treatment with indole-3-carbinol (25–125 μmol/l) was associated with significant inhibition of cell spread and invasion (Meng et al., 2000b). The results of this study also suggested that indole-3-carbinol inhibited cell attachment to a laminin substratum.

Other cellular effects
Antioxidant and anti-inflammatory mechanisms
Data derived from several experimental systems suggest that indole-3-carbinol and derived compounds are generally not highly efficient antioxidants. In two of the earliest studies, three in-vitro systems were used to analyse the ability of indole-3-carbinol to scavenge radical species (Shertzer et al., 1986, 1988). The systems involved phospholipid dissolved in chlorobenzene with peroxidation initiated by thermal and photodecomposition of azobisisobutyronitrile; sonicated phospholipid vesicles in phosphate buffer (pH 7.4) with peroxidation initiated by ferrous or ascorbate; and mouse liver microsomes containing an NADPH-regenerating system, with peroxidation initiated with carbon tetrachloride. Lipid peroxidation was measured in each of these systems by the

assay for thiobarbituric acid-reactive substances. In the first two systems, indole-3-carbinol was about 30% as efficient as α-tocopherol and butylhydroxytoluene but inhibited peroxidation in a dose-dependent manner. In the third system, indole-3-carbinol was more effective, with 50% inhibition at doses of 35–40 μmol/l, about one-third of the concentration that could be achieved in mouse liver after administration of 50 mg/kg bw by gavage.

In a limited study of antioxidant capacity, the scavenging capacity of indole-3-carbinol and 29 structurally related compounds was compared with that of α-tocopherol. None of the common plant-derived indoles occurring in the diet were as efficient as α-tocopherol in two cell-free soya bean phospholipid peroxidation assays (Tabor et al., 1991).

In an enzyme system consisting of peroxidase, hydrogen peroxide and 2,2´-azinobis(3-ethylbenzylthiazoline)-6-sulfonic acid, the ability of various indoles to scavenge the radicals of the last compound was examined. Indole-3-carbinol was effective at doses of 100–500 μmol/l, indole-3-aldehyde and indole-3-carboxylic acid were inactive, while indole-3-acetic acid had less activity than indole-3-carbinol (Arnao et al., 1996).

In a screen of 90 compounds in six chemoprevention assays, indole-3-carbinol was one of only eight compounds that was chemopreventive in all the assays (Sharma et al., 1994). The reagent was tested at concentrations up to its maximum solubility in the medium. It inhibited tyrosine kinase and ornithine decarboxylase activity, the former in a dose-dependent fashion. It also increased the levels of reduced GSH and effectively inhibited free radical production, carcinogen–DNA binding and poly(ADP-ribose)polymerase activity.

In another series of mechanism-based screens of potential chemopre-ventive agents, however, in which radical scavenging ability, antioxidant effects, inhibition of inducible nitric oxygen synthase, COX-1 and ornithine decarboxylase activity were tested, indole-3-carbinol showed only weak activity (Gerhäuser et al., 2003). In a survey of 14 compounds for possible protection against the toxicity of MNNG or methyl methane sulfonate in isolated rat hepatocytes by mechanisms including antioxidant capacity, indole-3-carbinol was one of the least active compounds (Shertzer et al., 1991).

Estrogen receptor and estrogen-associated effects

Many studies have shown effects on signalling through the estrogen receptor in a variety of cell types.

The effect of indole-3-carbinol on proliferation of an estrogen receptor-positive breast cell line, MCF-7, and an estrogen receptor-negative line, MDA-MB-231, was assessed and correlated with estrogen responsiveness and CYP1A1 activity (Tiwari et al., 1994). Indole-3-carbinol (50 μmol/l) inhibited the growth of MCF-7 but not MDA-MB-231 cells after a 48-h period of serum starvation and then stimulation with 17β-estradiol. Induction of CYP1A1 (by three- to fivefold with 500 μmol/l by 12 h) and 2-hydroxylation of estrogen (by fourfold) occurred only in the MCF-7 cell line, suggesting that indole-3-carbinol had no effect on estrogen receptor-negative cells in this respect. The basal levels of 16α-hydroxlation were higher in the MDA-MB-231 cells, indicating that these estrogen receptor-negative cells, which contain CYP1A1, still metabolize estradiol. Treatment with indole-3-carbinol alone at a concentration of 5, 50 or 500 μmol/l resulted in a dose-dependent decrease in the total number of MCF-7 cells (55% at 50 μmol/l, 85% at 500 μmol/l) and of soft agar colonies (94% at 500 μmol/l) after 5 days. The corresponding values for MDA-MB231 cells were 13%, 17% and 30%, respectively.

Indolo[3,2-b]carbazole at 1 μmol/l, a concentration which did not induce CYP1A1, had a number of antiestrogen effects in MCF-7 cells, including inhibition of estradiol-induced cell proliferation and uptake of tritiated thymidine, reduction of nuclear progesterone receptor levels and CAT activity in cells transfected with the estrogen-responsive vit-CAT plasmid. Indolo-[3,2-b]carbazole (100 nmol/l), in the absence of estradiol, caused a small but significant, increase in thymidine incorporation. Nuclear extracts from indolo[3,2-b]carbazole-treated cells had decreased estrogen receptor levels and reduced binding to an estrogen-responsive element in gel shift assays. Indolo[3,2-b]carbazole bound with low affinity to the estrogen receptor, eliciting weak estrogen-like activity (Liu et al., 1994). In this study, indole-3-carbinol (31–125 μmol/l) also caused a significant decrease in nuclear estrogen receptor levels, with no induction of CYP1A1. These results confirm that the anti-estrogenic effects of indole-3-carbinol and indolo[3,2-b]carbazole are mediated through pathways independent of altered estradiol metabolism.

In another study with MCF-7 cells, indole-3-carbinol (10^{-11}–10^{-6} mol/l) showed a steady increase in 2-hydroxylation of estradiol, the effect plateauing at 10^{-8} mol/l, with no significant change in 16α-hydroxylation (Niwa et al., 1994). No effect was observed in the estrogen receptor-negative lines T47D and MDA-MB-231. The altered metabolism was attributed at least partly to 3,3´-diindolylmethane, since indole-3-carbinol was found to be spontaneously converted after 48 h in modified Eagle medium at 37 °C .

Explant cultures were prepared from human mammary terminal duct lobular units obtained from surgical samples and treated with DMBA or benzo[*a*]pyrene (Telang *et al.*, 1997a). Both carcinogens decreased 2-hydroxy-estrone formation while increasing 16α-hydroxyestrone. After treatment with indole-3-carbinol at 50 µmol/l, the benzo[*a*]pyrene-treated explant cultures showed a 12-fold increase in the 2-:16α-hydroxy ratio. Similar results were obtained with 184-B5 mammary epithelial cells (Telang *et al.*, 1997a,c).

Bradlow *et al.* (1997), investigating the effect of organochlorine-based pesticides on the 2-:16α-hydroxy ratio in breast tumour cells, found a significant reduction only in estrogen receptor-positive MCF7 cells. In this cell line, indole-3-carbinol increased the ratio of 2-:16α-hydroxylation, when given alone or in combination with atrazine.

Indole-3-carbinol blocked the ability of estradiol to increase anchorage-independent growth in HPV-immortalized keratinocytes (Newfield *et al.*, 1998), an effect which was attributed to the ability of indole-3-carbinol to induce 2-hydroxylation of estradiol.

Chen, I. *et al.* (1998) reported that 3,3´-diindolylmethane at concentrations of 0.1–10 µmol/l did not affect the proliferative rate of MCF-7 cells, while cells co-treated with estradiol at 1 nmol/l had a concentration-dependent decrease in estradiol-induced proliferation. At a concentration of 50 mmol/l, the nuclear levels of estrogen receptor were reduced by 70–80%. After treatment with 3,3´-diindolylmethane at 10–50 µmol/l, binding of nuclear extracts from MCF-7 cells to the estrogen response element (ERE) was significantly reduced in gel shift assays.

In the cervical cancer cell line CaSki, estradiol increased expression of HPV-16, whereas indole-3-carbinol and 2-hydroxyestrone (the formation of which is increased by indole-3-carbinol) inhibited the estrogen-increased expression. Both compounds competed with estradiol for binding to the estrogen receptor (Yuan *et al.*, 1999).

2-(Indol-3-ylmethyl)-3,3´-diindolylmethane (LTr-1; 25 µmol/l) inhibited the growth of both estrogen receptor-positive MCF-7 and estrogen receptor-negative MDA-MB-231 breast cells by about 60%, but had no effect on the MCF-7 cells in the absence of estrogen. This finding was in contrast to that with 3,3´-diindolylmethane (see below), which markedly induced the growth of MCF-7 cells under estradiol-depleted conditions. 2-(Indol-3-yl-methyl)-3,3´-diindolylmethane appeared to be a weak ligand for the estrogen receptor (median inhibitory concentration, 70 µmol/l versus nanomolar concentrations of tamoxifen and estradiol) and efficiently inhibited estradiol-induced binding of the estrogen receptor to its DNA response element. Estradiol-induced transcription of pS2 was inhibited by approximately 50% by 10 µmol/l. 2-(Indol-3-ylmethyl)-3,3´-diindolylmethane activated the Ah receptor and expression of CYP1A1 but was a competitive inhibitor of EROD activity (median inhibitory concentration, 1 µmol/l) (Chang *et al.*, 1999).

3,3´-Diindolylmethane given for 7 days was a weak inhibitor of estradiol-induced proliferation of estrogen receptor-containing MCF-7 cells; however, at 10 µmol/l, it induced proliferation in the absence of steroid, to about 60% of the estradiol response. There was little effect on estrogen receptor-negative MDA-MB-231 cells. 3,3´-Diindolylmethane was a promoter-specific activator of the estrogen receptor in the absence of estradiol, but did not bind to the receptor (Riby *et al.*, 2000b). The agonist effects of 3,3´-diindolylmethane appeared to require the presence of a *cis*-acting DNA element, in addition to the core ERE consensus, and could be blocked by co-treatment with a protein kinase A inhibitor. The antagonist effects were less dependent on promoter context. These results suggest that 3,3´-diin-

dolylmethane is a selective activator of estrogen receptor function.

The main cyclic trimeric product of indole-3-carbinol, CT, was investigated for its effects on estrogen receptor signalling (Riby *et al.*, 2000a). It was a strong agonist of estrogen receptor function, stimulating the proliferation of estrogen receptor-positive MCF-7 cells (at concentrations between 10 nmol/l and 1 µmol/l) to a similar degree as estradiol. It had no such effect on estrogen receptor-negative MDA-MD-231 cells. CT displaced estradiol from the receptor in competitive binding assays (median effective concentration, about 1 µmol/l) and, in EMSA (at 10 or 100 nmol/l), increased estrogen receptor binding to an estrogen-responsive DNA element. CT (10 nmol/l to 1 µmol/l) activated transcription of an endogenous estrogen receptor-responsive gene, *pS2*, and of exogenous reporter genes after transfection into MCF-7 cells. Unlike indolo[3,2-*b*]carbazole, which was used as a positive control, no activation of Ah receptor-mediated pathways occurred, as indicated by induction of CYP1A1 activity, in agreement with previous results suggesting that CT binds weakly to the Ah receptor (Bjeldanes *et al.*, 1991). The conformation of CT is similar to that of 4-hydroxy-tamoxifen, suggesting an excellent fit into the estrogen receptor ligand binding site; however, the binding affinity was estimated to be two orders of magnitude lower (Riby *et al.*, 2000a). The authors suggested that the estrogenic activity of CT might account for the tumour promoting effect of indole-3-carbinol reported in liver and for the protective effect in mammary tissue.

Indole-3-carbinol (50–100 µmol/l) inhibited estradiol-activated expression of an ERE-containing luciferase reporter gene transfected into MCF-7, T47D or MDA-MB-231 breast cells or CaSki, SiHa or C33-A cervical cancer

Chapter 6

Carcinogenicity

Humans

In the epidemiological studies of cancer reviewed in section 4, some of the relative risks for high versus low consumption of cruciferous vegetables were above unity, and a few were significantly greater than 1.0: i.e., in one cohort study of colorectal cancer, one case–control study of breast cancer and one case–control study of thyroid cancer. These were extreme examples of estimates that tended to centre close to the null. None of these results was considered by the Working Group to represent evidence of carcinogenicity in humans.

Experimental studies

Cruciferous vegetables

The fact that control animals given cruciferous vegetables alone did not show tumour enhancement indicates that these vegetables alone are not carcinogenic. Nevertheless, in a few studies, dietary *Brassica* vegetables may have enhanced the tumour response in carcinogen-treated animals (Table 61).

Colon

In two studies, Temple and Basu (1987) and Temple and El-Khatib (1987) examined the potential inhibitory effect of dietary cabbage on the formation of colon tumours in female Swiss mice treated with dimethylhydrazine. Unexpectedly, cabbage elicited some enhancement of tumour response when given throughout the experiment or during carcinogen treatment, although these increases were not statistically significant.

Pancreas and gall-bladder

Birt *et al.* (1987) evaluated the ability of dried cabbage supplements in the diet to inhibit pancreatic carcinogenesis in hamsters. Pancreatic cancer was induced by treatment with N-nitroso-bis(2-oxopropyl)amine (BOP) at 40 mg/kg bw. Before receiving the carcinogen, the animals were given a low-fat diet containing 9% (w/w) dried cabbage; from 1 week after BOP treatment, cabbage was given in low- (at 9%) and high-fat (at 11%) diets. The high-fat cabbage-containing diet increased the yield of BOP-induced pancreatic ductule carcinoma (1.6 carcinomas per animal) in comparison with that observed in hamsters fed the low-fat diet cabbage-containing or a high-fat diet without cabbage (0.6–0.8 carcinomas per animal; $p < 0.05$). The incidence of BOP-induced gall-bladder adenocarcinoma was increased in cabbage-fed hamsters irrespective of dietary fat.

Skin

Birt *et al.* (1987) evaluated the ability of dietary dried cabbage supplements to inhibit skin tumorigenesis in mice. Skin tumours were induced in SENCAR mice with 10 nmol of 7,12-dimethyl-benz[a]anthracene (DMBA) and promoted beginning 1 week later by twice weekly applications of 2 μg of 12-O-tetradecanoylphorbol 13-acetate (TPA). Dried cabbage was incorporated into AIN semi-purified diets before DMBA and throughout TPA treatment. The skin papilloma yield was increased in DMBA-initiated TPA-promoted mice fed diets containing 10% cabbage, from 7.25 papillomas per mouse in mice given control diet to an average of 8.45 papillomas per mouse after 22 weeks of promotion ($p < 0.001$).

Spermatic cord and others

Srisangnam *et al.* (1980) fed diets containing dehydrated cabbage to weanling male C57BL/6 mice injected subcutaneously with 20 mg/kg bw of dimethylhydrazine at weekly intervals for 36 weeks. Diets known to be adequate in all nutrients for mice were modified to include ground dehydrated cabbage leaves to 10%, 20% and 40% of diet, protein, crude fibre and lipids being held at constant levels. The diets containing 10% or 20% cabbage enhanced dimethylhydrazine-induced tumorigenicity, while the diet containing cabbage at 40% had a protective effect, which was not significant. Tumours of the spermatic cord were the most frequent, with occasional kidney and liver tumours.

Glucosinolates

Morse *et al.* (1988) studied the effects of long-term dietary administration of sinigrin (2-propenyl glucosinolate) at 3 μmol/g of diet to Fischer 344 rats before and during treatment with 4-(methylnitrosamino)-1-(3-pyridyl)-1-butanone (NNK) (1.76 mg/kg subcutaneously three times a week for 20 weeks). After 104 weeks, there was no effect of sinigrin on tumorigenesis in liver, lung or nasal cavities; however, a significant increase in pancreatic tumours was observed in rats treated with both sinigrin and NNK.

Table 61. Enhancement of carcinogen-induced tumours by dietary cruciferous vegetables in experimental animals

Species, strain (sex)	Age at start (weeks)	No. of animals per group	Carcinogen, route, dose, duration	Cruciferous vegetable, amount, duration	Timing of treatment	Enhancement of tumour incidence (TI) or multiplicity (TM)	Summarized effect	Reference
Colon Mouse, ICR (F)	5–7	20–40	Dimethylhydrazine, starting at 17 mg/kg bw and then increasing by 21%, weekly × 8 (total, 291 mg/kg bw), s.c., killed 27 weeks after first dose	Cabbage, 12.8% of diet, purchased locally, starting 5 weeks before or after the carcinogen	Initiation, post-initiation or throughout	Adenoma TM: dimethylhydrazine alone, 1.85; + cabbage during initiation, 2.00; + cabbage after initiation, 0.92 ($p < 0.05$); + cabbage throughout, 2.00 Adenocarcinoma TM: dimethylhydrazine alone, 0.85; + cabbage during initiation, 1.15; + cabbage after initiation, 0.75; + cabbage throughout, 1.42	Cabbage increased colon tumours, particularly adeno-carcinomas, in initiation period but reduced adenomas in promotion period	Temple & Basu (1987)
Mouse, Swiss (M, F)	5–7	14–17	Dimethyl-hydrazine, starting at 23 mg/kg bw and then increasing weekly × 7, s.c., killed 17 weeks after first dose	Cabbage, 13% of diet, 21 weeks, purchased locally, starting 31 days before carcinogen	Through-out	Adenoma incidence (%) Females: dimethylhydrazine alone, 42.9; + cabbage, 62.5 Males: dimethylhydrazine alone, 47.0; + cabbage, 37.5 Adenocarcinoma TI (%) Females: dimethylhydrazine alone, 35.7; + cabbage, 68.7 Males: dimethylhydrazine alone, 64.7; + cabbage, 37.5 Total tumours per tumour-bearing mouse Females: dimethylhydrazine alone, 3.17; + cabbage, 4.92 Males: dimethylhydrazine alone, 3.08; + cabbage, 2.89	Although males were little affected by cabbage, females fed cabbage showed a tendency for increase in colon tumours	Temple & El-Khatib (1987)

Table 61 (contd)

Species, strain (sex)	Age at start (weeks)	No. of animals per group	Carcinogen, route, dose, duration	Cruciferous vegetable, amount, duration	Timing of treatment	Enhancement of tumour incidence (TI) or multiplicity (TM)	Summarized effect	Reference
Pancreas and gall-bladder								
Hamster, Syrian golden (M)	4	15–30	BOP, 40 mg/kg bw × 1 s.c., killed at 52 weeks	Dried cabbage, 9.1% of diet, starting 4 weeks before carcinogen or 10.9% starting 1 week after carcinogen	Through-out	Pancreatic ductule carcinomas per animal: high fat, 0.6; cabbage + high fat, 1.6 ($p < 0.05$) Gall-bladder adenocarcinoma TI (%): no cabbage, 3; cabbage, 12 ($p < 0.05$)	Cabbage diet enhanced pancreatic and gall-bladder tumours	Birt *et al.* (1987)
Skin								
Mouse, Sencar (F)	5	10–30	DMBA, 10 nmol × 1 + TPA, 2 µg twice per week beginning 1 week after DMBA, topically, killed at 24 weeks	Dried cabbage, 10% of diet, starting 4 weeks before carcinogen	Through-out	Skin papillomas per mouse: TPA, 7.25 after 22 weeks of promotion; cabbage + TPA, 8.45 ($p < 0.001$)	Cabbage diet enhanced skin tumours	Birt *et al.* (1987)
Spermatic cord and others								
Mouse, C57/Bl/6 (M)	Weanlin g	19–89	Dimethylhy-drazine, 20 mg/kg bw weekly × 36, s.c., killed at 36 weeks	Dehydrated cabbage, 10%, 20%, 40% of diet	Through-out	TI (%): dimethylhydrazine alone, 30.5; + 10% cabbage, 40.4; + 20% cabbage, 46.1; + 40% cabbage, 15.8 Spermatic cord TI (%): dimethylhydrazine alone, 23.2; + 10% cabbage, 29.8; + 20% cabbage, 34.9; + 40% cabbage, 15.8	Diets containing 10% and 20% cabbage enhanced dimethyl-hydrazine-induced tumorigenicity, while cabbage at 40% provided a protective effect	Srisangnam *et al.* (1980)

s.c., subcutaneously; DMBA, 7,12-dimethylbenz[a]anthracene; M, male; F, female; TPA, 12-O-tetradecanoyl-13-phorbol acetate; BOP, *N*-nitrosobis(2-oxo-propyl)amine

Isothiocyanates

Like most agents that disrupt or impair biological processes, isothiocyanates can also have adverse effects, including tumour promotion, weak tumorigenicity, genotoxicity and slight, transient organ toxicity. Whether an isothiocyanate inhibits or enhances tumorigenesis depends on its alkyl chain length, the animal species, the target organ, the time and duration of treatment, the dose and the carcinogen used to induce the tumours. The studies in which enhancement of carcinogenicity was observed are summarized in Table 62.

Tumour promotion

Oesophagus

Stoner et al. (1995) reported that oesophageal carcinogenesis was enhanced in male Fischer 344 rats by 6-phenylhexyl-ITC, a synthetic ITC, given in the diet for 2 weeks before challenge with N-nitrosomethylbenzylamine (NMBA) (0.5 mg/kg bw once a week for 15 weeks by subcutaneous injection), and continued in the diet for the remainder of the 21-week experimental period. 6-Phenylhexyl-ITC increased the number of NMBA-induced oesophageal tumours at all dietary concentrations (0.4, 1.0 and 2.5 µmol/g of diet), with significant increases at 1.0 and 2.5 µmol/g: the tumour multiplicity increased from 7.2 papillomas per oesophagus in controls given NMBA alone to 11.6 and 12.2, respectively. There was no effect on tumour incidence or size.

Colon

Dietary 6-phenylhexyl-ITC given in the diet at 640 or 320 mg/kg 2 weeks before treatment with azoxymethane (subcutaneous injection of 15 mg/kg bw, once a week for 2 weeks) and for the duration of the experiment (52 weeks) increased tumorigenicity in the intestine of male Fischer 344 rats (Rao et al., 1995). At the higher dietary concentration, the incidence of intestinal adenocarcinomas (small intestine and colon) was significantly increased (81% to 97%), as was the multiplicity of invasive and non-invasive adenocarcinomas of the colon (0.53 to 0.86 and 0.97 to 1.67, respectively). At the lower concentration of 6-phenylhexyl-ITC, the multiplicity of non-invasive adenocarcinomas was significantly increased in the colon (0.97 to 1.46) but not in the small intestine. The tumour volume in the colon was increased by approximately twofold (at 320 mg/kg) and 4.3-fold (at 640 mg/kg), and at the higher concentration the tumour size was significantly increased (tumours > 1 cm increased from 10 to 35). In addition, COX-2 and LOX activities were increased by approximately twofold at the higher concentration of 6-phenylhexyl-ITC in both colon mucosa and colon tumours.

Liver and urinary bladder

Phenethyl-ITC and benzyl-ITC were reported to have promoting activity on bladder carcinogenesis in male Fischer 344 rats (Hirose et al., 1998). Rats were pretreated with a single intraperitoneal injection of N-nitrosodiethylamine (NDEA) at 200 mg/kg bw and 2 days later were given drinking-water containing N-butyl-N-(4-hydroxybutyl)nitrosamine (BBN) for 4 weeks. Three days after the end of BBN treatment, phenethyl-ITC or benzyl-ITC was added to the powdered diet at 0.1%, and animals were maintained on this diet until they were killed at 32 weeks. The number of rats with papillary and nodular hyperplasia or carcinoma of the bladder was increased from 57% to 100% and from 24% to 100%, respectively, with both compounds. Phenethyl-ITC, but not benzyl-ITC, also significantly increased the number of altered liver cell foci > 0.5 mm in liver, from 1.05 to 1.45 per cm^2.

Using the same dosing schedule but varying the concentration of phenethyl-ITC, Ogawa et al. (2001) also found an increased incidence of papillary or nodular hyperplasia (73% to 100%) with phenethyl-ITC at a concentration of 0.1%, 0.05% or 0.01% in the diet and an increase in the frequency of dysplasia (33% to 73% and 100% at 0.01%, 0.05% and 0.1%, respectively). The frequency of transitional-cell carcinoma increased from 20% to 100% at 0.1% and 0.05%. More importantly, phenethyl-ITC at the two highest concentrations increased the incidence of invasive carcinoma from 0% to 67% and 93%. In the liver, both the number (per cm^2) and area (mm^2/cm^2) of GST-P$^+$ foci were increased with phenethyl-ITC at 0.1% and 0.05% of diet (in number from 5.8 to 17.8 and 11.9 and in area from 0.4 to 1.18 and 0.8, respectively).

Mammary gland

Lubet et al. (1997) found that phenethyl-ITC actually decreased the latency for mammary tumours in female Sprague-Dawley rats, slightly increased the tumour incidence and increased tumour multiplicity. Phenethyl-ITC was given to rats in the diet at a concentration of 1200 or 600 mg/kg, beginning 1 week before dosing with 12 mg of DMBA by gavage. Phenethyl-ITC at 1200 mg/kg also weakly induced hyperplasia in the bladders of all rats and increased the liver:body weight ratio. Using a different chemoprevention scheme, Ino et al. (1996) also found that benzyl-ITC lacked inhibitory activity for mammary tumorigenesis. Benzyl-ITC at 400 mg/kg in a high-fat diet (23.5% corn oil) was fed to Sprague-Dawley rats, beginning 1 week before dosing with the carcinogen 2-amino-1-methyl-6-phenylimidazo[4,5-b]pyridine (PhIP) at 100 mg/kg bw eight times over 16 days by gavage. One week after the final PhIP dose, the rats were given the high-fat diet only. After 31 weeks, rats given PhIP alone had a tumour incidence of 74.2% and a tumour

Table 62. Promoting effect of isothiocyanates (ITCs) on carcinogen-induced tumours in male Fischer 344 rats

Organ site	Age at start (weeks)	No. per group	Carcinogen, route, dose, duration	ITC, dose, route	Timing of treatment	Effect on tumour incidence (TI) or multiplicity (TM)	Reference
Oesopha-gus	6–7	15	NMBA, s.c., 0.5 mg/kg bw, once a week for 15 weeks	6-Phenylhexyl-ITC, 0.4, 1, 2.5 μmol/g diet	2 weeks before, during and after NMBA	At 21 weeks, no effect on TI; at 1 and 2.5 μmol/g, significantly enhanced TM	Stoner et al. (1995)
Colon	5	12–36	Azoxymethane, s.c., 15 mg/kg bw, once a week for 2 weeks	6-Phenylhexyl-ITC, 320 or 640 mg/kg diet	2 weeks before azoxymethane to termination at 52 weeks	At 640 mg/kg, significantly enhanced TI, TM and tumour volume At 320 mg/kg, increased TM and tumour volume	Rao et al. (1995)
Urinary bladder, liver	6	21	NDEA, i.p., 200 mg/kg bw once, after 2 days BBN, drinking-water, 0.05%, 4 weeks	Phenethyl-ITC, 0.1% or benzyl-ITC, 0.1% in diet for 32 weeks	3 days after BBN	Both ITCs increased incidences of papillary or nodular hyperplasia and carcinoma of bladder. Phenethyl-ITC, but not benzyl-ITC, increased foci in liver	Hirose et al. (1998)
Urinary bladder, liver	6	15	NDEA, i.p., 200 mg/kg bw, once, after 2 days BBN in drinking-water at 0.05%, 4 weeks	Phenethyl-ITC, 0.01%, 0.05%, 0.1%, in diet for 32 weeks	3 days after BBN	At 0.05% and 0.1%, significantly increased papillary or nodular lesions, dysplasia and carcinomas of bladder in carcinogen-promoted animals. Also weakly promoted hepato-carcinogenesis	Ogawa et al. (2001)

s.c., subcutaneously; i.p., intraperitoneally; NMBA, N-nitrosomethylbenzylamine; NDEA, N-nitrosodiethylamine; BBN, N-butyl-N-(4 hydroxybutyl)-nitrosamine multiplicity of 1.71, and those given benzyl-ITC and PhIP had an incidence of 62.5% and a multiplicity of 1.91; the mean size of tumours in benzyl-ITC-treated rats increased, although not statistically significantly, from 9.9 mm to 10.8 mm.

Carcinogenicity

Hirose *et al.* (1998) found that feeding a diet containing phenethyl-ITC or benzyl-ITC at 1000 mg/kg without carcinogen treatment increased the incidence of papillary or nodular hyperplasia in the bladder of Fischer 344 rats (from 0 to 100%) but did not increase the number of foci in the liver.

Similarly, Ogawa *et al.* (2001) found that phenethyl-ITC in the diet at 500 or 1000 mg/kg without carcinogen pretreatment increased the frequencies of simple hyperplasia (from 0 to 100%), papillary or nodular hyperplasia (from 0 to 100%) and dysplasia (from 0 to 53% and 80%).

Okazaki *et al.* (2002) found that benzyl-ITC in the diet at 100 or 1000 mg/kg resulted in an increased frequency of epithelial hyperplasia in the bladder and suggested that benzyl-ITC not only did not inhibit bladder carcinogenesis but might also have a weak carcinogenic effect.

In another study with phenethyl-ITC, Sugiura *et al.* (2003) reported that feeding Fischer 344 rats a diet containing phenethyl-ITC at 1000 mg/kg for 48 weeks or for 32 weeks with normal diet for 1, 3 or 7 days or 16 weeks before death resulted in high incidences of simple and papillary or nodular hyperplasia, dysplasia and carcinoma (transitional-cell carcinoma with squamous-cell carcinoma and adenocarcinoma components). Phen-ethyl-ITC at 1000 mg/kg of diet for 32 weeks and then basal diets increased the incidence of simple and papillary or nodular hyperplasia from 0 to 100% and that of dysplasia from 0 to 67% and 92% when animals were killed 7 days and 16

weeks after removal of phenethyl-ITC from the diet. Furthermore, the incidence of carcinoma increased from 0 to 33% and 58%, respectively. Treatment of animals for 48 weeks with phenethyl-ITC increased the incidence of simple and papillary or nodular hyperplasia and dysplasia from 0 to 100% and the incidence of carcinoma from 0 to 92% (11/12 animals). Although the area of bladder mucosa occupied by hyperplasia was reduced after removal of phenethyl-ITC after 32 weeks, the numbers of animals with dysplasia and carcinoma actually increased, showing tumour progression in the absence of phenethyl-ITC. The areas of hyperplasia that were reversible were those showing little atypia.

Allyl-ITC was administered at 12 or 25 mg/kg bw in corn oil five times per week by gavage to groups of 50 Fischer 344 rats and 50 B6C3F$_1$ mice of each sex for 103 weeks. Groups of 50 rats and 50 mice of each sex received corn oil alone and served as vehicle controls. Transitional-cell papillomas in the urinary bladder occurred in treated male rats with a statistically significant trend ($p < 0.05$; controls, 0/49; lower dose, 2/49, 4%; higher dose, 4/49, 8%). Administration of allyl-ITC also increased the prevalence of epithelial hyperplasia in the urinary bladder in male rats. No evidence of an association between administration of allyl-ITC and increased tumour incidence was seen in the mice (Dunnick *et al.*, 1982).

Indoles

The initial studies on the chemopreventive effects of indole-3-carbinol (Wattenberg & Loub, 1978; Bailey *et al.*, 1982) addressed its efficacy as a 'blocking agent', that is, when given before or during carcinogen treatment. These and subsequent studies showed that indole-3-carbinol is an effective chemopreventive agent

against a variety of chemical carcinogens and in a variety of target organs and animal models (see section 4). Studies of its efficacy against estrogen-driven cancers, especially breast cancer, have attracted special attention; however, with few exceptions, these studies did not address its efficacy in animals in which cancer had already been initiated, that is, post-initiation or 'suppression' effects. Several such studies suggest that certain protocols result in enhanced tumour response in carcinogen-treated animals (Table 63).

Protocol-dependent tumour promotion in liver and mammary gland

The first evidence that dietary indole-3-carbinol treatment might have deleterious consequences came from studies with models of colon and liver carcinogenesis. In a multi-factorial design for studying colon cancer (Pence *et al.*, 1986), indole-3-carbinol fed to mice before, during and after dimethylhydrazine was found to act synergistically with tallow and cholesterol to increase the tumour response. More direct evidence that indole-3-carbinol promotes tumours was provided by studies of liver carcinogenesis. While dietary co-treatment with indole-3-carbinol resuted in strong, dose-dependent decreases in aflatoxin B$_1$–DNA adduction and hepatocarcinogenesis in rainbow trout (Bailey *et al.*, 1982; Dashwood *et al.*, 1988, 1989b), subsequent treatment with indole-3-carbinol of trout previously initiated with aflatoxin B$_1$ resulted in potent tumour promotion (Bailey *et al.*, 1987; Dashwood *et al.*, 1990, 1991; Dashwood, 1998). These experiments provided reproducible evidence that indole-3-carbinol has multi-functional activity in vivo, with protocol-dependent potential to enhance as well as reduce cancer risk.

The finding of promotion in trout was confirmed and extended in

Table 63. Promoting effect of indole-3-carbinol on carcinogen-induced tumours in rats

Strain (sex), organ	Age at start (weeks)	No. per group	Carcinogen, route, dose, duration	Indole-3-carbinol dose, route	Timing of treatment	Effect observed on tumour incidence (TI) or multiplicity (TM)	Reference
Sprague-Dawley (M), liver	6	11–15	NDEA, 200 mg/kg bw, i.p.	0.25%, diet	2 weeks before or after NDEA for 6 weeks	Decreased hepatic GST-P⁺ foci before initiation; increased number and area after initiation	Kim et al. (1994)
Sprague-Dawley (M), multiple organs	6	10–20	NDEA, MNU, DHPN	0.25%, diet	1 week after carcinogen for 20 weeks	Significant GST-P⁺ foci promotion at week 24, non-significant liver adenoma promotion at week 52, significant enhancement of thyroid tumours at week 52	Kim et al. (1997)
Sprague-Dawley (F), multiple organs	54 days	20	DMBA, aflatoxin B₁, azoxy-methane	2000 mg/kg, diet, 25 weeks, weeks 5–30	After last carcinogen treatment on day 29	500% increase in hepatic GST-P⁺ foci	Stoner et al. (2002)
Sprague-Dawley (F), mammary gland	7	19	DMBA, 20 mg, orally	250 mg/kg bw, three times a week, 12 weeks	3 weeks after DMBA	No inhibition	Malejka-Giganti et al. (2000)
Sprague-Dawley (F), mammary gland	4	24–34	MNU, 50 mg/kg bw, i.p.	100 or 300 mg/kg, diet, 24 weeks	1 week after MNU	Increased TI and TM at 300 mg/kg bw	Kang et al. (2001)
Fischer 344 (M), colon	4–5	20–23	Dimethyl-hydrazine, 20 mg/kg bw, once a week, 5 weeks, s.c.	1000 mg/kg, 1 year, diet	1 week after last carcinogen treatment	No effect	Xu et al. (2001)

NDEA, N-nitrosodiethylamine; MNU, N-methyl-N-nitrosourea; DHPN, dihydroxy-di-N-propylnitrosamine; DMBA, 7,12-dimethylbenz[a]anthracene; i.p., intraperitoneally; S.C., subcutaneously; F, female; M, male

Chapter 7

Toxic effects

Adverse effects

The classic toxic effect of cruciferous vegetables is goitrogenicity, which has been described in cattle and humans and is caused by goitrin and other compounds derived from certain *Brassica* seeds.

Humans
Brassica vegetables
Owing to the high content of vitamin K in broccoli, drug interactions have been reported in patients receiving medication for hypoprothrombinaemia. Two such cases were reported in women who ate 230–450 g/day of broccoli (Kempin, 1983). One survey showed that most health-care professionals (> 87%) were aware of possible interactions between warfarin medication and the high content of vitamin K in certain *Brassica* vegetables, such as broccoli, whereas fewer [55%, read from figure] knew about the potential drug interaction with white cabbage (Couris *et al.*, 2000).

Drug interactions as a consequence of effects of cruciferous vegetables on xenobiotic metabolizing enzymes are also well known from controlled human intervention studies (see section 4 for more detail). In one study on the effects of eating 400 g/day of Brussels sprouts for 2 weeks on warfarin clearance, a 29% increase was observed (Ovesen *et al.*, 1988). The effect of eating Brussels sprouts and cabbage on the clearance of antipyrine, oxazepam and acetaminophen has also been assessed in controlled human intervention studies. The drugs were excreted significantly

faster (by 10–20%) after intervention with cruciferous vegetables at a level of 250 g/day (Pantuck *et al.*, 1979, 1984).

Endemic goitre was common in many countries in the past century and in many European countries as late as 1985. Only the Nordic countries and the United Kingdom had succeeded by that time in decreasing the prevalence (European Thyroid Association, 1985). Goitre can be controlled by compulsory addition of iodide to all household salt. Several studies were conducted after 1947 on the goitrogenic effects of dietary components and drugs by injecting volunteers with radioiodine and determining uptake into the thyroid by external counting (van Etten *et al.*, 1969a).

A goitrogenic effect of cruciferous vegetables was hypothesized on the basis of field observations of Tasmanian schoolchildren and the source of milk in their homes. The most likely source of the goitrogenic compounds in the diets of these children was the milk of cows given *Brassica* forage crops, particularly during the winter months (Clements, 1957).

In Finland, when goitre was common, it was suspected to be due to low dietary iodine intake in combination with consumption of milk from cows grazing on fields rich in cruciferous vegetation. In an experiment with 22 healthy volunteers (7 women, 15 men) aged 22–46 years, radioiodine uptake into the thyroid was determined while they drank 1.5–2 l of milk containing 0–20.3 µg/l of goitrin, 2.1–8.0 mg/l of SCN^- and 8–142 µg/l of I^- (Vilkki *et al.*, 1962). No effects were found on radioiodine uptake, plasma-bound iodine or total serum iodine. In an

experiment in which a single dose of 0.15–100 mg of goitrin was given to volunteers [number per group not given], a reduction in radioiodine uptake was seen at doses ≥ 50 mg.

Shortly after injection of ^{131}I and determinations of baseline uptake, groups of two men or women [sex not specified for each group] were given crystalline goitrin at one of six doses from 12.5 to 400 mg (Langer *et al.*, 1971). A dose-related decrease in radioiodine intake was observed, with 50% inhibition at around 300 mg [value read from curve]. In two further experiments described in the same publication, each individual served as his or her own control by undergoing two tests for radioiodine uptake 1 week apart. After a baseline test for radioiodine uptake 1 week earlier, six volunteers received 50 mg of crystalline goitrin, and 13 received 25 mg 1 h before the second test. A third group of 18 volunteers were given 10 mg of crystalline goitrin 12 h before and another 10 mg 1 h before the second test. Radioiodine uptake was statistically significantly decreased in the two former groups, whereas no decline was observed in the third group. In two individuals given 50 mg, uptake of radioiodine was completely blocked. Reduced iodine uptake by the thyroid gland was observed with the radioiodine test after a daily intake of 500–600 g of cabbage (raw, pickled, boiled or quick-steamed) for 2 weeks by a group of nine volunteers [previous work cited by Langer *et al.* (1971)]. Each individual served as his or her own control by comparison with a baseline test performed 6 months earlier.

In a parallel study of the effects of ingestion of 150 g of Brussels sprouts daily for 4 weeks by a group of three women and seven men, no effects were observed on serum concentrations of thyrotropic hormone, total or free thyroxine or total triiodothyronine (McMillan et al., 1986). The sprouts variety had been selected for its high content of progoitrin and glucobrassicin, and the daily doses of these compounds were confirmed by food analyses to be 99 mg and 105 mg, respectively; however, the daily intakes were decreased to 69 mg and 39 mg, respectively, by cooking. The intake of progoitrin in this study could have led to an intake of 14 mg of the goitrogenic goitrin. The authors speculated that the low (2.4%) residual activity of myrosinase in the sprouts decreased the formation of goitrogenic derivatives and was indirectly the cause of the null effect observed in this study.

Indoles

Groups of 20 women at high risk for breast cancer were assigned to 400 mg/day indole-3-carbinol or placebo for 3 months. They were interviewed monthly about any adverse effects, and blood samples were collected for extensive clinical chemistry. No systematic adverse effects were reported, and there was no effect on plasma bilirubin and albumin or on serum glutamyl ornithine transaminase, suggesting no effect on liver function. Also, plasma estrogen and the number of days between menses were unaffected (Bradlow et al., 1994).

In a double-blind placebo-controlled dose-ranging study, 57 women of an average age of 46.7 years (range, 22–74 years) who were at increased risk for breast cancer were randomized into groups of 7–10 and given indole-3-carbinol at a dose of 0–400 mg/day for 4 weeks (Wong et al., 1997). No toxicity or consistent adverse effects were reported.

In a prospective open-label trial, indole-3-carbinol was given to 18 patients aged 1.2–66 years with recurrent respiratory papillomatosis; the children received a weight-related dose of 5–10 mg/kg bw per day, while the adults took 200 mg twice a day for 8–24 months (average, 14.6 months). Symptoms of disequilibrium developed in three persons who took excessive doses, one of whom was a male volunteer given 800 mg/day for 10 days. Light tremor was also observed. These symptoms disappeared when the dose was decreased to 400 mg/day. Two girls aged 2.5 years and 12 years who accidentally took triple doses both experienced unsteadiness for periods of 8–24 h (Rosen et al., 1998).

Experimental animals
Acute toxicity
Glucosinolates and nitriles
The reported values for the median lethal dose (LD$_{50}$) of Brassica compounds in animals are shown in Table 64.

The acute toxic effects of subcutaneously injected Brassica glucosinolates and nitrites were studied in groups of 5–8 Holtzman rats of each sex, maintained on Teklad 4% mouse and rat diet and weighing 250–300 g (Nishie & Daxenbichler 1980). Some of the rats were pregnant. Indole-3-carbinol and 3-indolylacetonitrile induced sedation, ataxia, loss of righting reflex and sleep. In general, they were less toxic in pregnant females and more toxic in the younger male rats. Several other compounds were tested at only one or two doses, administered by a single or by two repeated subcutaneous injections. The kidneys, livers and adrenal and thyroid glands were examined histologically at necropsy or 12 days after dosing. 1-Cyano-3,4-epithiobutane (total dose, about 90 mg/kg bw) gave rise to increased renal weights and renal necrosis in pregnant dams, and signs

of restorative growth were observed in survivors. Abnormal thyroids were observed in non-pregnant females given acutely toxic doses (150–650 mg/kg bw) of epi-progoitrin, 3-indolylacetonitrile, S-1-cyano-2-hydroxy-3-butene or R-goitrin, in the form of hyperplastic cells, smaller follicles, foamy areas and scanty colloid, whereas the thyroids of pregnant females were largely unaffected by these compounds. Slightly hyperplastic thyroids were observed in pregnant and non-pregnant rats after near-lethal doses (100–700 mg/kg bw; see Table 64) of 1-cyano-3,4-epithiobutane, sinigrin (including oral administration), sinalbin hydrate, para-hydroxyphenylacetonitrile, iberin nitrile, 3-indolylacetonitrile and indole-3-carbinol. Iberin at an acutely toxic dose (100 mg/ kg bw) did not affect thyroid tissue in rats. Sporadic changes in liver and adrenal weights were found with the nitrites. 1-Cyano-3,4-epithiobutane consistently increased adrenal weights of males and pregnant female rats by 25–50% at a dose of 95 mg/kg bw.

In order to determine the lethal dose, high single doses of the compounds were administered subcutaneously to Sprague-Dawley rats. The rats were observed for 12 days after dosing, at which time they were killed. The mean LD$_{50}$ values were 90 mg/kg bw for iberin, 109 mg/kg bw for 1-cyano-3,4-epithiobutane, 200 mg/kg bw for S-1-cyano-2-hydroxy-3-butene and 255 mg/kg bw for 3-indolylacetonitrile; values could not be determined for indole-3-carbinol or para-hydroxyphenylacetonitrile, although their acute toxicity was similar to that of 3-indolylacetonitrile.

Isothiocyanates and derivatives
In the study of Nishie and Daxenbichler (1980), the mean LD$_{50}$ value for allyl-ITC was reported to be 92 mg/kg bw (see Table 64). Mildly abnormal thyroid tissues were

Table 64. Median lethal doses (LD$_{50}$) of *Brassica* compounds

Compound	Species, strain	Route of administration	Duration of follow-up	LD$_{50}$ (mg/kg bw)	Reference
1-Cyano-3,4-epithio-butane	Mouse	Oral	Not specified	178–240	van Etten *et al.* (1969a)
	Rat, Sprague-Dawley	Subcutaneous	12 days	109	Nishie & Daxenbichler (1980)
	Mouse	Oral	Not specified	170	van Etten *et al.* (1969a)
	Rat, Sprague-Dawley	Subcutaneous	12 days	200	Nishie & Daxenbichler (1980)
Allyl-ITC	Mouse (white)	Subcutaneous	14 days	80	Klesse & Lukoschek (1955)
	Rat	Oral		339	Jenner *et al.* (1964)
	Rat, Sprague-Dawley	Subcutaneous	12 days	92	Nishie & Daxenbichler (1980)
Phenethyl-ITC	Mouse (white)	Subcutaneous	14 days	250	Klesse & Lukoschek (1955)
	Mouse, Swiss-Webster	Subcutaneous	14 days	150	Lichtenstein *et al.* (1962)
		Oral	14 days	700	
		Intravenous	14 days	50	
Goitrin	Mouse	Oral	Not specified	1260–1415	van Etten *et al.* (1969a)
Iberin	Rat, Sprague-Dawley	Subcutaneous	12 days	90	Nishie & Daxenbichler (1980)
Indole-3-carbinol	Mouse, ICR	Oral	10 days cumulative	1670	Shertzer (1982)
		Intraperitoneal	10 days cumulative	500	
	Mouse, CD1	Oral	1 h	<750	Shertzer & Sainsbury (1991a)
	Rat, Wistar	Oral	10 days cumulative	1850	Shertzer (1982)
		Intraperitoneal	10 days cumulative	550	
	Rabbit, white	Oral	10 days cumulative	1400	
		Intraperitoneal	10 days cumulative	420	
3-Indolylacetonitrile	Rat, Sprague-Dawley	Subcutaneous	12 days	255	Nishie & Daxenbichler (1980)

observed in pregnant and non-pregnant rats after near-lethal doses. The LD_{50} of a 10% solution of allyl-ITC given subcutaneously in corn oil to mice was reported to be 80 mg/kg bw (IARC, 1985).

The acute toxicity of allyl-ITC in groups of five Fischer 344/N rats and five $B6C3F_1$ mice of each sex was examined in pilot studies before a long-term cancer bioassay (National Toxicology Program, 1982). After 16 days' administration of allyl-ITC in corn oil by gavage, growth retardation and dose-related signs of toxicity were seen at doses of 200 and 400 mg/kg bw in rats and 100–800 mg/kg bw in mice, evaluated on the basis of comparisons with the lowest dose (no controls). No female mice and only one male mouse survived the dose of 800 mg/kg bw.

Groups of five male and five female Osborne-Mendel rats were fasted for 18 h and then given a single high dose of allyl-ITC by gavage and observed for 14 days. An LD_{50} of 339 mg/kg bw (95% confidence interval, 318–361) was calculated (Jenner et al., 1964). The animals were described as scrawny, with porphyrin-like deposits around the eyes and nose and rough fur.

The LD_{50} values for phenethyl-ITC in mice were reported to be 700 mg/kg bw after oral administration and 50 mg/kg bw after intravenous injection. In the same species, the LD_{50} of phenethyl-ITC administered subcutaneously was reported to be 150 mg/kg bw (Lichtenstein et al., 1962) or 250 mg/kg bw (Klesse & Lukoschek, 1955).

In a study presented in an overview (van Etten et al., 1969a), the LD_{50} values in mice were 1260–1415 mg/kg bw for goitrin (R-5-vinyloxazolidine-2-thione), 169 mg/kg bw for S-1-cyano-2-hydroxy-3-butene and 178–240 mg/kg bw for S-1-cyano-2-hydroxy-3,4-epithiobutane.

Indoles

Preliminary LD_{50} values were determined by Shertzer (1982) in male ICR mice, Wistar rats and New Zealand white rabbits treated with indole-3-carbinol for 10 days (Table 64). Male ICR mice, weighing about 30 g bw, were maintained on Purina animal chow and dosed orally or intraperitoneally for 10 consecutive days. The LD_{50} in male ICR mice was estimated to be 500 mg/kg bw after intraperitoneal administration and 1670 mg/kg bw when given by gavage. In male Wistar rats (weighing 300 g), the LD_{50} values for intraperitoneal and oral administration were 550 mg/kg bw and 1850 mg/kg bw, respectively, whereas the LD_{50} values for rabbits (male New Zealand white, weighing about 2 kg) were 420 mg/kg bw when given intraperitoneally and 1400 mg/kg when administered orally. No further details about the experiments were given.

The acute toxicity of indole-3-carbinol was studied in groups of male CD-1 mice weighing 30–35 g, maintained on Teklad standard rodent diet for 7 days and then given indole-3-carbinol orally at 50 mg/kg bw per day (dissolved in corn oil, 1.5 µl/g bw) for 10 days (Shertzer & Sainsbury, 1991a). Indole-3-carbinol did not change the body weight or the liver:body weight ratio. The activity of several plasma enzymes was determined 2 and 24 h after a single oral dose of 50–500 mg/kg bw. Plasma creatine phospho-kinase activity was not changed at doses up to 500 mg/kg bw, indicating a lack of severe cardiotoxicity; however, indole-3-carbinol caused a dose-dependent increase in plasma ornithine transcarbamylase activity (at doses > 100 mg/kg bw) and alanine transaminase activity (at doses > 250 mg/kg bw), indicating a hepatotoxic effect, 24 h after treatment. Indole-3-carbinol decreased the hepatic GSH concentration in a dose-dependent manner 2 h after oral doses

> 100 mg/kg bw; the concentration had returned to background levels by 24 h at doses < 250 mg/kg bw. Leaking of hepatic enzymes into the bloodstream was seen at doses > 100 mg/kg bw. Neurological signs, including changes in posture and activity, were seen at doses ≥ 100 mg/kg bw 2 h after gavage. A dose of 500 mg/kg bw induced coma.

A single oral administration of indole-3-carbinol at a dose > 100 µmol per rat (15 mg/kg bw) to groups of four male Sprague-Dawley rats, 3–4 weeks old and maintained on a semi-purified diet for 7–8 days, led to toxic manifestations in the small intestine (Bradfield & Bjeldanes, 1987b).

Groups of six male guinea-pigs, weighing 400–500 g, were given two oral doses of indole-3-carbinol at 0.3 mg/kg bw per day for 4 days. The animals were killed after treatment on day 4, and four tissue samples were collected from the liver and lung of each animal and examined histopathologically. Indole-3-carbinol caused hepatic steatosis and interstitial pneumonia with septal hyperaemia (Gonzalez et al., 1986).

Short-term effects
Brassicas

Crambe oilseed meals processed to increase or decrease the levels of epi-progoitrin, goitrin or total nitriles were given at 10% in the feed to groups of five weanling rats for 90 days, and the weight and survival of the animals were recorded as a measure of toxicity (van Etten et al., 1969b). Fractions of epi-progoitrin (0.85%), R-goitrin (0.23%) and nitrile (0.1%) isolated from crambe seeds were mixed into the feed for additional groups. The nitrile-rich meals were the most toxic, leading to 100% mortality in a group fed 10% (w/w) meal treated to enrich nitriles, and a 40% reduction in body weight in a similar group in a second experiment. The weight of animals fed

0.1% nitrile fraction in the feed was only 17% that of controls (60% survival). Animals fed meal containing active myrosinase had only 40–60% weight gain and reduced survival. These meals had high concentrations of *epi*-progoitrin. The animals fed purified *epi*-progoitrin or *R*-goitrin reached 85% of the weight of controls.

Isothiocyanates and derivatives

WIST male rats weighing 70–90 g [number of animals per group not reported] were given allyl-ITC at a dose of 10, 20 or 40 mg/kg bw (5 days/week) by gavage for up to 6 weeks (Lewerenz *et al.*, 1988). The highest dose reduced body-weight gain and decreased blood glucose and serum globulin levels. Examination of the blood revealed an increased percentage of neutrophils and a decreased percentage of lymphocytes after treatment with the highest dose for 2 weeks. After 1–3 weeks, increased thymus, liver or adrenal weights (both relative and absolute) were found in all treated groups. Increasing the treatment period to 4 weeks resulted in no significant differences in thymus, liver or adrenal weights between treated and control animals. Renal dysfunction was indicated by increased urinary aspartate aminotransferase activity, reduced urine volume and changes in the specific gravity of the urine in the group of rats receiving the highest dose. Histopathological changes were observed in the kidneys of animals given 20 or 40 mg/kg bw per day and in the livers of animals at 40 mg/kg bw per day.

The toxicity of allyl-ITC after repeated doses was investigated in pilot studies before a long-term cancer bioassay in rats and mice of each sex. An experiment in which groups of five male and five female Fischer 344/N rats and B6C3F$_1$ mice received doses in corn oil of 25–400 mg/kg bw and 3–50 mg/kg bw, respectively, by gavage for 14 days resulted in 'adhesion of the stomach wall to the peritoneum' in rats and a dose-dependent thickening of the stomach mucosa in both species. Furthermore, mice given the highest dose developed thickening of the urinary-bladder wall. [The Working Group noted that histological details were not presented and that the significance of these findings is uncertain.] The doses of 200 and 400 mg/kg bw per day to rats and 50 mg/kg bw per day to mice were lethal. In a 13-week study in groups of 10 male and female Fischer 344/N rats and B6C3F$_1$ mice given a dose of 1.5, 3, 6, 12 or 25 mg/kg bw per day, no dose-related effects were observed on growth or gross morphology (National Toxicology Program, 1982).

Administration of phenethyl-ITC at a dose of 41, 82 or 122 mg/kg bw per day for 6 days by gavage to groups of 24 female and 24 male young A/J mice resulted in significantly reduced body-weight gains [absolute numbers not specified], hyperactivity, rough fur and emaciation (Adam-Rodwell *et al.*, 1993). A dose of 244 mg/kg bw per day was lethal after two to four doses and was discontinued.

The toxicity of benzyl-ITC was investigated in groups of 15 male rats weighing 85–110 g given the compound dissolved in sunflower oil at a dose of 50, 100 or 200 mg/kg bw per day by gavage for 4 weeks (Lewerenz *et al.*, 1992). Control rats were given the vehicle only. Body-weight gain and food consumption were decreased with increasing doses of benzyl-ITC. Haematological changes were observed at the highest dose, with increased serum cholesterol concentrations in all treated groups and decreased serum triglycerides at 200 mg/kg bw per day. Renal dysfunction was indicated by reduced urine volume, proteinuria and enhanced urinary lactate dehydrogenase activity.

Benzyl-ITC at 200 mg/kg bw per day caused histological changes in the ductus choledochus, liver, ileum and mesenteric lymph nodes. The weights of the thymus (at 100 and 200 mg/kg bw per day) and spleen (at 200 mg/kg bw per day) were decreased in relation to body weight, whereas the weights of all other organs were increased.

Even at a low dose of 7.5 mg/kg bw per day to ACI rats for 53 weeks, benzyl-ITC resulted in a decrease in weight gain of 8–9% as compared with control animals (Sugie *et al.*, 1991).

Morse *et al.* (1989a) examined the toxicity of phenethyl-ITC at 0, 0.75, 1.5, 3 or 6 μmol/g of diet in male Fischer 344 rats (weighing 100–120 g) in a 13-week study. Dietary administration of phenethyl-ITC did not produce any deleterious effects on survival, body weight or food intake. Clinical evaluation showed no adverse changes suggesting toxicity. In addition, no significant differences from control animals were found on gross examination at necropsy or by determination of relative organ weights. Histopathological analyses, however, revealed centribular and mid-zonal fatty metamorphosis in the livers of rats exposed to phenethyl-ITC at all doses tested.

Indoles

Groups of eight male Sprague-Dawley rats weighing 70 g were given a control diet or control diet containing either glucobrassicin at 0.5 g/kg [30 mg/kg bw per day], sinigrin, gluconapin, glucosinalbin or glucotropaeolin each at 1.0 g/kg [60 mg/kg bw per day] or progoitrin at 3.0 mg/kg [160 mg/kg bw per day] for 29 days. Before treatment, the animals were held on control diet for 2 days, for 1 day on control diet containing 50% of the final glucosinolate level and for 1 day on control diet containing 75% of the final glucosinolate level. The dietary glucosinolates did not affect feed intake or body-weight gain throughout the period. Only progoitrin affected the relative weights of the thyroid, liver and kidney (Vermorel et al., 1986).

The effect of indoles on body weight was investigated in groups of six male weanling Sprague-Dawley rats fed AIN76 diet containing indole-3-carbinol at 50, 500, 5000 or 7500 mg/kg ad libitum for 3 weeks (Babish & Stoewsand, 1978). Significantly lower body-weight gain was observed with 5000 mg/kg [1500 mg/kg bw per day] and 7500 mg/kg [2250 mg/kg bw per day], representing 85% and 59% of the weight gain of untreated controls, respectively. The relative liver weights were increased by 1.6- and 1.8-fold, respectively, in these two groups. In another study, indole-3-carbinol was given by gavage at 5, 25, 50, 100 or 200 mg per day for 6 weeks to female Sprague-Dawley rats from 43 days of age (Grubbs et al., 1995). The highest dose caused a 10% depression in body-weight gain and a 20% increase in liver weight. The modifying effect of indole-3-carbinol was investigated in a multi-organ carcinogenesis model in groups of 20 male Fischer 344 rats, 6 weeks of age, maintained on AIN-76A diet for 4 weeks and then switched to the same diet containing 0.5% indole-3-carbinol for 36 weeks [300 mg/kg bw per day]. An insignificant decrease in body weight was observed (Jang et al., 1991).

The effect of dietary indole-3-carbinol on liver and body weight was investigated in groups of six female C3H/OuJ adult mice, 80–100 days old, maintained on Purina basal diet with 10% corn oil for 3 days and then given the same diet containing indole-3-carbinol at 0, 1000, 3000 or 5000 mg/kg [120, 360 or 600 mg/kg bw per day] for 3 weeks (Bradlow et al., 1991). The average daily food consumption decreased significantly only in mice at the highest dose. The relative liver:body weight ratio increased with

dose. Additionally, groups of six female SW mice, 80–100 days of age, were maintained on Purina basal diet with 10% corn oil for 3 days and then given the same diet containing indole-3-carbinol at 0, 250, 1000 or 2500 mg/kg [30, 120 or 300 mg/kg bw per day] for 3 weeks. No difference in body weight was observed. A slight increase in the liver:body weight ratio was seen in treated animals, but there was no gross evidence of hepatic toxicity. Two groups of 10 male and 10 female C3H/OuJ mice, 21–28 days of age, were kept on control Purina semi-synthetic diet or the same diet containing indole-3-carbinol at 2000 mg/kg [240 mg/kg bw per day] for 6 months. The average body weights of the females in each group were recorded about every 10–15 days. No differences in body weight were observed.

Groups of seven male Sprague-Dawley rats were fed diets containing indole-3-carbinol at concentrations providing a dose of 0, 50, 100 or 150 mg/kg bw per day, 5 days/week for 7 weeks (Exon et al., 2001). The antibody response to an antigen challenge was significantly decreased at the highest dose. No effects were found on natural killer cell activity or delayed-type hypersensitivity.

Goitrogenic effects
Crucifers and unrefined fractions
A goitrogenic effect of crucifers was first noted after feeding Brassica seeds to rabbits (Chesney et al., 1928). Several years later, the effect was found to be due mainly to the formation of organic and inorganic isothiocyanates and goitrins (oxazolidinethiones) (Astwood et al., 1949). Goitrogenic effects in various domestic and laboratory animals have been reviewed (Fenwick et al., 1989; Mawson et al., 1994; Stoewsand, 1995).

Groups of 4–9 male Wistar rats were fed 10–15 g/day of a low-iodine

diet (0.5–0.8 µg/day) with about 40 g of cabbage or carrots (both vegetables contained negligible amounts of iodine), or cabbage or carrots alone, for 60 days (Langer & Stolc, 1965). The thyroid glands were significantly enlarged and contained significantly less iodine per gram of organ. Plasma-bound iodine was also significantly decreased.

Pigs appear to be vulnerable to rapeseed meal glucosinolates. Groups of 7–10 male and female pigs, initially weighing 20–25 kg, received their ordinary diet containing 2–15% unrefined rapeseed meal to replace skim milk powder (Nordfeldt et al., 1954). Thyroid and liver weights were increased in all treated animals. Adding an antibiotic (bacitracin), vitamin B_{12} or wheat bran to the diet did not alleviate the effects. Water extraction of the rapeseed meal significantly attenuated the effect.

Studies in pigs were reviewed by Mawson et al. (1994). A generally linear relationship was observed between glucosinolate intake from feed and thyroid weight at slaughter. Significant increases in thyroid weights were observed in pigs given feed with a total glucosinolate content of 2–3 mg/kg, particularly when progoitrin was one of the main glucosinolates.

Isothiocyanates and derivatives
The spontaneous formation of goitrin from 2-hydroxy-3-butenyl-ITC, resulting from degradation of progoitrogen catalysed by myrosinase, is one of the main causes of the goitrogenic action of rapeseed meal. Groups of eight female Sprague-Dawley rats given a diet containing about twice the minimal required iodine content were given 5-vinyl-2-thiooxazolidone intraperitoneally at a dose of 1–200 µg/day for 3 weeks (Elfving, 1980). Controls were injected with saline. Significant increases in thyroid weights were observed at doses > 5 µg/day. In the

thyroid, significantly increased ratios of 3′-monoiodothyronine:3,5-diiodothyronine and of 3,5,3′-triiodothyronine: 3,5,3′,5′-tetraiodothyronine were observed even at the lowest dose. Total ^{125}I uptake into the thyroid was unchanged at all doses, but iodine excretion into urine was decreased at the highest dose. The authors concluded that goitrin acts primarily on thyroxin biosynthesis.

Allyl-ITC has slight goitrogenic activity in rodents. Studies in rats (weighing 150–320 g) given allyl-ITC as a single dose of 2–4 mg in water by gavage showed 40–60% less iodine uptake into the thyroid gland. Oral administration of allyl-ITC at 2.5–5 mg/day for 60 days, however, did not decrease the total iodine content in the thyroid (Langer & Stolc, 1965).

The degree of goitrogenicity induced by allyl-ITC was found to be weaker than that induced by better-known goitrogens, such as thiouracil (Duncan, 1991).

Indoles
Groups of eight male Sprague-Dawley rats, weighing 70 g, were fed control diet or control diet complemented by glucobrassicin at 0.5 g/kg [30 mg/kg bw per day] for 29 days. Before treatment, the animals were given control diet for 2 days, then control diet containing 50% of the final glucosinolate level for 1 day and finally control diet containing 75% of the final glucosinolate level for 1 day. The animals were killed 29 days after the start of treatment. Neither thyroid weight nor thyroid hormone concentrations in the thyroid were affected (Vermorel et al., 1986).

Haemolytic effects
Kale fed to ruminants in considerable quantities for 1–3 weeks led to haemolytic anaemia due to its content of S-methylcysteine sulfoxide (Smith, 1980). Groups of 52 and 103 goats were fed kale containing S-methylcysteine sulfoxide at 99 or 154 mg/kg. Heinz bodies reached their peak level at 9 and 33 days of the feeding period, respectively, and serum haemoglobin reached minimal levels at 20 and 44 days, respectively. Additional groups of goats received different concentrations: 10 animals received a fractionated kale extract containing S-methylcysteine sulfoxide at 285 mg/kg, 97 animals received S-methylcysteine sulfoxide at 150 mg/kg, and 104 animals received S-methylcysteine sulfoxide at 195 mg/kg. The number of days required to attain maximal formation of Heinz bodies was 7, 35 and 21, and the number of days to reach the lowest haemoglobin level was 15, 42 and 35, respectively.

The metabolite of S-methylcysteine sulfoxide, dimethyl disulfide, precipitates GSH to initiate the formation of Heinz–Ehrlich bodies in erythrocytes. According to a recent review, ruminants, fowl and rats are also vulnerable to anaemia after being fed kale or dimethyl disulfide, but guinea-pigs and rabbits are refractory (Stoewsand, 1995). Dosing of rats with feed containing S-methylcysteine sulfoxide at 2–4% (w/w) elicited the effect, but it was reversible after about 14 days.

Reproductive effects
Decreased fertility has been described repeatedly in domestic animals given rapeseed meal as part of their feed. Mawson et al. (1994) summarized published and anecdotal evidence and concluded that rats and pigs are the most vulnerable species, whereas ruminants and chicken are less sensitive. Pigs may be affected by total rapeseed glucosinolate concentrations exceeding 4 mg/kg of feed, whereas rats appear to tolerate even less.

Groups of 3–12 pregnant Holzman rats were given Brassica glucosinolates and degradation products at doses close to the LD_{50} on day 8 or 9 of gestation, and the numbers of live fetuses and resorptions were examined at necropsy or at termination 12 days later (Nishie & Daxenbichler, 1980). A significant 48% increase in fetal resorption was observed after a single dose of 1-cyano-3,4-epithiobutane at 95 mg/kg bw given on day 8 of gestation, whereas two doses of 44 mg/kg bw on days 8 and 9 did not affect fetal survival. A significant 19% increase in fetal resorption was observed after two doses of allyl-ITC at 100 mg/kg bw on days 8 and 9 of gestation, whereas one-half of this dose on the same days had no effect. Administration of iberin at 100 mg/kg bw on day 8 of gestation increased fetal resorption by 29%. None of these compounds resulted in malformations. Significant changes in mean fetal weights were recorded with epigoitrin, S-1-cyano-2-hydroxy-3-butene, R-goitrin, 1-cyano-3,4-epithiobutane, sinigrin, iberin nitrile, 3-indolylacetonitrile, indole-3-carbinol and para-hydroxyphenylacetonitrile when given at near-lethal doses to the pregnant dams. Sinalbin hydrate given at 300–600 mg/kg bw to pregnant dams did not lead to increased altered fetal weights, fetal resorption or malformations.

The teratogenic activity of allyl-ITC was evaluated in mice, rats, hamsters and rabbits in a study performed by the Food and Drug Research Laboratories in 1973 (IARC, 1985). Allyl-ITC dissolved in corn oil was administered by gavage in all studies. Groups of 23–25 CD-1 mice were given 0, 0.3, 1.3, 6 or 28 mg/kg bw per day on days 6–15 of gestation, and fetuses were examined on day 17 for malformations. Groups of 25 Wistar rats received a dose of 0, 0.2, 0.85, 4 or 18.5 mg/kg bw per day on days 6–15 of gestation, and fetuses were examined for malformations on day 20. Groups of 25–27 golden hamsters received a dose of 0, 0.2, 1.1, 5.1 or 23.8 mg/kg bw per day on days 6–10 of gestation, and fetuses were examined for malformations on day 14. Groups of 11–14 Dutch-belted rabbits received a dose of 0, 0.123, 0.6, 2.8 or 12.3 mg/kg bw per day on days 6–18 of gestation, and fetuses were examined for malformations on day 29. No evidence of maternal toxicity or treatment-related malformations was found in any species. In mice, there appeared to be an increase in the number of dead and resorbed fetuses at the highest dose (28 mg/kg bw per day) (38/276 implantation sites had dead or resorbed fetuses, compared with 15/264 in the control group, and the average number of live pups per litter was 9.92 versus 11.3), although no statistical analysis of the data was presented.

Groups of pregnant Wistar rats were given allyl-ITC in corn oil by gavage at 0, 60 or 120 mg/kg bw per day on day 12 or 13 of gestation. Despite severe maternal toxicity at the higher dose, no adverse effect on the fetuses was reported (Ruddick et al., 1976).

Groups of pregnant Sprague-Dawley rats were given indole-3-carbinol at a dose of 0 (vehicle, corn oil:acetone 19:1), 1 or 100 mg/kg bw on day 15 of gestation (Wilker et al., 1996). Each observation group consisted of three to five litters of male offspring, standardized at 10 per litter after whelping. Ano–genital distance and crown–rump length were decreased significantly at the higher dose on day 1 after birth. Several markers of sperm count and abnormalities were affected on day 62 after birth at either or both doses, including daily sperm production and epididymal transit time.

Groups of 6–8 weaned female Sprague-Dawley rats, 23 days of age (weighing 55–60 g) were given indole-3-carbinol (0.05, 0.5, 1 or 1.5 g/kg bw per day), 3,3′-diindolylmethane (0, 100, 200 or 400 mg/kg bw per day) or vehicle (dimethyl sulfoxide) by gavage (Gao et al., 2002). Indole-3-carbinol at

doses > 0.5 mg/kg bw per day decreased body-weight gain after four daily doses, whereas 3,3′-diindolylmethane had no effect on weight. The latter compound slightly decreased ovarian weight gain after a challenge with 5 IU of equine chorionic gonadotropin and reduced the number of ova shed after 72 h by about 30% in all treated groups. [The Working Group noted that these changes were not statistically significant]. Indole-3-carbinol decreased both markers significantly and in a dose-dependent manner, even at the lowest dose tested. Furthermore, the time courses of serum luteinizing hormone, follicle-stimulating hormone and progesterone were significantly decreased by indole-3-carbinol, but these end-points were tested only at the highest dose.

Groups of juvenile (12–18-month-old) rainbow trout were given diets containing indole-3-carbinol (providing five doses between 25 and 2000 mg/kg bw per day) or 3,3′-diindolylmethane (2.5–250 mg/kg bw per day) or control feed for 2 weeks (Shilling et al., 2001). 3,3′-Diindolylmethane significantly increased vitellogenin production in the liver in a dose-dependent manner, showing saturation at around 25 mg/kg bw per day. In an additional experiment, the effect was shown to be additive to that of estradiol.

Cytotoxicity, genotoxicity and mutagenic and related effects

Cruciferous vegetables

Plants are known to contain a variety of bioactive substances with toxic effects that may be comparable to or greater than those of synthetic compounds (Ames et al., 1990a,b). Thus, some studies have shown that cruciferous vegetables are cytotoxic, genotoxic and mutagenic. Wakabayashi et al. (1985) reported on

the direct mutagenic effects of nitrite-treated Chinese cabbage and indoles in Salmonella typhimurium. They found that the contributions of indoles to the total mutagenic activity of nitrite-treated Chinese cabbage to S. typhimurium TA100 were 0.2% from indole-3-acetonitrile, 0.3% from 4-methoxyindole-3-acetonitrile and 17% from 4-methoxyindole-3-aldehyde (Wakabayashi et al., 1986). Tiedink et al. (1988) studied the potential of 30 vegetables to form biologically active N-nitroso compounds after treatment with nitrite under acidic conditions. Although all the treated extracts contained N-nitroso compounds, only half of the vegetables were mutagenic after nitrite treatment. Extracts of cruciferous vegetables showed the highest mutagenic effect with respect to the number of Salmonella revertants induced; however, there was no significant correlation between the level of glucosinolates in these vegetables and the number of revertants. Subsequent detailed studies on the role of glucosinolates in the formation of N-nitroso compounds showed that only indole glucosinolates are involved in the formation of mutagenic agents (Tiedink et al., 1991). Nevertheless, the contribution of these glucosinolates to the mutagenicity of nitrite-treated cruciferous vegetables appears to be negligible. For instance, although Brussels sprouts are one of the richest sources of indolyl glucosinolates (6.6 µmol/g of dry weight) they induced only 61 ± 2 revertants of S. typhimurium TA100 per 25 mg of dry matter, whereas radish, with an indolyl-glucosinolate concentration of 1 µmol/g of dry weight, induced 233 ± 63 revertants per 25 mg of dry matter (Tiedink et al., 1988). Tiedink et al. (1990) found that the individual contribution of indole-3-acetonitrile to the total mutagenicity of green cabbage extracts treated with nitrite was about 2%. The most abundant indole in the extract, indole-3-carboxyaldehyde, was not mutagenic. These studies therefore indicate that the contribution of indole compounds to the mutagenicity of cruciferous vegetables treated with nitrite is negligible.

The mutagenic effect of nitrosated indole compounds is not restricted to certain groups of indoles. Eight indole compounds, indole-3-acetonitrile, indole-3-carbinol, indole-3-acetamide, indole-3-acetic acid, 3-methylindole, indole-3-aldehyde, indole-3-carboxylic acid and indole, tested in *S. typhimurium* strains TA98 and TA100 and *Escherichia coli* WP2 uvr/PKM101 after nitrite treatment at pH 3 were mutagenic in all three strains in the absence of metabolic activation (at up to 0.5 µmol/plate). Indole-3-acetic acid had the strongest effect. Addition of a metabolic activation system decreased the effect (Sasagawa & Matsushima, 1991). None of the compounds was mutagenic without nitrite.

As the effect of vegetable extracts not treated with nitrite was not investigated in these studies, it is not clear whether other bioactive substances in cruciferous vegetables contributed to the observed effect. The genotoxicity and mutagenicity of eight cruciferous vegetables (Brussels sprouts, white cabbage, cauliflower, green cabbage, kohlrabi, broccoli, turnip and black radish) was tested in the *Salmonella*/microsome test, in the differential DNA repair assay with *E. coli* and in a test for chromosomal aberrations in Chinese hamster ovary cells (Kassie *et al.*, 1996). Brussels sprout juice had the strongest effect in all three assays, and exogenous metabolic activation was not required for induction of the genotoxic and mutagenic effects. Addition of Arochlor-induced rat liver microsomes reduced the mutagenicity of the juices to *S. typhimurium* TA100 by 20–50%. Tests carried out with two fractions of the juices, one containing isothiocyanate and the other phenolic

compounds, showed that 70–80% of the mutagenicity of the crude juice was due to the isothiocyanate-containing portion. No correlation was found, however, between the mutagenicity of the juices and their histidine or total isothiocyanate content. Charles *et al.* (2002) studied the cytotoxic effect of Brussels sprouts, cauliflower, red cabbage, broccoli and turnip towards Chinese hamster ovary cells. The concentration of the crude extracts that produced a 50% reduction in the number of cells relative to the control was < 10 µl/ml of medium for broccoli and Brussels sprouts, 10–50 µl/ml of medium for turnips and 50–100 µg/ml for cauliflower and red cabbage. In the same study, broccoli juice significantly induced chromosomal aberrations at a concentration of 30 µl/ml of medium.

Purified glucosinolates do not have significant genotoxicity in vitro. Chromosomal aberrations were induced in Chinese hamster ovary cells by sinigrin and gluconasturtiin at concentrations > 2 mg/ml of medium (Musk *et al.*, 1995a).

Isothiocyanates

Isothiocyanates are biologically reactive compounds as a result of the highly electrophilic central carbon atom of their –N=C=S group. They react with oxygen-, sulfur- or nitrogen-centred nucleophiles to give rise to thiocarbamates, dithiocarbamates or thiourea, respectively.

Studies on the cytomorphological changes induced by benzyl-ITC–GSH, (10 µmol/ml of medium) and allyl-ITC–GSH (25 µmol/ml) in RL-4 rat hepatocytes showed that these compounds cause considerable toxicity, characterized by blebbing of the cells (Bruggeman *et al.*, 1986; Temmink *et al.,* 1986). At higher concentrations, distinct patches of dense heterochromatin in the nucleus, complete degranulation of the endoplasmic reticulum, disappearance of polysomes, high-

amplitude swelling of the mitochondria, disappearance of blebs with simultaneous appearance of microvilli and concentration of intermediate filaments in the juxtanuclear region were observed. These changes are characteristic features of apoptosis, and it has been shown that isothiocyanates are potent inducers of apoptosis (see section 4). Addition of excess GSH or cysteine either abolished or diminished the cytotoxic effects of benzyl-ITC and allyl-ITC. The GSH and L-cysteine conjugates of benzyl-ITC and allyl-ITC gave effects comparable to the parent compounds, as a result of the reversibility of the reaction between thiols and isothiocyanates. In another study, in which the cytotoxic effect of benzyl-ITC and phenethyl-ITC was investigated in NR50 BALB/c mouse 3T3 fibroblasts (0.016–0.02 mmol/ml), heteropyknosis and vacuolization of the cytoplasm were observed (Babich *et al.*, 1993). Intravesicular instillation of benzyl-ITC and allyl-ITC (2.8 mg/kg bw) or the same molar quantity (37 µmol/kg bw) of benzyl-ITC metabolites conjugated either with GSH, cysteine–glycine, cysteine or mercapturic acid to the urinary bladder of Fischer 344 rats caused cytotoxicity. The effect of benzyl-ITC was greater than that of allyl-ITC. The benzyl-ITC metabolite mercapturic acid, which is thought to be the main final metabolite, had less effect than the other metabolites (Masutomi *et al.*, 2001).

The genotoxic and mutagenic effects of the predominant isothiocyanates contained in cruciferous vegetables are presented in Table 65. Ethyl-, *n*-butyl-, *tert*-butyl-, allyl-, benzyl- and cyclohexyl-ITCs were mutagenic to *S. typhimurium* TA100 after 1 h of preincubation at 37 °C (Yamaguchi, 1980). Allyl-ITC had the strongest effect. Sinigrin, the parent glucosinolate of allyl-ITC, was mutagenic to the same degree as allyl-ITC. Addition of exogenous metabolic

Table 65. Genotoxic and mutagenic effects of isothiocyanates (ITCs)

Isothio-cyanate	Concentration or dose	Genetic effect	Remarks	Reference
Allyl-ITC	100 µg/plate	Increase in number of *his*⁺ *S typhimurium* TA100 revertants	S9 mix did not influence mutagenicity; weak effect in TA98 but no effect in TA1535, TA1536, TA1537 or TA1538	Yamaguchi (1980)
	0.05–500 µg/plate	Not mutagenic in *S. typhimurium* TA100 or TA98	No effects with or without S9 mix	Kasamaki *et al.* (1982)
	5 nmol/ml medium	Significant increase in structural and numerical chromosomal aberrations in Chinese hamster B241 cells	Colonies consisting of a pile of small cells were observed; S9 mix did not influence the result	Neudecker & Henschler (1985)
	0.06–0.5 µl/plate	Fivefold increase in number of *his*⁺ *S. typhimurium* TA100 revertants	Mutagenic effect observed after preincubation for 2 h; mutagenicity only upon addition of S9 mix	Musk & Johnson (1993); Musk *et al.* (1995a)
	0.2–3 µg/ml medium	Did not induce chromosomal aberrations or sister chromatid exchange in Chinese hamster ovary cells; no effect in SV40-transformed Indian muntjac cells	Parent glucosinolate, sinigrin, induced chromosomal aberrations at 4.6 mg/ml medium	Kassie & Knasmüller (2000)
	12–200 µg/plate	Marginal increase in number of *S. typhimurium* TA100 and TA98 revertants	S9 mix decreased effect	
	1–25 µg/plate	Dose-dependent increase in reparable DNA damage in *E. coli* 343/753 (*uvrB/recA*)	Genotoxicity attenuated by rat liver S9 mix, rat liver homogenate, bovine serum albumin, human saliva, vitamins E and C, β-carotene and sodium benzoate	
	0.2–4 µg/ml medium	Induction of micronucleus formation in human-derived HepG2 cells	Allyl-ITC less potent than phenethyl-ITC	
	90–270 mg/kg bw	Induction of reparable DNA damage in *E. coli* 343/753 (*uvrB/recA*) in host-mediated assay in mice	Significant effect in liver, lung, colon, kidney and stomach	
	0.5–5 µmol/ml medium	Increased formation of 8-oxo-7,8-dihydro-2′-deoxy-guanosine in calf thymus DNA and human leukaemia cell line; increased DNA damage in *P53* tumour suppressor gene and *c-Ha-ras-1* proto-oncogene	No effect in hydrogen peroxide-resistant leukaemic cells; genotoxicity of allyl-ITC stronger than that of benzyl-ITC or phenethyl-ITC	Murata *et al.* (2000)
	10–50 nmol/ml medium	Induction of DNA strand breaks in human-derived HepG2 cells	Synergistic effect with benzo[a]pyrene	Uhl *et al.* (2003)
Benzyl-ITC	100 µg/plate	Increase in number of *his*⁺ *S. typhimurium* TA100 revertants	S9 mix did not influence mutagenicity; weak effect in TA98 but no effect in TA1535, TA1536, TA1537 or TA1538	Yamaguchi (1980)
	0.22–0.88 µg/ml medium	Dose-related increase in *his*⁺ *S. typhimurium* TA100 revertants		Musk & Johnson (1993)

Table 65 (contd)

Isothio-cyanate	Concentration or dose	Genetic effect	Remarks	Reference
	0.3–1.2 µg/ml medium	Dose-dependent induction of chromosomal aberrations and sister chromatid exchange in Chinese hamster ovary cells	Frequency of sister chromatid exchange much lower than that of chromosomal aberrations	Musk et al. (1995b)
	1–25 µg/ml medium	Dose-dependent increase in DNA strand breaks in Chinese hamster ovary cells	Loss of comet heads at highest concentration	
	12–200 µg/plate	Marginal increase in number of S. typhimurium TA100 and TA98 revertants	S9 mix decreased effect	Kassie et al. (1999)
	0.5–5.5 µg/ml medium	Dose-dependent increase in reparable DNA damage in E. coli 343/753 (uvrB/recA)	Effect attenuated by rat liver S9 mix, rat liver homogenate, bovine serum albumin, human saliva, vitamins E and C, β-carotene and sodium benzoate	
	0.2–4 µg/ml medium	Dose-dependent induction of micronuclei in human-derived HepG2 cells		
	0.5–10 µg/ml medium	Dose-dependent induction of DNA strand breaks in primary rat hepatocytes and gastric mucosa cells	Genotoxic effect in gastric mucosa cells completely attenuated upon incubation of benzyl-ITC with gastric mucus	
	90–270 mg/kg bw	Moderate induction of reparable DNA damage in E. coli 343/753 (uvrB/recA) in host-mediated assay in mice	Similar effects in liver, kidney, lung, stomach and intestine	
	110–220 mg/kg bw	Moderate increase in DNA strand breaks in rat gastric mucosa and colon in vivo	Strand break maximal 1 h after administration; after 4 h, it reached level in untreated animals	
	0.5–2 µmol/ml medium	Increased formation of 8-oxo-7,8-dihydro-2´-deoxyguanosine in calf thymus DNA and human leukaemia cell line; increased DNA damage in P53 tumour suppressor gene and c-Ha-ras-1 proto-oncogene	Benzyl-ITC more genotoxic than phenethyl-ITC but less genotoxic than allyl-ITC	Murata et al. (2000)
	2.5–10 nmol/ml medium	Dose-related increase in DNA strand breaks in human-derived HepG2 cells	Synergistically genotoxic with benzo[a]pyrene at low concentrations	Kassie et al. (2003b)
Phenethyl-ITC	0.44–1.3 µg/ml medium	Dose-related increase in chromatid gaps and rearrangements in SV40-transformed Indian muntjac cell line and increased frequency of chromosomal aberrations and sister chromatid exchange in Chinese hamster ovary cells		Musk & Johnson (1993); Musk et al. (1995a)

Table 65 (contd)

Isothiocyanate	Concentration or dose	Genetic effect	Remarks	Reference
	12–200 µg/ml medium	Marginal mutagenicity to *S. typhimurium* TA100 and TA98	Effect diminished by S9 mix	Kassie & Knasmüller (2000)
	1–25 µg/plate	Dose-dependent increase in reparable DNA damage in *E. coli* 343/753 (*uvrB/recA*)	Genotoxicity attenuated by rat liver S9 mix; rat liver homogenate, bovine serum albumin, human saliva, vitamins E and C, β-carotene and sodium benzoate	
	0.2–4 µg/ml medium	Induction of micronucleus formation in human-derived HepG2 cells	Allyl-ITC less potent than phenethyl-ITC	
	90–270 mg/kg bw	Non-significant induction of reparable DNA damage in *E. coli* 343/753 (*uvrB/recA*) in host-mediated assay in mice		
	0.5–2 µmol/ml medium	Increased formation of 8-oxo-7,8-dihydro-2′-deoxyguanosine in calf thymus DNA and human leukaemia cell line; increased DNA damage in *P53* tumour suppressor gene and *c-Ha-ras-1* proto-oncogene	Less genotoxic than allyl-ITC or benzyl-ITC	Murata *et al.* (2000)
	2.5–10 nmol/ml medium	Dose-related increase in DNA strand breaks in human-derived HepG2 cells	Synergistically genotoxic with benzo[a]pyrene at low concentrations	Kassie *et al.* (2003b)
Methyl-ITC	12–200 µg/mlplate	Marginal mutagenicity to *S. typhimurium* TA100 and TA98	Mutagenicity diminished by S9 mix	Kassie *et al.* (2001)
	0.5–4 µg/ml medium	Dose-dependent increase in reparable DNA damage in *E. coli* 343/753 (*uvrB/recA*)	Genotoxicity attenuated by rat liver S9 mix; human saliva, bovine serum albumin and gastric juice	
	0.5–4 µg/ml medium	Dose-related increase in micronucleus frequency in human-derived HepG2 cells		
	3.6–5.4 µg/ml medium	Dose-related induction of DNA strand breaks in human-derived HepG2 cells		
	90 mg/kg bw	Moderate induction of reparable DNA damage in *E. coli* 343/753 (*uvrB/recA*) in host-mediated assay in mice	Significant effect in liver	

S9 mix, 9000 × *g* supernatant of rodent liver

activation did not change the effect. The effect of allyl-ITC in *S. typhimurium* TA98 was weak, and no effect was seen in TA1535, TA1536, TA1537 or TA1538. In another study (Neudecker & Henschler, 1985), allyl-ITC had clear mutagenic effects only after preincubation for 120 min. Although exogenous metabolic activation was a prerequisite for mutagenicity, an excess reduced the mutagenic potency. Other workers reported only borderline mutagenic effects of allyl-ITC (Eder *et al.*, 1980), benzyl-ITC, phenethyl-ITC and methyl-ITC (Kassie *et al.*, 1999; Kassie & Knasmüller, 2000; Kassie *et al.*, 2001) in the standard test. In all these studies, addition of an exogenous metabolic activation system abolished the effect almost completely. Allyl-ITC was not mutagenic in *S. typhimurium* TA98 or TA100 in the presence or absence of metabolic activation (Kasamaki *et al.*, 1982).

Benzyl-ITC, allyl-ITC, phenethyl-ITC and methyl-ITC induced reparable DNA damage in *E. coli* in vitro and in vivo and DNA strand breaks and cytogenetic effects in various mammalian cells (Kasamaki *et al.*, 1982; Musk & Johnson, 1993; Musk *et al.*, 1995a,b; Kassie *et al.*, 1999; Kassie & Knasmüller, 2000; Kassie *et al.*, 2001, 2003b; Uhl *et al.*, 2003) (Table 65). Benzyl-ITC was the most potent of all the isothiocyanates. Allyl-ITC was more genotoxic than phenethyl-ITC in the bacterial assay, but the latter was more potent in cytogenetic tests. In an assay for differential DNA repair with *E. coli* in vivo, the pattern of genotoxicity was similar to that found in vitro, the effect of phenethyl-ITC being the weakest. The doses of isothiocyanates required to induce moderate genotoxic effects in mice were much higher (90–270 mg/kg bw) than those required for the highly cytotoxic and genotoxic effects in vitro. A similar observation was made in comet assays with benzyl-ITC, which weakly induced DNA damage at doses of 110 and 220 mg/kg bw, with a maximum effect 1 h after exposure; by 4 h after exposure, the damage was reduced to the level of that in untreated controls (Kassie *et al.*, 1999). The reduction in the effect of isothiocyanates in vivo could be due to non-specific binding to proteins, as witnessed by the pronounced reduction in the mutagenicity and genotoxicity of the compounds with addition of liver homogenate, an exogenous metabolic activation system, bovine serum albumin or saliva. Moreover, radical scavengers might also contribute to the weak effect of the compounds in vivo, as vitamin E and C, β-carotene and sodium benzoate reduced isothiocyanate-induced differential DNA damage in vitro. The effect of benzyl-ITC on gastric mucosa cells was drastically diminished by incubation of the compound with gastric mucus, corroborating the result observed in the differential DNA repair assay with *E. coli*.

The cytotoxic and genotoxic effects of isothiocyanates might be related to their potential to induce formation of reactive oxygen intermediates. Treatment of rat liver epithelial (RL34) cells with benzyl-ITC or allyl-ITC (10 nmol/ml) resulted in an immediate increase in reactive oxygen intermediates, which corresponded to induction of class πGST P1 (Nakamura *et al.*, 2000b). Depletion of GSH by diethyl maleate significantly increased the production of isothiocyanate-induced reactive oxygen intermediates (hydrogen peroxide, lipid hydroperoxide and peroxynitrite) and accelerated isothiocyanate-induced GST activity, while treatment of cells with GSH inhibited both reactions. Whereas benzyl-ITC was the most potent inducer of reactive oxygen intermediates, the effect of allyl-ITC was intermediate, and phenyl-ITC did not induce these compounds. Kassie and colleagues (1999, 2001) reported that benzyl-ITC, allyl-ITC, phenethyl-ITC and methyl-ITC induced thiobarbituric acid-reactive substances, indicators of lipid peroxidation, in HepG2 cells exposed to 0.5–4 μg/ml of the compounds for 1 h, the order of potency of induction being benzyl-ITC > allyl-ITC = methyl-ITC > phenethyl-ITC. In another study on the induction of reactive oxygen intermediates, allyl-ITC induced a significantly higher level of 8-oxodG in hydrogen peroxide-susceptible human myelogenous leukaemia cells than their resistant counterparts (Murata *et al.*, 2000). In the same study, the authors compared induction by allyl-ITC, benzyl-ITC and phenethyl-ITC of 8-oxodG in calf thymus DNA and DNA damage in ^{32}P-labelled DNA fragments obtained from the human *P53* tumour suppressor gene and the *c-Ha-ras-1* proto-oncogene. All the isothiocyanates caused Cu[II]-mediated formation of DNA damage and 8-oxodG, the order of potency being allyl-ITC > benzyl-ITC > phenethyl-ITC. Catalase and the Cu[II]-specific chelator bathocuproine, reduced 8-oxodG formation, suggesting the involvement of hydrogen peroxide and Cu[I], respectively. Superoxide dismutase was also inhibitory, indicating participation of superoxide in the DNA damage.

Another possible mechanism of the cytotoxicity and genotoxicity of isothiocyanates may be oxidative desulfuration of the compounds to reactive isocyanates by cytochrome P450 enzymes. Arochlor-inducible cytochrome P450 enzymes convert phenyl-ITC, benzyl-ITC, phenethyl-ITC and methyl-ITC to the respective isocyanates (Lee, 1992, 1996). Phenyl-ITC underwent the most metabolic conversion, followed by benzyl-ITC and phenethyl-ITC; methyl-ITC was only weakly metabolized. Isocyanates are reactive electrophilic agents capable of modifying nucleic acids in vitro and in vivo and cause chromosome aberrations, sister chromatid exchange, mutations and cancer (Mason et al., 1987; Bucher et al., 1989).

Exposure of Chinese hamster B241 cells to allyl-ITC at 5 pmol/ml for 24 h and further cultivation for generations caused transformation of the cells (Kasamaki et al., 1987). Subsequent isolation and subcutaneous injection of the anchorage-independent cell population resulted in tumour formation after 3–8 months. In another study, phenethyl-ITC failed to transform BALB/c 3T3 cells but enhanced the cell transforming potential of benzo[a]pyrene (Perocco et al., 2002).

Indoles

With the exception of one report in which indole-3-carbinol was found to be cytotoxic to BALB/c 3T3 mouse fibroblasts at a concentration of 1 nmol/ml (Babich et al., 1993), none of the studies of indole compounds contained in cruciferous vegetables has shown them to be genotoxic or mutagenic. After treatment with nitrite, however, most indole compounds become mutagenic. The first report on the mutagenicity of nitrite-treated indole-compounds was that of Wakabayashi et al. (1985).

Vegetables are the main sources of dietary nitrate (Meah et al., 1994).

Reduction of ingested nitrate to nitrite by bacteria in the oral cavity and reaction of nitrite with ingested vegetables at the acidic pH of the stomach may lead to formation of mutagenic indole compounds, which may be risk factors for stomach cancer. To shed light on the possible association between the risk for stomach cancer and exposure to nitrosated indoles, rats were given high doses of these compounds, and effects on the stomach mucosa were examined. 1-Nitrosoindole-3-acetonitrile, a nitrosated form of indole-3-acetonitrile, at 100 mg/kg bw caused the formation of DNA adducts in the forestomach and glandular stomach (Yamashita et al., 1988), whereas indole-3-acetonitrile did not. 1-Nitrosoindole-3-acetonitrile also induced replicative DNA synthesis and ornithine decarboxylase activity in the gastric mucosa of rats treated at doses of 40–300 mg/kg bw (Furihata et al., 1987), suggesting that the compound has tumour promoting activity.

Indolo[3,2-b]carbazole has some structural and functional properties in common with the tumour promoter 2,3,7,8-tetrachlorodibenzo-para-dioxin (TCDD), and some of the cellular changes induced by this indole in vitro might favour tumour promotion rather than chemoprevention. During carcino-

genesis, the level of gap junction proteins is generally reduced, and Herrmann et al. (2002) found inhibition of gap-junction intracellular communication between primary rat hepatocytes co-cultured with a rat liver epithelial cell line, WB-F344, in response to indolo[3,2-b]carbazole at 0.1 nmol/ml for 8 or 12 h, with maximum inhibition after 24–48 h. Both plasma membrane staining and the mRNA levels of connexin 32 were reduced.

Prostaglandin E2 is believed to contribute to formation of tumours by increasing cell proliferation, preventing apoptosis and facilitating angiogenesis, particularly in the colon. In a study of the regulation of prostaglandin E2 in a colon carcinoma cell line, HCA7, Sherratt et al. (2003) found that indolo[3,2-b]carbazole at 1 nmol/ml for 6 h increased COX-2 mRNA by 2.8-fold. Co-treatment with interleukin-1β increased the mRNA levels even further. Subsequent increases in prostaglandin E2 were also observed.

The Working Group concluded that exposure to indole compounds as a result of consumption of cruciferous vegetables does not appear to have adverse genetic effects.

Chapter 8

Summary

Cruciferous vegetables

Cruciferous vegetables belong to the botanical family Brassicaceae. The greatest consumption of cruciferous vegetables has been reported to be that of adults in China, who may eat more than 100 g per day. Other Asian populations also have a relatively large consumption of cruciferous vegetables, ranging from 40 to 80 g per day. The average cruciferous vegetable intake in North America is reported to be 25–30 g per day. The consumption in European countries varies substantially, intake in some countries in central and northern Europe being more than 30 g per day and that in some southern European countries being less than 15 g per day. This pattern differs from that for the consumption of all vegetables, which shows a decreasing gradient from south to north in Europe. Relatively small amounts of cruciferous vegetables, 15 g per day or less, are reported to be eaten in South Africa and some countries in South America, and less than 20 g per day in India.

Overall, cruciferous vegetable intake would appear to account for 10–15% of total vegetable intake, ranging from almost 25% in countries with high consumption to only 5% in countries with low consumption. In 2000, cruciferous vegetables represented 25% of all vegetables produced in eastern Europe, about 10% of those produced in Australia, eastern and South-East Asia and western Europe, and less than 10% of those produced in the rest of the world. Between 1962 and 2002, there was a decreasing trend in the production of cruciferous vegetables in Australia, New Zealand and western Europe.

Glucosinolates, isothiocyanates and indoles

Isothiocyanate and indole compounds are derived from consumption of cruciferous vegetables and manufactured products, including condiments, sauerkraut and *kimchi*. Although these two groups of compounds appear to be structurally unrelated, they are both derived from degradation of glucosinolates, the characteristic sulfur-containing glycosides found in cruciferous vegetables. After tissue disruption, glucosinolates are degraded by the action of β-thioglucosidases, commonly known as myrosinases.

Although over 90 different naturally occurring isothiocyanates (ITCs) have been described, people commonly consume only about six: 4-methylsulfinylbutyl- (sulforaphane), 2-propenyl- (allyl), 3-butenyl-, 4-pentenyl-, 3-methylsulfinylpropyl- (iberin) and phenethyl-ITC. Sulforaphane is derived predominantly from broccoli but can also be obtained from rocket (*Eruca sativa*). 2-Propenyl- and 3-butenyl-ITC and iberin are derived from consumption of cultivars of *B. oleracea*. 3-Butenyl- and 4-pentenyl-ITC are derived from consumption of leafy *B. rapa* crops, particularly Chinese cabbage. 2-Propenyl-ITC is also derived from leafy mustard vegetables. Phenethyl-ITC is derived from watercress and to a lesser extent from root crops such as turnips and rutabaga. Benzyl-ITC is relatively rare in the diet, being obtained from cress (*Lepidium*) species. 6-Methylsulfinyl-hexyl-ITC is derived from *wasabi*.

Six indole glucosinolates have been identified in cruciferous vegetables. Of these, only two are found frequently in the diet: 3-indolylmethyl glucosinolate (glucobrassicin) and 1-methoxy-3-indolylmethyl glucosinolate (neoglucobrassicin) These are found in most cruciferous vegetables. Indole glucosinolates degrade mainly to indole-3-carbinol, which condenses to form 3-3´-diindolylmethane, or to 1-methoxy-indole-3-carbinol. Further condensation reactions may occur, particularly in the acid conditions of the stomach, to produce a series of oligomeric products. Indole glucosinolates can also react with ascorbic acid to form ascorbigen.

Four factors determine exposure of the human gastrointestinal tract to isothiocyanates and indoles: (1) the genetics of glucosinolate biosynthesis within the crop plant, which determines the chemical structure of the degradation products and partially determines the overall amount; (2) abiotic and biotic environmental factors, which can influence the overall amounts of glucosinolates and degradation products produced by the plant; (3) post-harvest storage, processing and cooking; and (4) the myrosinase-like activity of the intestinal microbial flora.

Metabolism, kinetics and genetic variation

Humans

Ingested isothiocyanates are metabolized principally through the mercapturic acid pathway and excreted in urine as dithiocarbamates, mainly in the form of *N*-acetylcysteine conjugates. The initial reaction with glutathione (GSH) may be either spontaneous or may be catalysed by GSH transferases (GSTs). The role of GST polymorphisms in exposure of tissues to isothiocyanates and excretion of isothiocyanates remains unresolved. Analytical methods, especially the cyclocondensation assay, have enabled quantification of isothiocyanates in cruciferous vegetables and of isothiocyanates and their dithiocarbamate metabolites (isothiocyanate equivalents) in human fluids, including blood and urine. The total quantity of urinary isothiocyanate equivalents has been shown to be a reliable marker of human dietary intake of these compounds and to correlate positively with the consumption of cruciferous vegetables.

After intake of indole-3-carbinol, several condensation products are formed, either in the acid environment of the stomach or in the near-neutral environment of the large intestine. 3,3′-Diindolylmethane can be detected in plasma and urine of volunteers given indole-3-carbinol.

Experimental systems

Only limited information is available on the metabolic fate of isothiocyanate compounds, indoles and the nitrile forms in animals fed cruciferous vegetables. The fate of several purified isothiocyanates, including benzyl-, phenethyl- and allyl-ITCs and sulforaphane, has been investigated in rodents. The main route of metabolism of isothiocyanates involves conjugation with GSH and excretion via the mercapturic acid pathway, but minor pathways, such as hydrolysis, oxidation–reduction, ring hydroxylation and alkyl-chain degradation, may be used, depending on the structure of the compound. Analysis of urinary metabolites has shown that there are species differences in the metabolism of isothiocyanates. Studies with radio-labelled isothiocyanates show that these compounds are readily absorbed into blood and tissues and are eliminated almost completely within 24–48 h of oral administration.

Little information is available on the metabolism and distribution of indoles in animals fed cruciferous vegetables. The fate of purified indole-3-carbinol has been examined in rats and trout, whereas the fate of ascorbigen has been studied only in mice. Purified indole glucosinolates have also been studied. The primary indole-3-carbinol derivatives in liver, intestine and serum are 3,3′-diindolylmethane, indolo[3,2-*b*]carbazole and other oligomeric acid condensation products, at ratios and amounts that vary with species and tissue. It is these compounds, not parent indole-3-carbinol, that are believed to be responsible for the organ-specific changes in carcinogen-, endogenous estrogen- and drug-metabolizing enzymes that can occur after ingestion of indole-3-carbinol.

Cruciferous vegetables, isothiocyanates and indoles modulate phase I and phase II enzymes in animals. The modulating effects of isothiocyanates are complex, as they depend on many factors, including species, tissue, treatment protocol, dose and enzyme specificity. Isothiocyanates usually inhibit cytochrome P450 enzymes, whereas indoles can have either inhibitory or stimulatory effects. The mechanism of inhibition of cytochrome P450 enzymes by isothiocyanates and indoles may involve both competitive and non-competitive binding of target enzymes. Studies of structure–activity relationships have shown that aromatic isothiocyanate compounds with longer alkyl chains or greater lipophilicity have enhanced inhibitory action against these enzymes. These studies have resulted in identification of some isothiocyanates that are remarkably powerful inhibitors of cytochrome P450 enzymes.

Cancer preventive effects

Humans

Studies were considered in this evaluation only if the reports provided estimates of risk along with statistical confidence intervals for estimated consumption of all cruciferous vegetables or for specific cruciferous vegetables. The summaries below include only those studies that met these criteria (see Figures 17–24, pp. 94–97).

Most of the epidemiological studies relating cruciferous vegetable intake to cancer risk also included measures of the intake of many other vegetables. Few studies found inverse associations with cancer that were stronger for cruciferous vegetables than for all vegetables. In interpreting the evidence, therefore, it should be recognized that the evidence often was based on analyses of subgroups by vegetable type, and that confounding of cruciferous vegetable intake by total vegetable intake was possible. In only a few studies (especially those of thyroid cancer) was an association with cruciferous vegetable intake the primary hypothesis. When cohort studies were available, they were given more weight, because of the potential biases in sampling or recall that are associated with case–control studies.

Oral cavity and pharynx

One cohort study and three case–control studies gave inconsistent findings.

Oesophagus

Only one case–control study was available, in which no association with Chinese cabbage consumption was found.

Stomach

Three cohort and nine case–control studies were available; most showed inverse associations with cruciferous vegetable intake. Overall, there was a non-significant inverse association in the cohort studies and a statistically significant inverse association in the case–control studies.

Colon and rectum

Six cohort and five case–control studies of colorectal cancer were available. Overall, there was no association in the cohort studies, with as many positive as inverse associations. Four of the case–control studies showed inverse associations with cruciferous vegetable intake, and one case–control study on isothiocyanate intake showed a non-significant inverse association. Overall, there was a statistically significant association. In addition, one cohort and four case–control studies of colorectal adenomas were available. The cohort study showed no association; one of the case–control studies showed statistically significant inverse associations with cruciferous vegetable intake, but one showed a non-significant positive association in women.

Pancreas

One cohort and two case–control studies were available. The cohort study showed no association. Both case–control studies showed inverse associations with cruciferous vegetable intake.

Larynx

Two case–control studies were available; one showed a positive association with cruciferous vegetable intake in women.

Lung

Five cohort and six case–control studies were available; most showed inverse associations with cruciferous vegetable intake, and the results were statistically significant in three cohort studies. In a pooled analysis of cohort studies, however, no association with broccoli or cabbage consumption was found. One cohort and two case–control studies showed statistically significant inverse associations between dietary or urinary isothiocyanate concentration and lung cancer. Overall, there was a statistically significant inverse association in both the cohort and the case–control studies.

Breast

One cohort and eight case–control studies were available; most, as well as a pooled analysis of seven cohort studies, showed no association with cruciferous vegetable intake. In one large case–control study, however, a statistically significant inverse association was found. In addition, a statistically significant inverse association with urinary isothiocyanate concentration was observed in one case–control study. Overall, the cohort study showed an association close to null, while the case–control studies showed a statistically significant inverse association.

Cervix

In two case–control studies, inverse associations with cruciferous vegetable intake were reported, one being statistically significant.

Endometrium

Three case–control studies were available; one showed a statistically significant inverse association with cruciferous vegetable intake.

Ovary

Three case–control studies were available; one showed a statistically significant inverse association with cruciferous vegetable intake.

Prostate

Three cohort and four case–control studies were available. There was no association observed in the cohort studies. In two of the case–control studies, statistically significant inverse associations with cruciferous vegetable intake were reported. In one of these, the association was stronger for advanced disease.

Urinary bladder

Two cohort and one case–control studies were available. In one cohort study, a statistically significant inverse association with cruciferous vegetable intake was reported, and a non-significant inverse association was found in the case–control study.

Kidney

Five case–control studies were available; in two, a statistically significant inverse association with cruciferous vegetable intake was reported, but one was limited to a subgroup. In a pooled analysis of four case–control studies, a statistically significant inverse association was found only among non-smokers.

Brain

One case–control study of childhood brain cancer was available; it showed no inverse association with the cruciferous vegetable intake of the mother during pregnancy.

Thyroid

In a collaborative re-analysis of 11 case–control studies, no association was found. One case–control study showed a statistically significant inverse association with cruciferous vegetable intake, and another showed a non-significant inverse association in females only. In another, an inverse association was found for Brussels sprouts, but a positive association was found with cabbage and cauliflower intake.

Non-Hodgkin lymphoma

Two cohort studies were available; in one, a statistically significant inverse association with cruciferous vegetable intake was reported. No association was found in the other.

Interaction with glutathione S-transferase gene polymorphism

Eight studies were conducted to investigate the effect of GST gene polymorphism on the association between intake of cruciferous vegetables or isothiocyanates and cancer. Four of these were conducted in Chinese populations, and in two of the studies a urinary biomarker of isothiocyanate was used. In four studies on lung cancer (one cohort, three case–control) and a single case–control study on breast cancer, a more consistent inverse association between isothiocyanate or cruciferous vegetable intake and cancer risk was found for individuals null for the GSTM1 or GSTT1 genotype. The difference in odds ratios between subgroups defined by GST genotype was statistically significant in some, but not all, studies. This effect of GST gene polymorphism was observed in both smokers and non-smokers and was more consistent in studies in which urinary isothiocyanate concentration was used as the exposure variable than in those in which self-reported food frequency was used to assess dietary intake.

Intermediate effect biomarkers

In humans, intake of cruciferous vegetables, isothiocyanates and indoles has been shown to modulate biotransformation enzymes, which can lead to enhancement of both bioactivation and detoxification of various carcinogens and alterations in steroid hormone metabolism. Studies involving inter-mediate effect biomarkers could not, however, be interpreted in relation to cancer risk. Consequently, intermediate effects were not used for evaluating the chemopreventive effects of cruciferous vegetables, isothiocyanates or indoles in humans.

Experimental animals
Cruciferous vegetables

In experimental animals treated with carcinogens, dietary intake of cruciferous vegetables in amounts similar to those eaten by human populations have been shown to inhibit neoplastic and preneoplastic changes, especially in the colon, mammary gland and liver. These inhibitory effects were most apparent when the vegetables were given simultaneously with the carcinogen or throughout the experiment. Mustard seed was shown to inhibit skin carcinogenesis as well as transplacental or translactational carcinogenesis in mouse models; wasabi was shown to inhibit stomach tumorigenesis; and dietary cabbage and collards both decreased lung metastasis from injected mammary cancer cells.

Glucosinolates

Sinigrin (2-propenyl glucosinolate), which yields allyl-ITC, reduced the total number of colonic aberrant crypt foci induced by dimethylhydrazine and the incidence of hepatic tumours induced by N-nitrosodiethylamine in rats.

Isothiocyanates

Both naturally occurring and synthetic isothiocyanates have been evaluated for their preventive effects against carcinogen-induced tumours in rats, mice and hamsters. The isothiocyanates were administered to rodents by various routes, usually at more than one dose and in protocols to determine their efficacy as either 'blocking' (anti-initiation) or 'suppressing' (anti-promotion or progression) agents.

Phenethyl-ITC potently inhibited tumour development in the oesophagus when administered in the diet before, during and after treatment with N-nitrosomethylbenzylamine (NMBA), although it did not inhibit tumour development in rats pre-initiated with this carcinogen. Dietary phenethyl-ITC inhibited the total number of aberrant crypt foci in rat colon when administered before and after azoxymethane, whereas its N-acetylcysteine conjugate inhibited colon tumour development when given after but not before azoxymethane. In another study, phenethyl-ITC was ineffective in reducing the number of azoxy-methane-induced aberrant crypt foci in rat colon. Phenethyl-ITC was highly effective in blocking 4-(methylnitro-samino)-1-(3-pyridyl)-1-butanone (NNK)- induced lung tumours in rats. Dietary phenethyl-ITC did not affect the incidence or multiplicity of mammary tumours induced in rats by 7,12-dimethylbenz[a]anthracene (DMBA) and did not reduce the number of papillomas induced in rat urinary bladder by N-butyl-N-(4-hydroxybutyl)-nitrosamine (BBN).

Phenethyl-ITC potently inhibited lung tumours in mice when administered orally before treatment with NNK. Thiol and N-acetylcysteine conjugates of phenethyl-ITC were also effective. Phenethyl-ITC was ineffective when given after NNK. It did not prevent benzo[a]pyrene-induced tumours in mice, but benzyl-ITC and phenethyl-ITC administered in combination reduced the number of lung tumours induced by a combination of NNK and benzo[a]pyrene. Phenethyl-ITC did not inhibit lung tumours induced in mice by environmental tobacco smoke. It inhibited the development of forestomach tumours in mice given benzo[a]pyrene. When administered in the diet before and after N-nitrosodiethylamine, phenethyl-ITC inhibited the formation of foci and adenomas in mouse liver.

Phenethyl-ITC was a highly effective inhibitor of lung tumours induced in hamsters by *N*-nitrosobis(2-oxopropyl)amine (BOP). When administered orally before treatment of hamsters with BOP, phenethyl-ITC reduced pancreatic tumour development.

Benzyl-ITC administered in the diet before, during and after NMBA treatment moderately inhibited oesophageal tumour development in rats. Dietary benzyl-ITC inhibited induction of tumours in the small intestine and colon of rats by methylazoxymethanol and inhibited DMBA-induced mammary tumours in rats. Benzyl-ITC administered by gavage inhibited tumours of the forestomach in mice treated with benzo[a]pyrene in one study, but not in another. It did not inhibit lung tumours induced in mice by NNK but was effective against tumours induced by benzo[a]pyrene and other polycyclic aromatic hydrocarbons.

3-Phenylpropyl-ITC potently inhibited induction of oesophageal tumours in rats when administered in the diet before, during and after NMBA treatment. When administered orally to mice before treatment with NNK, 3-phenylpropyl-ITC potently inhibited lung tumour formation. It was a highly effective inhibitor of BOP-induced lung tumours in hamsters but was ineffective in inhibiting BOP-induced tumours in hamster pancreas when administered before the carcinogen.

Oral administration of sulforaphane inhibited mammary tumorigenesis induced in rats by DMBA. Dietary sulforaphane inhibited benzo[a]pyrene-induced forestomach tumours in *nrf2* competent mice but not in *nrf2* null mice.

In studies with synthetic isothiocyanates, 6-phenylhexyl-ITC was highly effective in blocking NNK-induced lung tumours in rats. When given in the diet, it also reduced the number of papillomas induced in rat urinary bladder by BBN. 4-Phenylbutyl-ITC administered in the diet of rats before, during and after NMBA moderately inhibited oesophageal tumour development. 6-Phenylhexyl-, 4-phenylbutyl- and 5-phenylpentyl-ITC administered orally to mice before treatment with NNK potently inhibited lung tumours. The thiol and *N*-acetylcysteine conjugates of 6-phenylhexyl-ITC were also effective. 4-Phenylbutyl-ITC was a highly effective inhibitor of BOP-induced lung tumours in hamsters but was only moderately effective in inhibiting BOP-induced tumours in hamster pancreas when administered before the carcinogen. Dietary α-naphthyl-ITC inhibited both hepatocellular carcinoma development and nodular hyperplasia in the livers of rats exposed to *meta*-toluylenediamine, *N*-ethionine or *N*-2-fluorenylacetamide. In structure–function studies, the synthetic isothiocyanates 1-hexyl-ITC, 2-hexyl-ITC, 1-dodecyl-ITC, 1,2-diphenethyl-ITC and 2,2-diphenethyl-ITC inhibited NNK-induced lung tumours in mice, but 4-oxo-4-(3-pyridyl)butyl-ITC and 4-(3-pyridyl)butyl-ITC were ineffective.

Indoles

Indole-3-carbinol reduced the tumour response in a range of species and target organs and acted against most carcinogens examined when applied before and during the period of carcinogen administration as a blocking agent. For instance, concomitant treatment provided dose-responsive inhibition of hepatocellular carcinoma in rats or rainbow trout receiving aflatoxin B$_1$. At sufficient doses, indole-3-carbinol either suppressed or blocked mammary tumorigenesis induced in rats, usually with DMBA as the initiating agent. The compound effectively inhibited lung tumours in mice initiated with tobacco-specific nitrosamines as well as DMBA-induced skin carcinogenesis in mice. Prolonged treatment also reduced the number of 'spontaneous' mammary tumours in BALB/cfC3H mice harbouring the murine mammary tumour virus, cervical cancer in mice transgenic for human papilloma virus-16 and uterine adenocarcinoma in female Donyu rats.

3.3′-Diindolylmethane blocked tumour initiation in several models, including DMBA-initiated rat mammary tumours and benzo[a]pyrene-initiated forestomach tumours in mice. It also suppressed mammary tumour progression in rats previously initiated with DMBA.

Intermediate effect biomarkers

Whole cruciferous vegetables, extracts and isothiocyanates have been shown to modulate intermediate biomarkers of effect in a variety of experimental animal models. The effect on expression of phase I and II enzymes and on the formation of DNA adducts is generally consistent with predictions from in-vitro studies and with inhibition of tumours in animal models. The rather limited data on the antioxidant properties of cruciferous vegetables are, however, difficult to interpret. Extracts of cruciferous vegetables have been shown to have antioxidant effects in vivo, but other vegetables may also have these effects. Some glucosinolate breakdown products can selectively modulate cell proliferation and induce apoptosis in initiated cells in vivo, and these phenomena may provide a mechanism for tumour suppression.

The results of studies on the inhibition of carcinogen–DNA adduct formation in vivo by indole-3-carbinol have been remarkably consistent, inhibition being seen with a variety of carcinogens in several animal species (rat, mouse, rainbow trout), independently of the method used to quantify DNA adducts. In addition, indole-3-carbinol inhibited DNA adduct formation in both target and non-target organs and in peripheral white blood cells.

In almost all studies in rats in which enzyme markers of chemoprevention of carcinogenesis by indole-3-carbinol were evaluated, the markers predicted the outcome (inhibition of tumour formation). In several cases, induction of enzymes (phase I or phase II) by indole-3-carbinol could also be related to inhibition of carcinogen–DNA adduct formation, which is a more generally accepted intermediate marker of chemopreventive effects. Evaluation of enzyme markers appeared to be less useful in the rainbow trout model of aflatoxin B_1-induced liver tumours.

While the limitations of the trout model for aflatoxin B_1-induced liver carcinogenesis are well known, it has proven to be useful in studying inhibition of carcinogenesis by indole-3-carbinol, not only because of the extreme sensitivity of the trout liver to aflatoxin B_1, but also because it facilitates the study of dose–response relationships. The main chemopreventive property of indole-3-carbinol in this system is as an anti-initiator. It appears to act in this manner in rodents mainly by inducing pathways involved in the detoxification of carcinogens, thereby reducing the availability of substrate for activation pathways leading to DNA adduct formation.

There is little evidence from experiments in animals that the urinary 16α-hydroxyestrone:2-hydroxyestrone ratio could be used as a biomarker of an anti-estrogenic or anticarcinogenic effect of indole-3-carbinol.

In-vitro studies

Cruciferous vegetable juices prepared from homogenates induced NAD(P)H:-quinone oxidoreductase, a marker of phase II enzyme induction, due in part to the isothiocyanates and indoles formed from glucosinolates during homogenization. Isothiocyanates induce this quinone reductase by transcriptionally activating gene expression through the anti-oxidant response element, mediated by the transcription factor Nrf2, which is negatively regulated by Keap-1. Isothiocyanates are selective inhibitors of cytochrome P450 enzymes involved in carcinogen metabolic activation. The combination of inhibition of cytochrome P450s, induction of phase II enzymes such as GSTs and induction of NAD(P)H:-quinone oxidoreductase plays an important role in the chemopreventive effects of isothiocyanates in animals.

Isothiocyanates bind non-enzymatically and reversibly to protein and non-protein thiols; the reaction with GSH is also catalysed by GSTs. Isothiocyanate–GSH conjugates are expelled from cells, thereby depleting GSH, inducing oxidative stress and favouring the formation of isothiocyanate–protein adducts (thiocarbamoylated proteins). These adducts are implicated in the induction of enzyme expression associated with the activation of apoptosis. Apoptosis is associated with activation of caspases, MAP kinases—especially JNK-1—and mitochondrial dysfunction. Changes in function and enhanced proteasomal destruction of thiocarbamoylated proteins might mediate these effects.

Indole-3-carbinol and its derived compounds activate a range of drug-metabolizing enzymes, in particular CYP1A1. These compounds alter the metabolism of estrogen, increasing the 2-OH product and decreasing the 16α-OH product, thus decreasing proliferation of estrogen-responsive cells. They inhibit growth and induce apoptosis in a range of cell types, both estrogen receptor-positive and -negative. These effects are often more marked in tumour cells than in their non-tumorigenic counterparts. The expression of many proteins relevant to growth inhibition and apoptosis can be modified by indole-3-carbinol and 3,3´-diindolylmethane. Derivatives of indol-3-carbinol are generally more potent than the parent compound. In vitro, indolo[3,2-b]carbazole appears to have the least favourable profile for a chemopreventive agent.

Other beneficial effects

Two large cohort studies showed a statistically significant inverse association between consumption of cruciferous vegetables and coronary heart disease and ischaemic stroke. One of the studies also showed an inverse association between broccoli consumption and cataract.

Isothiocyanates have been found to be effective bacteriostatic and bactericidal agents, and this characteristic has been used in food preservation. A recent study showed evidence of an effect of sulforaphane against Helicobacter pylori in a human cell line.

Carcinogenicity

Humans

Studies in humans do not provide evidence that cruciferous vegetables are carcinogenic.

Experimental animals

There is no evidence that cruciferous vegetables per se are carcinogenic, although a few studies provide some evidence that dietary cabbage might enhance tumour responses in the colon, pancreas, skin and spermatic cord of animals treated with carcinogens.

A number of studies in experimental animals showed that isothiocyanates can not only inhibit but also enhance chemically induced tumorigenesis in rats. Phenethyl-ITC and benzyl-ITC increased chemically induced preneoplastic lesions and tumours in rat bladder, and phenethyl-ITC increased the frequency of altered foci in the liver. When given to hamsters in the diet after initiation, it increased the frequency of dysplastic lesions in the pancreas. The mechanisms of the enhancing effects of these two compounds have not been determined. The synthetic 6-phenylhexyl-ITC enhanced carcinogenesis in rat oesophagus and colon. The enhancement in the oesophagus appeared to be due to toxic effects leading to increased cell proliferation, as the compound increased tumour size and the activities of both COX-2 and LOX enzymes.

Isothiocyanates can also elicit carcinogenic effects in untreated animals. In a number of studies, phenethyl-ITC induced preneoplastic lesions and tumours, and allyl-ITC induced preneoplastic lesions and papillomas in rat bladder. Treatment with benzyl-ITC led to the development of preneoplastic bladder lesions. The mechanisms of these adverse effects have not been determined.

In a number of studies, prolonged treatment of carcinogen-treated animals with indole-3-carbinol enhanced, rather than suppressed, the tumour response in some organs, especially liver. Dietary indole-3-carbinol promoted hepatocellular carcinoma when given to trout previously initiated with aflatoxin B_1. The potency of indole-3-carbinol for this adverse effect exceeded its potency as a blocking agent, was proportional to the duration and dose, with no evident threshold, and was not reversed after treatment was stopped. Prolonged dietary administration of indole-3-carbinol to rats post-initiation promoted hepatic GST-P⁺ biomarkers and enhanced thyroid tumour development. In a separate study in rats, administration of indole-3-carbinol post-initiation resulted in modest suppression of mammary tumour and aberrant crypt foci formation in the colon but strongly promoted hepatic GST-P⁺ foci in the same animals. Studies in trout and rodents and in cultured mammalian cells in vitro showed that indole-3-carbinol or derived metabolites can have estrogenic as well as anti-estrogenic behaviour, depending on the organ, cell type, biomarker or pathway being examined. This may be one basis for the bi-directional behaviour of indole-3-carbinol in tumorigenesis.

Toxic effects

Humans

There is little evidence of acute effects in humans after ingestion of cruciferous vegetables. Reversible drug interactions have been described that are due either to the high vitamin K content of several *Brassica* vegetables or to modulation of the activities of enzymes responsible for the metabolism of xenobiotics. The possible contribution of goitrogenic compounds present in seeds, roots and leaves of cruciferous vegetables to endemic goitre in many parts of the world remains controversial. There is some evidence that intake of certain glucosinolates at a level exceeding 50 mg per day might have goitrogenic effects, but the complex interactions between long-term intake of possible goitrogens from cruciferous vegetables and dietary intake of iodine and possibly other nutrients are not well understood.

Experimental animals and in vitro

Animal species differ significantly in their sensitivity to the various toxic compounds formed from glucosinolates. Acute and subacute toxic effects are observed mainly in the thyroid, liver and kidney. Rats and pigs are more sensitive than other species to goitrogenic compounds, and effects on the thyroid have been described at doses of 3–5 µg per kg bw per day of goitrin (5-vinyl-2-thiooxazolidone). The mechanism of this action appears to be unrelated to iodine uptake into the thyroid.

Several isothiocyanates have been shown to be cytotoxic, genotoxic and mutagenic in vitro in both prokaroyotes and eukaryotes. The doses required to induce DNA damage in rats and mice in vivo were, however, several orders of magnitude higher than the amounts found in human diets.

The available information on the mutagenicity of indoles is limited to nitrosated indoles. As vegetables are rich in nitrates, it is highly likely that nitrosated indoles are formed in the stomach.

Chapter 9

Evaluation

Humans

The effects of cruciferous vegetables on human cancer risk have been assessed in many epidemiological studies. The conclusions that can be drawn from the current body of evidence are as follows:

There is *limited* evidence that eating cruciferous vegetables reduces the risk for cancers of the stomach and lung.

There is *inadequate* evidence that eating cruciferous vegetables reduces the risk for cancers at all other sites.

There is *inadequate* evidence to assess the independent effects on human cancer risk of isothiocyanates and indoles, as opposed to their combined effects with other compounds in cruciferous vegetables.

Experimental animals

The effects of cruciferous vegetables and of the compounds they contain on carcinogen-induced cancer have been assessed in many experimental animal models. The conclusions are difficult to generalize to all compounds in the classes of isothiocyanates and indoles, however, as differences are found by cancer site, the carcinogen used and species. The conclusions that can be drawn from the current body of evidence are as follows:

There is *sufficient* evidence that intake of cruciferous vegetables reduces the occurrence of cancer in experimental animal models. The strongest evidence for risk reduction comes from studies in which *Brassica* species were fed in amounts equivalent to human consumption during carcinogen administration and constantly thereafter, with reductions in the occurrence of cancers of the colon, mammary gland and liver.

There is *sufficient* evidence that intake of phenethyl-, benzyl- or 3-phenylpropylisothiocyanate reduces the occurrence of cancer in experimental animal models.

There is *sufficient* evidence that intake of indole-3-carbinol or 3,3′-diindolylmethane reduces the occurrence of cancer in experimental animal models.

There is *limited* evidence that intake of glucosinolates or sulforaphane reduces the occurrence of cancer in experimental animal models.

Some of these compounds have also been shown to increase tumour growth in some experimental animal systems.

Overall evaluation

Cruciferous vegetables are an important part of the diet in many parts of the world and constitute between 5% and 25% of all vegetable intake in different countries. These vegetables are also important because they contain glucosinolates, a group of compounds not found in other vegetables. Glucosinolates degrade to isothiocyanates and indoles, two classes of compound that have been shown both in vitro and in experimental animals to affect cancer risk. Although most of the effects of isothiocyanates and indoles are consistent with benefits with respect to human cancer risk, many studies showed no effect and some showed effects that could be interpreted as adverse. In epidemiological studies, cruciferous vegetables have been found to be associated with reduced risks for cancers at some sites.

In summary, the weight of the available evidence supports the following conclusions:

1. Compounds contained in cruciferous vegetables could affect cancer risk by several mechanisms: by altering the activity of various metabolizing enzymes and by affecting cellular mechanisms important in cancer development.

2. Cruciferous vegetables and compounds contained therein can have anti-cancer effects in many animal cancer models. These effects vary by compound, by experimental conditions and by species; adverse effects have been seen under some conditions.

3. Human consumption of cruciferous vegetables has been shown to be associated with modest reductions in the risks for cancers at some sites, although the reductions are no greater than those observed with total vegetable intake.

Summary of evidence for cancer preventive effects of cruciferous vegetables, isothiocyanates and indoles

	Degree of evidence for cancer preventive effect	Site and species
Humans		
Cruciferous vegetables	Limited	Lung, stomach
Experimental animals		
Cruciferous vegetables	Sufficient	Colon, mammary gland, liver (rat, mouse)
Glucosinolates	Limited	Colon, liver (rat)
Isothiocyanates		
Phenethyl-	Sufficient	Lung (rat, mouse, hamster); oesophagus (rat); liver (mouse); forestomach (mouse); pancreas (hamster)
Benzyl-	Sufficient	Oesophagus, colon, mammary gland (rat); lung, forestomach (mouse)
3-Phenylpropyl-	Sufficient	Oesophagus (rat); lung (mouse, hamster)
α-Naphthyl-	Limited	Liver (rat)
Sulforaphane	Limited	Colon, mammary gland (rat); forestomach (mouse)
Indoles		
Indole-3-carbinol	Sufficient	Liver (rat, trout); colon (rat); mammary gland (rat, mouse); cervix (rat); lung, skin (mouse)
3,3′-Diindolylmethane	Sufficient	Mammary gland (rat); forestomach (mouse)

Chapter 10
Recommendations

Research recommendations

Research done to date suggests that cruciferous vegetables contain constituents that reduce cancer risk. Governments, voluntary organizations and the private sector should continue to invest in research to elucidate the roles of these foods and their constituents in cancer risk reduction. Research is needed in particular in the following areas.

1. **Improve our understanding of the basic metabolism in both animals and humans of the compounds contained in cruciferous vegetables. In particular, there is a need to:**
   - better understand the pharmacokinetics, pharmacodynamics and pharmacogenetics of isothiocyanates and indoles. This information is needed to relate knowledge of effects in vitro and in animals to those in humans.
   - develop methods to quantify the levels of specific isothiocyanates, their conjugates and indoles in plasma. This information is needed to aid understanding of their cancer preventive potential and to relate their function in humans to that in animals and in vitro.
   - better understand the interactions between isothiocyanates, indoles and other nutrients contained in cruciferous vegetables, especially in animal models, in which the compounds have typically been studied alone.
   - better understand the influence of the ingestion of intact glucosinolates on the delivery of isothiocyanates and indoles to the lower gastrointestinal tract;
   - better understand the influence of intestinal bacterial flora on the metabolism of compounds contained in cruciferous vegetables;
   - better understand the biological significance of the effects of cruciferous vegetables and compounds therein on changes in cell growth, apoptosis and proliferation in vitro, in animals and in humans;
   - better understand the role of polymorphisms of glutathione *S*-transferases and other metabolizing enzymes in the metabolism of isothiocyanates and other compounds in cruciferous vegetables;
   - conduct short-term dietary interventions in humans to assess the impact of glutathione *S*-transferase polymorphisms on isothiocyanate metabolism and excretion;
   - create additional transgenic animals to elucidate the roles of specific genes in metabolizing compounds in cruciferous vegetables.

2. **Improve estimates of intake of cruciferous vegetables and their constituents in epidemiological studies. In particular, there is a need to:**
   - conduct studies to understand variations within the same food in the levels of isothiocyanates and indoles, which appear to be sensitive to soil, climate, growing conditions, food processing and preparation;
   - improve dietary assessment methods for cruciferous vegetables to include information on storage, processing and cooking methods, which can substantially modify their nutrient content;
   - develop and validate better biomarkers of intake of cruciferous vegetables and of supplements of compounds present in cruciferous vegetables. As these biomarkers might well include isothiocyanate or indole excretion products, proper interpretation will require careful attention to effects on the timing of excretion of factors such as metabolizing gene polymorphisms or other cancer risk factors.
   - use an optimized method to assess glucosinolate intake in large-scale epidemiological studies with stratification for genetic polymorphisms for relevant metabolic and response genes.

3. **Conduct short-term interventions to assess the effect of cruciferous vegetable intake on validated intermediate markers of effect, such as precancerous tissue changes, alteration of gene expression, DNA damage, or other markers known to lie in the causal pathway to cancer.**

4. **Conduct phase 2 trials in humans to begin to evaluate the agents derived from cruciferous vegetables that have been shown to be chemopreventive in animal systems.**

5. **Conduct studies to better understand the possible benefits of cruciferous vegetables or the compounds they contain on infectious agents important to human cancer risk, including human papillomavirus and *Helicobacter pylori*.**

6. **Conduct studies to better understand the potential toxicity of compounds contained in or derived from cruciferous vegetables, including nitriles, which are formed during the degradation of glucosinolates, and compounds formed during the metabolism of isothiocyanates and indoles.**

- Better describe the functional importance of modulation of phase I and phase II enzymes in terms of risk and prevention of cancers at various sites. This information is needed to understand the general risks and benefits of compounds contained in foods but is also important for understanding the potential adverse interactions of high doses of foods or derived compounds delivered in supplements in the metabolism of prescription drugs.
- Develop better methods to determine risk:benefit ratios for compounds such as indole-3-carbinol that potentially have both beneficial and adverse effects. Such methods are needed for the proper design of human clinical trials.
- Better understand the potential long-term effects of the goitrogenic compounds contained in cruciferous vegetables on thyroxin biosynthesis in humans.

Public health recommendations

We recommend that governments and nongovernmental organizations promote and support the intake of cruciferous vegetables as part of a diet containing a variety of fruits and vegetables for cancer risk reduction and health promotion. We further recommend that:

1. Cruciferous vegetables should not be promoted in preference to other vegetables, in either public education messages or in agricultural policies.

2. On the basis of concern about toxicity and uncertain benefits, it is inadvisable to consume nutritional supplements containing high levels of compounds derived from cruciferous vegetables or analogous synthetic compounds. Similar caution should be exercised in the consumption of modified cruciferous vegetables designed to contain substantially increased concentrations of such compounds.

References

Adam-Rodwell, G., Morse, M.A. & Stoner, G.D. (1993) The effects of phenethyl isothiocyanate on benzo[a]pyrene-induced tumours and DNA adducts in A/J mouse lung. *Cancer Lett.*, **71**, 35–42

Adesida, A., Edwards, L.G. & Thornalley, P.J. (1996) Inhibition of human leukaemia 60 cell growth by mercapturic acid metabolites of phenylethyl isothiocyanate. *Food Chem. Toxicol.*, **34**, 385–392

Agudo, A., Estève, M.G., Pallarés, C., Martínez-Ballarín, I., Fabregat, X., Malats, N., Machengs, I., Badia, A. & González, C.A. (1997) Vegetable and fruit intake and the risk of lung cancer in women in Barcelona, Spain. *Eur. J. Cancer*, **33**, 1256–1261

Agudo, A., Slimani, N., Ocké, M.C., Naska, A., Miller, A.B., Kroke, A., Bamia, C., Karalis, D., Vineis, P., Palli, D., Bueno-de-Mesquita, H.B., Peeters, P.H., Engeset, D., Hjartaker, A., Navarro, C., Martinez, G.C., Wallstrom, P., Zhang, J.X., Welch, A.A., Spencer, E., Stripp, C., Overvad, K., Clavel-Chapelon, F., Casagrande, C. & Riboli, E. (2002) Consumption of vegetables, fruit and other plant foods in the European Prospective Investigation into Cancer and Nutrition (EPIC) cohorts from 10 European countries. *Public Health Nutr.*, **5**, 1179–1196

Alavanja, M.C., Brown, C.C., Swanson, C. & Brownson, R.C. (1993) Saturated fat intake and lung cancer risk among nonsmoking women in Missouri. *J. Natl Cancer Inst.*, **85**, 1906–1916

Almendingen, K., Hofstad, B., Trygg, K., Hoff, G., Hussain, A. & Vatn, M. (2001) Current diet and colorectal adenomas: A case–control study including different sets of traditionally chosen control groups. *Eur. J. Cancer Prev.*, **10**, 395–406

Amat-Guerri, F., Martinez-Utrilla, R. & Pascual, C. (1984) Condensation of 3-hydroxymethylindoles with 3-substituted indoles. Formation of 2,3´-methylenediindole derivatives. *Chem. Res.*, **5**, 160–161

Ames, B.N., Profet, M. & Gold, L.S. (1990a) Dietary pesticides (99.99% all natural). *Proc. Natl Acad. Sci. USA*, **87**, 7777–7781

Ames, B.N., Profet, M. & Gold, L.S. (1990b) Nature's chemicals and synthetic chemicals: Comparative toxicology. *Proc. Natl Acad. Sci. USA*, **87**, 7782–7786

Anderton, M.J., Jukes, R., Lamb, J.H., Manson, M.M., Gescher, A., Steward, W.P. & Williams, M.L. (2003) Liquid chromatographic assay for the simultaneous determination of indole-3-carbinol and its acid condensation products in plasma. *J. Chromatogr. B Analyt. Technol. Biomed. Life Sci.*, **787**, 281–291

Arif, J.M., Gairola, C.G., Kelloff, G.J., Lubet, R.A. & Gupta, R.C. (2000) Inhibition of cigarette smoke-related DNA adducts in rat tissues by indole-3-carbinol. *Mutat. Res.*, **452**, 11–18

Armstrong, R.W., Imrey, P.B., Lye, M.S., Armstrong, M.J., Yu, M.C. & Sani, S. (1998) Nasopharyngeal carcinoma in Malaysian Chinese: Salted fish and other dietary exposures. *Int. J. Cancer*, **77**, 228–235

Arnao, M.B., Sanchez-Bravo, J. & Acosta, M. (1996) Indole-3-carbinol as a scavenger of free radicals. *Biochem. Mol. Biol. Int.*, **39**, 1125–1134

Arneson, D.W., Hurwitz, A., McMahon, L.M. & Robaugh, D. (1999) Presence of 3,3´-diindolylmethane in human plasma after oral administration of indole-3-carbinol. *Proc. Am. Assoc. Cancer Res.*, **40**, 2833

Arora, A. & Shukla, Y. (2003) Modulation of vinca-alkaloid induced P-glycoprotein expression by indole-3-carbinol. *Cancer Lett.*, **189**, 167–173

Ashok, B.T., Chen, Y., Liu, X., Bradlow, H.L., Mittelman, A. & Tiwari, R.K. (2001) Abrogation of estrogen-mediated cellular and biochemical effects by indole-3-carbinol. *Nutr. Cancer*, **41**, 180–187

Ashok, B.T., Chen, Y.G., Liu, X., Garikapaty, V.P., Seplowitz, R., Tschorn, J., Roy, K., Mittelman, A. & Tiwari, R.K. (2002) Multiple molecular targets of indole-3-carbinol, a chemopreventive anti-estrogen in breast cancer. *Eur. J. Cancer Prev.*, **11** (Suppl. 2), S86–S93

Astwood, E.B., Greer, M.A. & Ettlinger, M.G. (1949) I-5-Vinyl-2-thiooxazolidone, an antithyroid compound from yellow turnip and from Brassica seeds. *J. Biol. Chem.*, **181**, 121–130

Atalah, E., Urteaga, C. & Rebolledo, A. (2001) [Dietary behaviour and risk for the most common cancers in Chile.] *Rev. Chil. Nutr.*, **28**, 277–283 (in Spanish)

Auborn, K.J., Abramson, A., Bradlow, H.L., Sepkovic, D. & Mullooly, V. (1998) Estrogen metabolism and laryngeal papillomatosis: A pilot study on dietary prevention. *Anticancer Res.*, **18**, 4569–4573

Auborn, K.J., Fan, S., Rosen, E.M., Goodwin, L., Chandraskaren, A., Williams, D.E., Chen, D. & Carter, T.H. (2003) Indole-3-carbinol is a negative regulator of estrogen. *J. Nutr.*, **133**, 2470S–2475S

Babich, H., Borenfreund, E. & Stern, A. (1993) Comparative cytotoxicities of selected minor dietary non-nutrients with chemopreventive properties. *Cancer Lett.*, **73**, 127–133

Babish, J.G. & Stoewsand, G.S. (1978) Effect of dietary indole-3-carbinol on the induction of the mixed-function oxidases of rat tissue. *Food Cosmet. Toxicol.*, **16**, 151–155

Baghurst, P.A., McMichael, A.J., Slavotinek, A.H., Baghurst, K.I., Boyle, P. & Walker, A.M. (1991) A case–control study of diet and cancer of the pancreas. *Am. J. Epidemiol.*, **134**, 167–179

Bailey, G., Taylor, M., Selivonchick, D., Eisele, T., Hendricks, J., Nixon, J., Pawlowski, N. & Sinnhuber, R. (1982) Mechanisms of dietary modification of aflatoxin B1 carcinogenesis. *Basic Life Sci.*, **21**, 149–165

Bailey, G.S., Hendricks, J.D., Shelton, D.W., Nixon, J.E. & Pawlowski, N.E. (1987) Enhancement of carcinogenesis by the natural anticarcinogen indole-3-carbinol. *J. Natl Cancer Inst.*, **78**, 931–934

Bailey, G.S., Dashwood, R.H., Fong, A.T., Williams, D.E., Scanlan, R.A. & Hendricks, J.D. (1991) Modulation of mycotoxin and nitrosamine carcinogenesis by indole-3-

Cram, E.J., Liu, B.D., Bjeldanes, L.F. & Firestone, G.L. (2001) Indole-3-carbinol inhibits CDK6 expression in human MCF-7 breast cancer cells by disrupting Sp1 transcription factor interactions with a composite element in the *CDK6* gene promoter. *J. Biol. Chem.*, **276**, 22332–22340

Cramer, D.W., Kuper, H., Harlow, B.L. & Titus-Ernstoff, L. (2001) Carotenoids, antioxidants and ovarian cancer risk in pre- and postmenopausal women. *Int. J. Cancer*, **94**, 128–134

D'Agostini, F., Balansky, R.M., Izzotti, A., Lubet, R.A., Kelloff, G.J. & De Flora, S. (2001) Modulation of apoptosis by cigarette smoke and cancer chemopreventive agents in the respiratory tract of rats. *Carcinogenesis*, **22**, 375–380

Dashwood, R.H. (1998) Indole-3-carbinol: Anticarcinogen or tumour promoter in Brassica vegetables? *Chem.-Biol. Interactions*, **110**, 1–5

Dashwood, R.H. & Xu, M. (2003) The disposition and metabolism of 2-amino-3-methylimidazo-[4,5-*f*]quinoline in the Fischer 344 rat at high versus low doses of indole-3-carbinol. *Food Chem. Toxicol.*, **41**, 1185–1192

Dashwood, R.H., Arbogast, D.N., Fong, A.T., Hendricks, J.D. & Bailey, G.S. (1988) Mechanisms of anti-carcinogenesis by indole-3-carbinol: Detailed *in vivo* DNA binding dose–response studies after dietary administration with aflatoxin B1. *Carcinogenesis*, **9**, 427–432

Dashwood, R.H., Uyetake, L., Fong, A.T., Hendricks, J.D. & Bailey, G.S. (1989a) *In vivo* disposition of the natural anti-carcinogen indole-3-carbinol after po administration to rainbow trout. *Food Chem. Toxicol.*, **27**, 385–392

Dashwood, R.H., Arbogast, D.N., Fong, A.T., Pereira, C., Hendricks, J.D. & Bailey, G.S. (1989b) Quantitative inter-relationships between aflatoxin B$_1$ carcinogen dose, indole-3-carbinol anti-carcinogen dose, target organ DNA adduction and final tumor response. *Carcinogenesis*, **10**, 175–181

Dashwood, R.H., Fong, A.T., Hendricks, J.D. & Bailey, G.S. (1990) Tumor dose–response studies with aflatoxin B1 and the ambivalent modulator indole-3-

carbinol: Inhibitory versus promotional potency. *Basic Life Sci.*, **52**, 361–365

Dashwood, R.H., Fong, A.T., Williams, D.E., Hendricks, J.D. & Bailey, G.S. (1991) Promotion of aflatoxin B1 carcinogenesis by the natural tumour modulator indole-3-carbinol: Influence of dose, duration, and intermittent exposure on indole-3-carbinol promotional potency. *Cancer Res.*, **51**, 2362–2365

Dashwood, R.H., Fong, A.T., Arbogast, D.N., Bjeldanes, L.F., Hendricks, J.D. & Bailey, G.S. (1994) Anticarcinogenic activity of indole-3-carbinol acid products: Ultrasensitive bioassay by trout embryo microinjection. *Cancer Res.*, **54**, 3617–3619

Davey Smith, G. & Ebrahim, S. (2003) 'Mendelian randomization': Can genetic epidemiology contribute to understanding environmental determinants of disease? *Int. J. Epidemiol.*, **32**, 1–22

Daxenbichler, M.E., Spencer, G.F., Carlson, D.G., Rose, G.B., Brinker, A.M. & Powell, R.G. (1991) Glucosinolate composition of seeds from 297 species of wild plants. *Phytochemistry*, **30**, 2623–2638

Delaquis, P.J. & Sholberg, P.L. (1997) Antimicrobial activity of gaseous allyl isothiocyanate. *J. Food Prot.*, **60**, 943–947

DeMarini, D.M., Hastings, S.B., Brooks, L.R., Eischen, B.T., Bell, D.A., Watson, M.A., Felton, J.S., Sandler, R. & Kohlmeier, L. (1997) Pilot study of free and conjugated urinary mutagenicity during consumption of pan-fried meats: Possible modulation by cruciferous vegetables, glutathione *S*-transferase-M1, and *N*-acetyltransferase-2. *Mutat. Res.*, **381**, 83–96

Deneo-Pellegrini, H., Boffetta, P., De Stefani, E., Ronco, A., Brennan, P. & Mendilaharsu, M. (2002) Plant foods and differences between colon and rectal cancers. *Eur. J. Cancer Prev.*, **11**, 369–375

Deng, X.S., Tuo, J., Poulsen, H.E. & Loft, S. (1998) Prevention of oxidative DNA damage in rats by Brussels sprouts. *Free Radicals Res.*, **28**, 323–333

Denissenko, M.F., Pao, A., Tang, M. & Pfeifer, G.P. (1996) Preferential formation of benzo[a]pyrene adducts at lung cancer mutational hotspots in P53. *Science*, **274**, 430–432

Department of Health and Human Services (2000) *Nutrition and Your Health: Dietary Guidelines for Americans*, 5th Ed. (Home and Garden Bulletin No. 232), Washington DC

De Stefani, E., Boffetta, P., Oreggia, F., Brennan, P., Ronco, A., Deneo-Pellegrini, H. & Mendilaharsu, M. (2000) Plant foods and risk of laryngeal cancer: A case–control study in Uruguay. *Int. J. Cancer*, **87**, 129–132

De Stefani, E., Correa, P., Boffetta, P., Ronco, A., Brennan, P., Deneo-Pellegrini, H. & Mendilaharsu, M. (2001) Plant foods and risk of gastric cancer: A case–control study in Uruguay. *Eur. J. Cancer Prev.*, **10**, 357–364

Dinkova-Kostova, A.T., Massiah, M.A., Bozak, R.E., Hicks, R.J. & Talalay, P. (2001) Potency of Michael reaction acceptors as inducers of enzymes that protect against carcinogenesis depends on their reactivity with sulfhydryl groups. *Proc. Natl Acad. Sci. USA*, **98**, 3404–3409

Du, L., Lykkesfeldt, J., Olsen, C.E. & Halkier, B.A. (1995) Involvement of cytochrome P450 in oxime production in glucosinolate biosynthesis as demonstrated by an *in vitro* microsomal enzyme system isolated from jasmonic acid-induced seedlings of *Sinapis alba* L. *Proc. Natl Acad. Sci. USA*, **92**, 12505–12509

Duncan, A.J. (1991) Glucosinolates. In: D'Mello, J.P., Duffus, C.M. & Duffus, J.H., eds, *Toxic Substances in Crop Plants*, London, Royal Society of Chemistry, pp. 126–145

Dunnick, J.K., Prejean, J.D., Haseman, J., Thompson, R.B., Giles, H.D. & McConnell, E.E. (1982) Carcinogenesis bioassay of allyl isothiocyanate. *Fundam. Appl. Toxicol.*, **2**, 114–120

Eder, E., Neudecker, T., Lutz, D. & Henschler, D. (1980) Mutagenic potential of allyl and allylic compounds. Structure–activity relationship as determined by alkylating and direct *in vitro* mutagenic properties. *Biochem. Pharmacol.*, **29**, 993–998

Eisele, T.A., Bailey, G.S. & Nixon, J.E. (1983) The effect of indole-3-carbinol, an aflatoxin B1 hepatocarcinoma inhibitor, and other indole analogs on the rainbow trout hepatic mixed function oxidase system. *Toxicol. Lett.*, **19**, 133–138

Eklind, K.I., Morse, M.A. & Chung, F.L. (1990) Distribution and metabolism of the natural anticarcinogen phenethyl isothiocyanate in A/J mice. *Carcinogenesis*, **11**, 2033–2036

Ekström, A.M., Serafini, M., Nyrén, O., Hansson, L.E., Ye, W. & Wolk, A. (2000) Dietary antioxidant intake and the risk of cardia cancer and noncardia cancer of the intestinal and diffuse types: A population-based case–control study in Sweden. *Int. J. Cancer*, **87**, 133–140

El Bayoumy, K., Upadhyaya, P., Desai, D.H., Amin, S., Hoffmann, D. & Wynder, E.L. (1996) Effects of 1,4-phenyl-enebis-(methylene)selenocyanate, phenethyl iso-thiocyanate, indole-3-carbinol, and d-limo-nene individually and in combination on the tumorigenicity of the tobacco-specific nitrosamine 4-(methylnitrosamino)-1-(3-pyridyl)-1-butanone in A/J mouse lung. *Anticancer Res.*, **16**, 2709–2712

Elfoul, L., Rabot, S., Khelifa, N., Quinsac, A., Duguay, A. & Rimbault, A. (2001) Formation of allyl isothiocyanate from sinigrin in the digestive tract of rats monoassociated with a human colonic strain of *Bacteroides thetaiotaomicron*. *FEMS Microbiol. Lett.*, **197**, 99–103

Elfving, S. (1980) Studies on the naturally occurring goitrogen 5-vinyl-2-thiooxazolidone. Metabolism and antithyroid effect in the rat. *Ann. Clin. Res.*, **12** (Suppl. 28), 1–47

Elmore, E., Luc, T.T., Steele, V.E. & Redpath, J.L. (2001) Comparative tissue-specific toxicities of 20 cancer preventive agents using cultured cells from 8 different normal human epithelia. *In Vitro Mol. Toxicol.*, **14**, 191–207

van Etten, C.H. & Tookey, H.L. (1979) Glucosinolates in cruciferous plants. In: Rosenthal, G.A. & Jansen, D.H., eds, *Herbivores, Their Interaction with Secondary Plant Metabolites*, New York, Academic Press, pp. 507–520

van Etten, C.H., Daxenbichler, M.E. & Wolff, I.A. (1969a) Natural glucosinolates (thioglucosides) in foods and feeds. *J. Agric. Food Chem.*, **17**, 483–491

van Etten, C.H., Gagne, W.E., Robbins, D.J., Booth, A.N., Daxenbichler, M.E. & Wolff, I.A. (1969b) Biological evaluation of

crambe-D seed meals and derived products by rat feeding. *Cereal Chem.*, **46**, 145–155

European Thyroid Association (1985) Goitre and iodine deficiency in Europe. Report of the Subcommittee for the Study of Endemic Goitre and Iodine Deficiency. *Lancet*, **i**, 1289–1293

Ewertz, M. & Gill, C. (1990) Dietary factors and breast-cancer risk in Denmark. *Int. J. Cancer*, **46**, 779–784

Exon, J.H., South, E.H., Magnuson, B.A. & Hendrix, K. (2001) Effects of indole-3-carbinol on immune responses, aberrant crypt foci, and colonic crypt cell proliferation in rats. *J. Toxicol. Environ. Health*, **62**, 561–573

Fahey, J.W., Zhang, Y. & Talalay, P. (1997) Broccoli sprouts: An exceptionally rich source of inducers of enzymes that protect against chemical carcinogens. *Proc. Natl Acad. Sci. USA*, **94**, 10367–10372

Fahey, J.W., Zalcmann, A.T. & Talalay, P. (2001) The chemical diversity and distribution of glucosinolates and isothiocyanates among plants. *Phytochemistry*, **56**, 5–51

Fahey, J.W., Haristoy, X., Dolan, P.M., Kensler, T.W., Scholtus, I., Stephenson, K.K., Talalay, P. & Lozniewski, A. (2002) Sulforaphane inhibits extracellular, intracellular, and antibiotic-resistant strains of *Helicobacter pylori* and prevents benzo[a]pyrene-induced stomach tumours. *Proc. Natl Acad. Sci. USA*, **99**, 7610–7615

FAOSTAT (2000) Available at http://apps.fao.org/page/collections?subset=agriculture, under 'Food Balance Sheets'

Fares, F.A., Ge, X., Yannai, S. & Rennert, G. (1998) Dietary indole derivatives induce apoptosis in human breast cancer cells. *Adv. Exp Med. Biol.*, **451**, 153–157

Faris, M., Kokot, N., Latinis, K., Kasibhatla, S., Green, D.R., Koretzky, G.A. & Nel, A. (1998) The c-Jun N-terminal kinase cascade plays a role in stress-induced apoptosis in Jurkat cells by up-regulating Fas ligand expression. *J. Immunol.*, **160**, 134–144

Faulkner, K., Mithen, R. & Williamson, G. (1998) Selective increase of the potential anticarcinogen 4-methylsulphinylbutyl glucosinolate in broccoli. *Carcinogenesis*, **19**, 605–609

Fenwick, G.R. & Heaney, R.K. (1983) Glucosinolates and their breakdown products in cruciferous crops, foods, and feeding stuffs. *Food Chem.*, **11**, 1–23

Fenwick, G.R., Heaney, R.K. & Mullin, W.J. (1983) Glucosinolates and their breakdown products in food and food plants. *Crit. Rev. Food Sci. Nutr.*, **18**, 123–201

Fenwick, G.R., Heaney, R.K. & Mawson, R., eds (1989) *Glucosinolates*, Boca Raton, Florida, CRC Press, Inc.

Feskanich, D., Ziegler, R.G., Michaud, D.S., Giovannucci, E.L., Speizer, F.E., Willett, W.C. & Colditz, G.A. (2000) Prospective study of fruit and vegetable consumption and risk of lung cancer among men and women. *J. Natl Cancer Inst.*, **92**, 1812–1823

Fimognari, C., Nüsse, M., Cesari, R., Iori, R., Cantelli-Forti, G. & Hrelia, P. (2002a) Growth inhibition, cell-cycle arrest and apoptosis in human T-cell leukemia by the isothiocyanate sulforaphane. *Carcinogenesis*, **23**, 581–586

Fimognari, C., Nüsse, M., Berti, F., Iori, R., Cantelli-Forti, G. & Hrelia, P. (2002b) Cyclin D3 and p53 mediate sulforaphane-induced cell cycle delay and apoptosis in non-transformed human T lymphocytes. *Cell. Mol. Life Sci.*, **59**, 2004–2012

Finley, J.W. & Davis, C.D. (2001) Selenium (Se) from high-selenium broccoli is utilized differently than selenite, selenate and selenomethionine, but is more effective in inhibiting colon carcinogenesis. *Biofactors*, **14**, 191–196

Finley, J.W., Davis, C.D. & Feng, Y. (2000) Selenium from high selenium broccoli protects rats from colon cancer. *J. Nutr.*, **130**, 2384–2389

Finley, J.W., Ip, C., Lisk, D.J., Davis, C.D., Hintze, K.J. & Whanger, P.D. (2001) Cancer-protective properties of high-selenium broccoli. *J. Agric. Food Chem.*, **49**, 2679–2683

Firestone, G.L. & Bjeldanes, L.F. (2003) Indole-3-carbinol and 3-3´-diindolylmethane antiproliferative signaling pathways control cell-cycle gene transcription in human breast cancer cells by regulating promoter-Sp1 transcription factor interactions. *J. Nutr.*, **133**, 2448S–2455S

Fong, A.T., Hendricks, J.D., Dashwood, R.H., Van Winkle, S., Lee, B.C. & Bailey, G.S. (1988) Modulation of diethylnitrosamine-induced hepatocarcinogenesis and O^6-ethylguanine formation in rainbow trout by indole-3-carbinol, β-naphthoflavone, and Aroclor 1254. *Toxicol. Appl. Pharmacol.*, **96**, 93–100

Fong, A.T., Swanson, H.I., Dashwood, R.H., Williams, D.E., Hendricks, J.D. & Bailey, G.S. (1990) Mechanisms of anti-carcinogenesis by indole-3-carbinol. Studies of enzyme induction, electrophile-scavenging, and inhibition of aflatoxin B$_1$ activation. *Biochem. Pharmacol.*, **39**, 19–26

Foo, H.L., Gronning, L.M., Goodenough, L., Bones, A.M., Danielsen, B., Whiting, D.A. & Rossiter, J.T. (2000) Purification and characterisation of epithiospecifier protein from *Brassica napus*: Enzymic intramolecular sulphur addition within alkenyl thiohydroximates derived from alkenyl glucosinolate hydrolysis. *FEBS Lett.*, **468**, 243–246

Fowke, J.H., Longcope, C. & Hebert, J.R. (2000) *Brassica* vegetable consumption shifts estrogen metabolism in healthy postmenopausal women. *Cancer Epidemiol. Biomarkers Prev.*, **9**, 773–779

Fowke, J.H., Fahey, J.W., Stephenson, K.K. & Hebert, J.R. (2001) Using isothiocyanate excretion as a biological marker of *Brassica* vegetable consumption in epidemiological studies: Evaluating the sources of variability. *Public Health Nutr.*, **4**, 837–846

Fowke, J.H., Chung, F.L., Jin, F., Qi, D., Cai, Q., Conaway, C., Cheng, J.-R., Shu, X.-O., Gao, Y.-T. & Zheng, W (2003) Urinary isothiocyanate levels, Brassica, and human breast cancer. *Cancer Res.*, **63**, 3980–3986.

Franceschi, S., Bidoli, E., Baron, A.E., Barra, S., Talamini, R., Serraino, D. & La Vecchia, C. (1991a) Nutrition and cancer of the oral cavity and pharynx in north-east Italy. *Int. J. Cancer*, **47**, 20–25

Franceschi, S., Levi, F., Negri, E., Fassina, A. & La Vecchia, C. (1991b) Diet and thyroid cancer: A pooled analysis of four European case–control studies. *Int. J. Cancer*, **48**, 395–398

Frazier, A.L., Ryan, C.T., Rockett, H., Willett, W.C. & Colditz, G.A. (2003) Adolescent diet and risk of breast cancer. *Breast Cancer Res.*, **5**, R59–R64

Frydoonfar, H.R., McGrath, D.R. & Spigelman, A.D. (2003) The effect of indole-3-carbinol and sulforaphane on a prostate cancer cell line. *Aust. N.Z J. Surg.*, **73**, 154–156

Furihata, C., Sato, Y., Yamakoshi, A., Takimoto, M. & Matsushima, T. (1987) Inductions of ornithine decarboxylase and DNA synthesis in rat stomach mucosa by 1-nitrosoindole-3-acetonitrile. *Jpn. J. Cancer Res.*, **78**, 432–435

Futakuchi, M., Hirose, M., Miki, T., Tanaka, H., Ozaki, M. & Shirai, T. (1998) Inhibition of DMBA-initiated rat mammary tumour development by 1-O-hexyl-2,3,5-trimethylhydroquinone, phenylethyl isothiocyanate, and novel synthetic ascorbic acid derivatives. *Eur. J. Cancer Prev.*, **7**, 153–159

Galanti, M.R., Hansson, L., Bergström, R., Wolk, A., Hjartaker, A., Lund, E., Grimelius, L. & Ekbom, A. (1997) Diet and the risk of papillary and follicular thyroid carcinoma: A population-based case–control study in Sweden and Norway. *Cancer Causes Control*, **8**, 205–214

Gamet-Payrastre, L., Lumeau, S., Gasc, N., Cassar, G., Rollin, P. & Tulliez, J. (1998) Selective cytostatic and cytotoxic effects of glucosinolates hydrolysis products on human colon cancer cells *in vitro*. *Anticancer Drugs*, **9**, 141–148

Gamet-Payrastre, L., Li, P., Lumeau, S., Cassar, G., Dupont, M.A., Chevolleau, S., Gasc, N., Tulliez, J. & Terce, F. (2000) Sulforaphane, a naturally occurring isothiocyanate, induces cell cycle arrest and apoptosis in HT29 human colon cancer cells. *Cancer Res.*, **60**, 1426–1433

Gao, Y.T., McLaughlin, J.K., Gridley, G., Blot, W.J., Ji, B.T., Dai, Q. & Fraumeni, J.F., Jr (1994) Risk factors for esophageal cancer in Shanghai, China. II. Role of diet and nutrients. *Int. J. Cancer*, **58**, 197–202

Gao, X., Petroff, B., Oluola, O., Georg, G., Terranova, P. & Rozman, K. (2002) Endocrine disruption by indole-3-carbinol and tamoxifen: Blockage of ovulation. *Toxicol. Appl. Pharmacol.*, **183**, 179–188

Garrote, L.F., Herrero, R., Reyes, R.M., Vaccarella, S., Anta, J.L., Ferbeye, L., Muñoz, N. & Franceschi, S. (2001) Risk factors for cancer of the oral cavity and oropharynx in Cuba. *Br. J. Cancer*, **85**, 46–54

Garte, S., Gaspari, L., Alexandrie, A.K., Ambrosone, C., Autrup, H., Autrup, J.L., Baranova, H., Bathum, L., Benhamou, S., Boffetta, P., Bouchardy, C., Breskvar, K., Brockmoller, J., Cascorbi, I., Clapper, M.L., Coutelle, C., Daly, A., Dell'Omo, M., Dolzan, V., Dresler, C.M., Fryer, A., Haugen, A., Hein, D.W., Hildesheim, A., Hirvonen, A., Hsieh, L.L., Ingelman-Sundberg, M., Kalina, I., Kang, D., Kihara, M., Kiyohara, C., Kremers, P., Lazarus, P., Le Marchand, L., Lechner, M.C., Van Lieshout, E.M., London, S., Manni, J.J., Maugard, C.M., Morita, S., Nazar-Stewart, V., Noda, K., Oda, Y., Parl, F.F., Pastorelli, R., Persson, I., Peters, W.H., Rannug, A., Rebbeck, T., Risch, A., Roelandt, L., Romkes, M., Ryberg, D., Salagovic, J., Schoket, B., Seidegard, J., Shields, P.G., Sim, E., Sinnet, D., Strange, R.C., Stucker, I., Sugimura, H., To-Figueras, J., Vineis, P., Yu, M.C. & Taioli, E. (2001) Metabolic gene polymorphism frequencies in control populations. *Cancer Epidemiol. Biomarkers Prev.*, **10**, 1239–1248

Gaziano, J.M., Manson, J.E., Branch, L.G., Colditz, G.A., Willett, W.C. & Buring, J.E. (1995) A prospective study of consumption of carotenoids in fruits and vegetables and decreased cardiovascular mortality in the elderly. *Ann. Epidemiol.*, **5**, 255–260

Ge, X., Yannai, S., Rennert, G., Gruener, N. & Fares, F.A. (1996) 3,3′-Diindolylmethane induces apoptosis in human cancer cells. *Biochem. Biophys. Res. Commun.*, **228**, 153–158

Ge, X., Fares, F.A. & Yannai, S. (1999) Induction of apoptosis in MCF-7 cells by indol-3-carbinol is independent of p53 and bax. *Anticancer Res.*, **19**, 3199–3203

Gerhäuser, C., You, M., Liu, J., Moriarty, R.M., Hawthorne, M., Mehta, R.G., Moon, R.C. & Pezzuto, J.M. (1997) Cancer chemopreventive potential of sulforamate, a novel analogue of sulforaphane that induces phase 2 drug-metabolizing enzymes. *Cancer Res.*, **57**, 272–278

Gerhäuser, C., Klimo, K., Heiss, E., Neumann, I., Gamal-Eldeen, A., Knauft, J., Liu, G.Y., Sitthimonchai, S. & Frank, N. (2003) Mechanism-based in vitro screening of potential cancer chemopreventive agents. *Mutat. Res.*, **523–524**, 163–172

Getahun, S.M. & Chung, F.L. (1999) Conversion of glucosinolates to isothiocyanates in humans after ingestion of cooked watercress. *Cancer Epidemiol. Biomarkers Prev.*, **8**, 447–451

Giamoustaris, A. & Mithen, R. (1996) Genetics of aliphatic glucosinolates. 4. Side-chain modification in *Brassica oleracea*. *Theor. Appl. Genet.*, **93**, 1006–1010

Gillner, M., Bergman, J., Cambillau, C., Fernstrom, B. & Gustafsson, J.A. (1985) Interactions of indoles with specific binding sites for 2,3,7,8-tetrachlorodibenzo-p-dioxin in rat liver. *Mol. Pharmacol.*, **28**, 357–363

Giovannucci, E., Ascherio, A., Rimm, E.B., Stampfer, M.J., Colditz, G.A. & Willett, W.C. (1995) Intake of carotenoids and retinol in relation to risk of prostate cancer. *J. Natl Cancer Inst.*, **87**, 1767–1776

Godlewski, C.E., Boyd, J.N., Sherman, W.K., Anderson, J.L. & Stoewsand, G.S. (1985) Hepatic glutathione S-transferase activity and aflatoxin B$_1$-induced enzyme altered foci in rats fed fractions of Brussels sprouts. *Cancer Lett.*, **28**, 151–157

Gonzalez, J.M., Yusta, B., Garcia, C. & Carpio, M. (1986) Pulmonary and hepatic lesions in experimental 3-hydroxymethylindole intoxication. *Vet. Hum. Toxicol.*, **28**, 418–420

Gonzalez, C.A., Sanz, J.M., Marcos, G., Pita, S., Brullet, E., Saigi, E., Badia, A. & Riboli, E. (1991) Dietary factors and stomach cancer in Spain: A multi-centre case–control study. *Int. J. Cancer*, **49**, 513–519

Goodman, M.T., Hankin, J.H., Wilkens, L.R., Lyu, L.C., McDuffie, K., Liu, L.Q. & Kolonel, L.N. (1997) Diet, body size, physical activity, and the risk of endometrial cancer. *Cancer Res.*, **57**, 5077–5085

Goosen, T.C., Kent, U.M., Brand, L. & Hollenberg, P.F. (2000) Inactivation of cytochrome P450 2B1 by benzyl isothiocyanate, a chemopreventative agent from cruciferous vegetables. *Chem. Res. Toxicol.*, **13**, 1349–1359

Goosen, T.C., Mills, D.E. & Hollenberg, P.F. (2001) Effects of benzyl isothiocyanate on rat and human cytochromes P450: Identification of metabolites formed by P450 2B1. *J. Pharmacol. Exp. Ther.*, **296**, 198–206

Görler, K., Krumbiegel, G. & Mennicke, W.H. (1982) The metabolism of benzyl isothiocyanate and its cysteine conjugate in guinea-pigs and rabbits. *Xenobiotica*, **12**, 535–542

Graham, S., Marshall, J., Mettlin, C., Rzepka, T., Nemoto, T. & Byers, T. (1982) Diet in the epidemiology of breast cancer. *Am. J. Epidemiol.*, **116**, 68–75

Graser, G., Schneider, B., Oldham, N.J. & Gershenzon, J. (2000) The methionine chain elongation pathway in the biosynthesis of glucosinolates in *Eruca sativa* (Brassicaceae). *Arch. Biochem. Biophys.*, **378**, 411–419

Gridley, G., McLaughlin, J.K., Block, G., Blot, W.J., Winn, D.M., Greenberg, R.S., Schoenberg, J.B., Preston-Martin, S., Austin, D.F. & Fraumeni, J.F., Jr (1990) Diet and oral and pharyngeal cancer among blacks. *Nutr. Cancer*, **14**, 219–225

Grootwassink, J., Reed, D.W. & Kolenovsky, A.D. (1994) Immunopurifica-tion and immunocharacterization of the glucosinolate biosynthetic enzyme thiohydroximate *S*-glucosyltransferase. *Plant Physiol.*, **105**, 425–433

Grose, K.R. & Bjeldanes, L.F. (1992) Oligomerization of indole-3-carbinol in aqueous acid. *Chem. Res. Toxicol.*, **5**, 188–193

Grubbs, C.J., Steele, V.E., Casebolt, T., Juliana, M.M., Eto, I., Whitaker, L.M., Dragnev, K.H., Kelloff, G.J. & Lubet, R.L. (1995) Chemoprevention of chemically-induced mammary carcinogenesis by indole-3-carbinol. *Anticancer Res.*, **15**, 709–716

Guo, L.K. & Poulton, J.E. (1994) Partial purification and characterization of *Arabidopsis thaliana* UDPG:thiohydroximate glucosyltransferase. *Phytochemistry*, **36**, 1133–1138

Guo, Z., Smith, T.J., Wang, E., Sadrieh, N., Ma, Q., Thomas, P.E. & Yang, C.S. (1992) Effects of phenethyl isothiocyanate, a carcinogenesis inhibitor, on xenobiotic-metabolizing enzymes and nitrosamine metabolism in rats. *Carcinogenesis*, **13**, 2205–2210

Guo, Z., Smith, T.J., Wang, E., Eklind, K.I., Chung, F.L. & Yang, C.S. (1993) Structure–activity relationships of arylalkyl isothiocyanates for the inhibition of 4-(methylnitrosamino)-1-(3-pyridyl)-1-butanone metabolism and the modulation of xenobiotic-metabolizing enzymes in rats and mice. *Carcinogenesis*, **14**, 1167–1173.

Guo, D., Schut, H.A., Davis, C.D., Snyderwine, E.G., Bailey, G.S. & Dashwood, R.H. (1995) Protection by chlorophyllin and indole-3-carbinol against 2-amino-1-methyl-6-phenylimidazo[4,5-*b*]pyridine (PhIP)-induced DNA adducts and colonic aberrant crypts in the F344 rat. *Carcinogenesis*, **16**, 2931–2937

Hagiwara, A., Yoshino, H., Ichihara, T., Kawabe, M., Tamano, S., Aoki, H., Koda, T., Nakamura, M., Imaida, K., Ito, N. & Shirai, T. (2002) Prevention by natural food anthocyanins, purple sweet potato color and red cabbage color, of 2-amino-1-methyl-6-phenylimidazo[4,5-*b*]pyridine (PhIP)-associated colorectal carcinogenesis in rats initiated with 1,2-dimethylhydrazine. *J. Toxicol. Sci.*, **27**, 57–68

Halkier, B.A. & Du, L.C. (1997) The biosynthesis of glucosinolates. *Trends Plant Sci.*, **2**, 425–431

Hall, C., McCallum, D., Prescott, A. & Mithen, R. (2001) Biochemical genetics of glucosinolate modification in *Arabidopsis* and *Brassica*. *Theor. Appl. Genet.*, **102**, 369–374

Hallquist, A., Hardell, L., Degerman, A. & Boquist, L. (1994) Thyroid cancer: Reproductive factors, previous diseases, drug intake, family history and diet. A case–control study. *Eur. J. Cancer Prev.*, **3**, 481–488

Hamilton, S. & Teel, R. (1996) Effects of isothiocyanates on cytochrome P450 1A1 and 1A2 activity and on the mutagenicity of heterocyclic amines. *Anticancer Res.*, **16**, 3597–3602

Hankinson, O. (1995) The aryl hydrocarbon receptor complex. *Annu. Rev. Pharmacol. Toxicol.*, **35**, 307–340

Hansen, M., Moller, P. & Sorensen, H. (1995) Glucosinolates in broccoli stored under controlled atmosphere. *J. Am. Soc. Hortic. Sci.*, **120**, 1069-1074

Hansen, C.H., Du, L., Naur, P., Olsen, C.E., Axelsen, K.B., Hick, A.J., Pickett, J.A. & Halkier, B.A. (2001) CYP83b1 is the oxime-metabolizing enzyme in the glucosinolate pathway in *Arabidopsis*. *J. Biol. Chem.*, **276**, 24790–24796

Hansson, L.E., Nyren, O., Bergström, R., Wolk, A., Lindgren, A., Baron, J. & Adami, H.O. (1993) Diet and risk of gastric cancer. A population-based case–control study in Sweden. *Int. J. Cancer*, **55**, 181–189

Harrison, L.E., Zhang, Z.F., Karpeh, M.S., Sun, M. & Kurtz, R.C. (1997) The role of dietary factors in the intestinal and diffuse histologic subtypes of gastric adenocarcinoma: A case–control study in the US. *Cancer*, **80**, 1021–1028

Hasegawa, T., Nishino, H. & Iwashima, A. (1993) Isothiocyanates inhibit cell cycle progression of HeLa cells at G2/M phase. *Anticancer Drugs*, **4**, 273–279

Hashim, S., Banerjee, S., Madhubala, R. & Rao, A.R. (1998) Chemoprevention of DMBA-induced transplacental and translactational carcinogenesis in mice by oil from mustard seeds (*Brassica* spp.). *Cancer Lett.*, **134**, 217–226

Hayes, J.D. & McMahon, M. (2001) Molecular basis for the contribution of the antioxidant responsive element to cancer chemoprevention. *Cancer Lett.*, **174**, 103–113

Hayes, J.D. & Strange, R.C. (2000) Glutathione S-transferase polymorphisms and their biological consequences. *Pharmacology*, **61**, 154–166

Hayes, J.D., Pulford, D.J., Ellis, E.M., McLeod, R., James, R.F., Seidegard, J., Mosialou, E., Jernstrom, B. & Neal, G.E. (1998) Regulation of rat glutathione S-transferase A5 by cancer chemopreventive agents: Mechanisms of inducible resistance to aflatoxin B1. *Chem.–Biol. Interactions*, **111–112**, 51–67

Hayes, J.D., Ellis, E.M., Neal, G.E., Harrison, D.J. & Manson, M.M. (1999) Cellular response to cancer chemopreventive agents: Contribution of the antioxidant responsive element to the adaptive response to oxidative and chemical stress. *Biochem. Soc. Symp.*, **64**, 141–168

He, Y.H. & Schut, H.A. (1999) Inhibition of DNA adduct formation of 2-amino-1-methyl-6-phenylimidazo[4,5-*b*]pyridine and 2-amino-3-methylimidazo[4,5-*f*]quinoline by dietary indole-3-carbinol in female rats. *J. Biochem. Mol. Toxicol.*, **13**, 239–247

He, Y.H., Smale, M.H. & Schut, H.A. (1997) Chemopreventive properties of indole-3-carbinol (I3C): Inhibition of DNA adduct formation of the dietary carcinogen, 2-amino-1-methyl-6-phenylimidazo [4,5-*b*]pyridine (PhIP), in female F344 rats. *J. Cell. Biochem.*, **27** (Suppl.), 42–51

He, Y.H., Friesen, M.D., Ruch, R.J. & Schut, H.A. (2000) Indole-3-carbinol as a chemopreventive agent in 2-amino-1-methyl-6-phenylimidazo[4,5-*b*]pyridine (PhIP) carcinogenesis: Inhibition of PhIP–DNA adduct formation, acceleration of PhIP metabolism, and induction of cytochrome P450 in female F344 rats. *Food Chem. Toxicol.*, **38**, 15–23

Hecht, S.S. (1995) Chemoprevention by isothiocyanates. *J. Cell. Biochem.*, **22**, 195–209

Hecht, S.S. (1997) Approaches to chemoprevention of lung cancer based on carcinogens in tobacco smoke. *Environ. Health Perspect.*, **105** (Suppl. 4), 955–963

Hecht, S.S. (1999) Tobacco smoke carcinogens and lung cancer. *J Natl Cancer Inst*, **91**, 1194–1210

Hecht, S.S. (2000) Inhibition of carcinogenesis by isothiocyanates. *Drug Metab. Rev.*, **32**, 395–411

Hecht, S.S., Chung, F.L., Richie, J.P., Jr, Akerkar, S.A., Borukhova, A., Skowronski, L. & Carmella, S.G. (1995) Effects of watercress consumption on metabolism of a tobacco-specific lung carcinogen in smokers. *Cancer Epidemiol. Biomarkers Prev.*, **4**, 877–884

Hecht, S.S., Trushin, N., Rigotty, J., Carmella, S.G., Borukhova, A., Akerkar, S. & Rivenson, A. (1996a) Complete inhibition of 4-(methylnitrosamino)-1-(3-pyridyl)-1-butanone-induced rat lung tumorigenesis and favorable modification of biomarkers by phenethyl isothiocyanate. *Cancer Epidemiol. Biomarkers Prev.*, **5**, 645–652

Hecht, S.S., Trushin, N., Rigotty, J., Carmella, S.G., Borukhova, A., Akerkar, S., Desai, D., Amin, S. & Rivenson, A. (1996b) Inhibitory effects of 6-phenylhexyl isothiocyanate on 4-(methylnitrosamino)-1-(3-pyridyl)-1-butanone metabolic activation and lung tumorigenesis in rats. *Carcinogenesis*, **17**, 2061–2067

Hecht, S.S., Carmella, S.G. & Murphy, S.E. (1999) Effects of watercress consumption on urinary metabolites of nicotine in smokers. *Cancer Epidemiol. Biomarkers Prev.*, **8**, 907–913

Hecht, S.S., Kenney, P.M., Wang, M., Trushin, N. & Upadhyaya, P. (2000) Effects of phenethyl isothiocyanate and benzyl isothio-cyanate, individually and in combination, on lung tumorigenesis induced in A/J mice by benzo[*a*]pyrene and 4-(methylnitrosamino)-1-(3-pyridyl)-1-butanone. *Cancer Lett.*, **150**, 49–56

Hecht, S.S., Kenney, P.M., Wang, M. & Upadhyaya, P. (2002) Benzyl isothiocyanate: An effective inhibitor of polycyclic aromatic hydrocarbon tumorigenesis in A/J mouse lung. *Cancer Lett.*, **187**, 87–94

Hecht, S. S., Carmella, S. G., Kenney, P. M., Low, S. H., Arakawa, K., and Yu, M.C. (2004) Effects of cruciferous vegetable consumption on urinary metabolites of the tobacco-specific lung carcinogen 4-(methylnitrosamino)-1-(3-pyridyl)-1-butanone in Singapore Chinese. *Cancer Epidemiol. Biomarkers Prev.*, **13**, 997–1004

Heiss, E., Herhaus, C., Klimo, K., Bartsch, H. & Gerhäuser, C. (2001) Nuclear factor kB is a molecular target for sulforaphane-mediated anti-inflammatory mechanisms. *J. Biol. Chem.*, **276**, 32008–32015

Hemminki, K. (1993) DNA adducts, mutations and cancer. *Carcinogenesis*, **14**, 2007–2012

Herrmann, S., Seidelin, M., Bisgaard, H.C. & Vang, O. (2002) Indolo[3,2-*b*]carbazole inhibits gap junctional intercellular communication in rat primary hepatocytes and acts as a potential tumour promoter. *Carcinogenesis*, **23**, 1861–1868

Hill, C.B., Williams, P.H., Carlson, D.G. & Tookey, H.L. (1987) Variation in glucosinolates in oriental Brassica vegetables. *J. Am. Soc. Hortic. Sci.*, **112**, 309–313

Hiraku, Y., Yamashita, N., Nishiguchi, M. & Kawanishi, S. (2001) Catechol estrogens induce oxidative DNA damage and estradiol enhances cell proliferation. *Int. J. Cancer*, **92**, 333–337

Hirohashi, S. (1998) Inactivation of the E-cadherin-mediated cell adhesion system in human cancers. *Am. J. Pathol.*, **153**, 333–339

Hirose, M., Yamaguchi, T., Kimoto, N., Ogawa, K., Futakuchi, M., Sano, M. & Shirai, T. (1998) Strong promoting activity of phenylethyl isothiocyanate and benzyl isothiocyanate on urinary bladder carcinogenesis in Fischer 344 male rats. *Int. J. Cancer*, **77**, 773–777

Hoff, G., Moen, I.E., Trygg, K., Frolich, W., Foerster, A., Vatn, M., Sauar, J. & Larsen, S.

(1988) Colorectal adenomas and food. A prospective study of change in volume and total mass of adenomas in man. *Scand. J. Gastroenterol.*, **23**, 1253–1258

Hong, C., Firestone, G.L. & Bjeldanes, L.F. (2002a) Bcl-2 family-mediated apoptotic effects of 3,3´-diindolylmethane (DIM) in human breast cancer cells. *Biochem. Pharmacol.*, **63**, 1085–1097

Hong, C., Kim, H.A., Firestone, G.L. & Bjeldanes, L.F. (2002b) 3,3´-Diindolyl-methane (DIM) induces a G_1 cell cycle arrest in human breast cancer cells that is accompanied by Sp1-mediated activation of p21[WAF1/CIP1] expression. *Carcinogenesis*, **23**, 1297–1305

Horn, T.L., Reichert, M.A., Bliss, R.L. & Malejka-Giganti, D. (2002) Modulations of P450 mRNA in liver and mammary gland and P450 activities and metabolism of estrogen in liver by treatment of rats with indole-3-carbinol. *Biochem. Pharmacol.*, **64**, 393–404

Howell, P.M., Sharpe, A.G. & Lydiate, D.J. (2003) Homoeologous loci control the accumulation of seed glucosinolates in oilseed rape (*Brassica napus*). *Genome*, **46**, 454–460

Howells, L.M., Gallacher-Horley, B., Houghton, C.E., Manson, M.M. & Hudson, E.A. (2002) Indole-3-carbinol inhibits protein kinase B/Akt and induces apoptosis in the human breast tumor cell line MDA MB468 but not in the nontumorigenic HBL100 line. *Mol. Cancer Ther.*, **1**, 1161–1172

Hrncirik, K., Valusek, J. & Velisek, J. (2001) Investigation of ascorbigen as a breakdown product of glucobrassicin autolysis in *Brassica* vegetables. *Eur. Food Res. Technol.*, **212**, 576–581

Hsing, A.W., McLaughlin, J.K., Schuman, L.M., Bjelke, E., Gridley, G., Wacholder, S., Chien, H.T. & Blot, W.J. (1990) Diet, tobacco use, and fatal prostate cancer: Results from the Lutheran Brotherhood cohort study. *Cancer Res.*, **50**, 6836–6840

Hsing, A.W., McLaughlin, J.K., Chow, W.H., Schuman, L.M., Co Chien, H.T., Gridley, G., Bjelke, E., Wacholder, S. & Blot, W.J. (1998) Risk factors for colorectal cancer in a prospective study among US white men. *Int. J. Cancer*, **77**, 549–553

Hu, J., Nyrén, O., Wolk, A., Bergström, R., Yuen, J., Adami, H.O., Guo, L., Li, H., Huang, G., Xu, X., Zhao, F., Chen, Y., Wang, C., Qin, H., Hu, C. & Li, Y. (1994) Risk factors for oesophageal cancer in northeast China. *Int. J. Cancer*, **57**, 38–46

Hu, J., Mao, Y., Dryer, D. & White, K. (2002) Risk factors for lung cancer among Canadian women who have never smoked. *Cancer Detect. Prev.*, **26**, 129–138

Huang, Q., Lawson, T.A., Chung, F.L., Morris, C.R. & Mervish, S.S. (1993) Inhibition by phenylethyl and phenylhexyl isothiocyanate of metabolism of and DNA methylation by *N*-nitrosomethylamylamine in rats. *Carcinogenesis*, **14**, 749–754

Huang, C., Ma, W.Y., Li, J., Hecht, S.S. & Dong, Z. (1998) Essential role of p53 in phenethyl isothiocyanate-induced apoptosis. *Cancer Res.*, **58**, 4102–4106

Huang, X.E., Tajima, K., Hamajima, N., Xiang, J., Inoue, M., Hirose, K., Tominaga, S., Takezaki, T., Kuroishi, T. & Tokudome, S. (2000) Comparison of lifestyle and risk factors among Japanese with and without gastric cancer family history. *Int. J. Cancer*, **86**, 421–424

Huber, W.W., McDaniel, L.P., Kaderlik, K.R., Teitel, C.H., Lang, N.P. & Kadlubar, F.F. (1997) Chemoprotection against the formation of colon DNA adducts from the food-borne carcinogen 2-amino-1-methyl-6-phenylimidazo[4,5-*b*]pyridine (PhIP) in the rat. *Mutat. Res.*, **376**, 115–122.

Hudson, E.A., Howells, L., Ball, H.W., Pfeifer, A.M. & Manson, M.M. (1998) Mechanisms of action of indole-3-carbinol as a chemopreventive agent. *Biochem. Soc. Trans.*, **26**, S370

Hudson, E.A., Howells, L.M., Gallacher-Horley, B., Fox, L.H., Gescher, A. & Manson, M.M. (2003) Growth-inhibitory effects of the chemopreventive agent indole-3-carbinol are increased in combination with the polyamine putrescine in the SW480 colon tumour cell line. *BMC Cancer*, **3**, 2

IARC (1985) *IARC Monographs on the Carcinogenic Risk of Chemicals to Humans*, Vol. 36, *Allyl Compounds, Aldehydes, Epoxides, and Peroxides*, Lyon, IARCPress, pp. 55–68

IARC (2003) *IARC Handbooks on Cancer Prevention*, Volume 8, *Fruit and Vegetables*, Lyon, IARCPress

Ino, N., Sugie, S., Ohnishi, M. & Mori, H. (1996) Lack of inhibitory effect of benzyl isothiocyanate on 2-amino-1-methyl-6-phenylimidazo [4,5-b]pyridine (PhIP)-induced mammary carcinogenesis in rats. *J. Toxicol. Sci.*, **21**, 189–194

Ioannou, Y.M., Burka, L.T. & Mattews, H.B. (1984) Allyl isothiocyanate: Comparative disposition in rats and mice. *Toxicol. Appl. Pharmacol.*, **75**, 173–181

Ippoushi, K., Itou, H., Azuma, K. & Higashio, H. (2002) Effect of naturally occurring organosulfur compounds on nitric oxide production in lipopolysaccharide-activated macrophages. *Life Sci.*, **71**, 411–419

Ishizaki, H., Brady, J.F., Ning, S.M. & Yang, C.S. (1990) Effect of phenethyl isothiocyanate on microsomal N-nitrosodimethylamine metabolism and other monooxygenase activities. *Xenobiotica*, **20**, 255–264

Ito, N., Hiasa, Y., Konishi, Y. & Marugami, M. (1969) The development of carcinoma in liver of rats treated with *m*-toluylenediamine and the synergistic and antagonistic effects with other chemicals. *Cancer Res.*, **29**, 1137–1145

Ito, L.S., Inoue, M., Tajima, K., Yamamura, Y., Kodera, Y., Hirose, K., Takezaki, T., Hamajima, N., Kuroishi, T. & Tominaga, S. (2003) Dietary factors and the risk of gastric cancer among Japanese women: A comparison between the differentiated and non-differentiated subtypes. *Ann. Epidemiol.*, **13**, 24–31

Itoh, K., Chiba, T., Takahashi, S., Ishii, T., Igarashi, K., Katoh, Y., Oyake, T., Hayashi, N., Satoh, K., Hatayama, I., Yamamoto, M. & Nabeshima, Y. (1997) An Nrf2/small Maf heterodimer mediates the induction of phase II detoxifying enzyme genes through antioxidant response elements. *Biochem. Biophys. Res. Commun.*, **236**, 313–322

Itoh, K., Wakabayashi, N., Katoh, Y., Ishii, T., Igarashi, K., Engel, J.D. & Yamamoto, M. (1999) Keap1 represses nuclear activation of antioxidant responsive elements by Nrf2 through binding to the amino-terminal Neh2 domain. *Genes Dev.*, **13**, 76–86

Jain, J.C., Grootwassink, J.W., Kolenovsky, A.D. & Underhill, E.W. (1990) Purification and properties of 3´-phosphoadenosine-5´-

phosphosulfate desulfoglucosinolate sulfo-transferase from *Brassica-Juncea* cell cultures. *Phytochemistry*, **29**, 1425–1428

Jain, M.G., Hislop, G.T., Howe, G.R. & Ghadirian, P. (1999) Plant foods, antioxidants, and prostate cancer risk: Findings from case–control studies in Canada. *Nutr. Cancer*, **34**, 173–184

Jang, J.J., Cho, K.J., Lee, Y.S. & Bae, J.H. (1991) Modifying responses of allyl sulfide, indole-3-carbinol and germanium in a rat multi-organ carcinogenesis model. *Carcinogenesis*, **12**, 691–695

Jenner, P.M., Hagan, E.C., Taylor, J.M., Cook, E.L. & Fitzhugh, O.G. (1964) Food flavourings and compounds of related structure. I. Acute oral toxicity. *Food Cosmet. Toxicol.*, **2**, 327-343

Jensen, C.R., Mogensen, V.O., Mortensen, G., Fieldsend, J.K., Milford, G.F., Andersen, M.N. & Thage, J.H. (1996) Seed glucosinolate, oil and protein contents of field-grown rape (*Brassica napus* L.) affected by soil drying and evaporative demand. *Field Crops Res.*, **47**, 93–105

Jeon, K.I., Rih, J.K., Kim, H.J., Lee, Y.J., Cho, C.H., Goldberg, I.D., Rosen, E.M. & Bae, I. (2003) Pretreatment of indole-3-carbinol augments TRAIL-induced apoptosis in a prostate cancer cell line, LNCaP. *FEBS Lett.*, **544**, 246–251

Ji, Y & Morris, M.E. (2003) Determination of phenethyl isothiocyanate in human plasma and urine by ammonia derivatisation and liquid chromatography–tandem mass spectrometry. *Anal. Biochem.*, **323**, 39–47

Ji, B.T., Chow, W.H., Yang, G., McLaughlin, J.K., Zheng, W., Shu, X.O., Jin, F., Gao, R.N., Gao, Y.T. & Fraumeni, J.F., Jr (1998) Dietary habits and stomach cancer in Shanghai, China. *Int. J. Cancer*, **76**, 659–664

Jiang, Z.Q., Chen, C., Yang, B., Hebbar, V. & Kong, A.N. (2003) Differential responses from seven mammalian cell lines to the treatments of detoxifying enzyme inducers. *Life Sci.*, **72**, 2243–2253

Jiao, D., Eklind, K.I., Choi, C.I., Desai, D.H., Amin, S.G. & Chung, F.L. (1994) Structure–activity relationships of isothiocyanates as mechanism-based inhibitors of 4-(methylnitrosamino)-1-(3-pyridyl)-1-butanone-induced lung tumorigenesis in A/J mice. *Cancer Res.*, **54**, 4327–4333

Jiao, D., Conaway, C.C., Wang, M.H., Yang, C.S., Koehl, W. & Chung, F.L. (1996) Inhibition of *N*-nitrosodimethylamine demethylase in rat and human liver microsomes by isothiocyanates and their glutathione, L-cysteine, and *N*-acetyl-L-cysteine conjugates. *Chem. Res. Toxicol.*, **9**, 932–938

Jiao, D., Smith, T.J., Yang, C.S., Pittman, B., Desai, D., Amin, S. & Chung, F.L. (1997) Chemopreventive activity of thiol conjugates of isothiocyanates for lung tumorigenesis. *Carcinogenesis*, **18**, 2143–2147

Jiao, D., Yu, M.C., Hankin, J.H., Low, S.H. & Chung, F.L. (1998) Total isothiocyanate contents in cooked vegetables frequently consumed in Singapore. *J. Agric. Food Chem.*, **46**, 1055–1058

Jin, L., Qi, M., Chen, D.Z., Anderson, A., Yang, G.Y., Arbeit, J.M. & Auborn, K.J. (1999) Indole-3-carbinol prevents cervical cancer in human papilloma virus type 16 (HPV16) transgenic mice. *Cancer Res.*, **59**, 3991–3997

Johnston, C.S., Taylor, C.A. & Hampl, J.S. (2000) More Americans are eating '5 a day' but intakes of dark green and cruciferous vegetables remain low. *J. Nutr.*, **130**, 3063–3067

Jongen, W.M., Topp, R.J., Wienk, K.J. & Homan, E.C. (1989) Modulating effects of naturally occurring indoles on SCE induction depend largely on the type of mutagen. *Mutat. Res.*, **222**, 263–269

Joshipura, K.J., Ascherio, A., Manson, J.E., Stampfer, J.J., Rimm, E.B., Speizer, F.E., Hennekens, C.H., Spiegelman, D. & Willett, W.C. (1999) Fruit and vegetable intake in relation to risk of ischemic stroke. *JAMA*, **282**, 1233–1239

Joshipura, K.J., Hu, F.B., Manson, J.E., Stampfer, M.J., Rimm, E.B., Speizer, F.E., Colditz, G., Ascherio, A., Rosner, B., Spiegelman, D. & Willett, W.C. (2001) The effect of fruit and vegetable intake on risk for coronary heart disease. *Ann. Intern. Med.*, **134**, 1106–1114

Jowsey, I. R., Jiang, Q., Itoh, K., Yamamoto, M. & Hayes, J. D. (2003) Expression of the aflatoxin B_1-8,9-epoxide-metabolizing murine glutathione *S*-transferase a3 subunit is regulated by the Nrf2 transcription factor through an antioxidant response element. *Mol. Pharmacol.*, **64**, 1018–1028

Kabat, G.C., Chang, C.J., Sparano, J.A., Sepkovie, D.W., Hu, X.P., Khalil, A., Rosenblatt, R. & Bradlow, H.L. (1997) Urinary estrogen metabolites and breast cancer: A case–control study. *Cancer Epidemiol. Biomarkers Prev.*, **6**, 505–509

Kall, M.A., Vang, O. & Clausen, J. (1996) Effects of dietary broccoli on human *in vivo* drug metabolizing enzymes: Evaluation of caffeine, oestrone and chlorzoxazone metabolism. *Carcinogenesis*, **17**, 793–799

Kang, J.S., Kim, D.J., Ahn, B., Nam, K.T., Kim, K.S., Choi, M. & Jang, D.D. (2001) Post-initiation treatment of indole-3-carbinol did not suppress *N*-methyl-*N*-nitrosourea induced mammary carcinogenesis in rats. *Cancer Lett.*, **169**, 147–154

Kasamaki, A., Takahashi, H., Tsumura, N., Niwa, J., Fujita, T. & Urasawa, S. (1982) Genotoxicity of flavoring agents. *Mutat. Res.*, **105**, 387–392

Kasamaki, A., Yasuhara, T. & Ursawa, S. (1987) Neoplastic transformation of Chinese hamster cells *in vitro* after treatment with flavouring agents. *J. Toxicol. Sci.*, **12**, 383–396

Kassahun, K., Davis, M., Hu, P., Martin, B. & Baillie, T. (1997) Biotransformation of the naturally occurring isothiocyanate sulforaphane in the rat: Identification of phase I metabolites and glutathione conjugates. *Chem. Res. Toxicol.*, **10**, 1228–1233

Kassie, F. & Knasmüller, S. (2000) Genotoxic effects of allyl isothiocyanate (AITC) and phenethyl isothiocyanate (PEITC). *Chem.–Biol. Interactions*, **127**, 163–180

Kassie, F., Parzefall, W., Musk, S., Johnson, I., Lamprecht, G., Sontag, G. & Knasmüller, S. (1996) Genotoxic effects of crude juices from Brassica vegetables and juices and extracts from phytopharmaceutical preparations and spices of cruciferous plants origin in bacterial and mammalian cells. *Chem.–Biol. Interactions*, **102**, 1–16

Kassie, F., Pool-Zobel, B., Parzefall, W. & Knasmüller, S. (1999) Genotoxic effects of benzyl isothiocyanate, a natural chemopreventive agent. *Mutagenesis*, **14**, 595–604

Kassie, F., Laky, B., Nobis, E., Kundi, M. & Knasmüller, S. (2001) Genotoxic effects of methyl isothiocyanate. *Mutat. Res.*, **490**, 1–9

Kassie, F., Rabot, S., Uhl, M., Huber, W., Qin, H.M., Helma, C., Schulte-Hermann, R. & Knasmüller, S. (2002) Chemoprotective effects of garden cress (*Lepidium sativum*) and its constituents towards 2-amino-3-methyl-imidazo[4,5-f]quinoline (IQ)-induced genotoxic effects and colonic preneoplastic lesions. *Carcinogenesis*, **23**, 1155–1161

Kassie, F., Uhl, M., Rabot, S., Grasl-Kraupp, B., Verkerk, R., Kundi, M., Chabicovsky, M., Schulte-Hermann, R. & Knasmüller, S. (2003a) Chemoprevention of 2-amino-3-methylimidazo[4,5-*f*]quinoline (IQ)-induced colonic and hepatic preneoplastic lesions in the Fischer 344 rat by cruciferous vegetables administered simultaneously with the carcinogen. *Carcinogenesis*, **24**, 255–261

Kassie, F., Laky, B., Gminski, R., Mersch-Sundermann, V., Scharf, G., Lhoste, E. & Knasmuller, S. (2003b) Effects of garden and water cress juice and their constituents, benzyl and phenethyl isothiocyanates, towards benzo(a)pyrene-induced DNA damage: A model study with the single cell gel electrophoresis/Hep G2 assay. *Chem.–Biol. Interactions*, **142**, 285–296.

Katchamart, S. & Williams, D.E. (2001) Indole-3-carbinol modulation of hepatic monooxygenases CYP1A1, CYP1A2 and FMO1 in guinea pig, mouse and rabbit. *Comp. Biochem. Physiol. C Toxicol. Pharmacol.*, **129**, 377–384

Katchamart, S., Stresser, D.M., Dehal, S.S., Kupfer, D. & Williams, D.E. (2000) Concurrent flavin-containing monooxygenase down-regulation and cytochrome P-450 induction by dietary indoles in rat: Implications for drug–drug interaction. *Drug Metab. Disposition*, **28**, 930–936

Katdare, M., Osborne, M.P. & Telang, N.T. (1998) Inhibition of aberrant proliferation and induction of apoptosis in pre-neoplastic human mammary epithelial cells by natural phytochemicals. *Oncol. Rep.*, **5**, 311–315

Katsouyanni, K., Trichopoulos, D., Boyle, P., Xirouchaki, E., Trichopoulou, A., Lisseos, B., Vasilaros, S. & MacMahon, B. (1986) Diet and breast cancer: A case–control study in Greece. *Int. J. Cancer*, **38**, 815–820

Keck, A.S., Staack, R. & Jeffery, E.H. (2002) The cruciferous nitrile crambene has bioac-tivity similar to sulforaphane when administered to Fischer 344 rats but is far less potent in cell culture. *Nutr. Cancer*, **42**, 233–240

Keck, A.S., Qiao, Q. & Jeffery, E.H. (2003) Food matrix effects on bioactivity of broccoli-derived sulforaphane in liver and colon of F344 rats. *J. Agric. Food Chem.*, **51**, 3320–3327

Kempin, S.J. (1983) Warfarin resistance caused by broccoli. *N. Engl. J. Med.*, **308**, 1229–1230

Ketterer, B. (1998) Dietary isothiocyanates as confounding factors in the molecular epidemiology of colon cancer. *Cancer Epidemiol. Biomarkers Prev.*, **7**, 645–646

Kim, D.J., Lee, K.K., Han, B.S., Ahn, B., Bae, J.H. & Jang, J.J. (1994) Biphasic modifying effect of indole-3-carbinol on diethylnitrosamine-induced preneoplastic glutathione S-transferase placental form-positive liver cell foci in Sprague-Dawley rats. *Jpn. J. Cancer Res.*, **85**, 578–583

Kim, D.J., Han, B.S., Ahn, B., Hasegawa, R., Shirai, T., Ito, N. & Tsuda, H. (1997) Enhancement by indole-3-carbinol of liver and thyroid gland neoplastic development in a rat medium-term multiorgan carcinogenesis model. *Carcinogenesis*, **18**, 377–381

Kim, D.J., Shin, D.H., Ahn, B., Kang, J.S., Nam, K.T., Park, C.B., Kim, C.K., Hong, J.T., Kim, Y.B., Yun, Y.W., Jang, D.D. & Yang, K.H. (2003) Chemoprevention of colon cancer by Korean food plant components. *Mutat. Res.*, **523–524**, 99–107

Kirlin, W.G., Cai, J., DeLong, M.J., Patten, E.J. & Jones, D.P. (1999a) Dietary compounds that induce cancer preventive phase 2 enzymes activate apoptosis at comparable doses in HT29 colon carcinoma cells. *J. Nutr.*, **129**, 1827–1835

Kirlin, W.G., Cai, J., Thompson, S.A., Diaz, D., Kavanagh, T.J. & Jones, D.P. (1999b) Glutathione redox potential in response to differentiation and enzyme inducers. *Free Radicals Biol. Med.*, **27**, 1208–1218

Kishida, T., Beppu, M., Nashiki, K., Izumi, T. & Ebihara, K. (2000) Effect of dietary soy isoflavone aglycones on the urinary 16α-to-2-hydroxyestrone ratio in C3H/HeJ mice. *Nutr. Cancer*, **38**, 209–214

Kjaerheim, K., Gaard, M. & Andersen, A. (1998) The role of alcohol, tobacco, and dietary factors in upper aerogastric tract cancers: A prospective study of 10,900 Norwegian men. *Cancer Causes Control*, **9**, 99–108

Klesse, P. & Lukoschek, P. (1955) [Studies on the bacteriostatic effects of some mustard oils]. *Arzneimittelforschung*, **5**, 505–507 (in German)

Kneller, R.W., McLaughlin, J.K., Bjelke, E., Schuman, L.M., Blot, W.J., Wacholder, S., Gridley, G., CoChien, H.T. & Fraumeni, J.F., Jr (1991) A cohort study of stomach cancer in a high-risk American population. *Cancer*, **68**, 672–678

Knize, M.G., Kulp, K.S., Salmon, C.P., Keating, G.A. & Felton, J.S. (2002) Factors affecting human heterocyclic amine intake and the metabolism of PhIP. *Mutat. Res.*, **506–507**, 153–162

Kojima, T., Tanaka, T. & Mori, H. (1994) Chemoprevention of spontaneous endometrial cancer in female Donryu rats by dietary indole-3-carbinol. *Cancer Res.*, **54**, 1446–1449

Kolm, R.H., Danielson, U.H., Zhang, Y., Talalay, P. & Mannervik, B. (1995) Isothiocyanates as substrates for human glutathione transferases: Structure–activity studies. *Biochem. J.*, **311** (Part 2), 453–459

Kolonel, L.N., Hankin, J.H., Wilkens, L.R., Fukunaga, F.H. & Hinds, M.W. (1990) An epidemiologic study of thyroid cancer in Hawaii. *Cancer Causes Control*, **1**, 223–234

Kolonel, L.N., Hankin, J.H., Whittemore, A.S., Wu, A.H., Gallagher, R.P., Wilkens, L.R., John, E.M., Howe, G.R., Dreon, D.M., West, D.W. & Paffenbarger, R.S., Jr (2000) Vegetables, fruits, legumes and prostate cancer: A multiethnic case–control study. *Cancer Epidemiol. Biomarkers Prev.*, **9**, 795–804

Koo, L.C. (1988) Dietary habits and lung cancer risk among Chinese females in Hong Kong who never smoked. *Nutr. Cancer*, **11**, 155–172

Kore, A.M., Jeffery, E.H. & Wallig, M.A. (1993) Effects of 1-isothiocyanato-3-(methylsulfinyl)propane on xenobiotic metabolizing enzymes in rats. *Food Chem. Toxicol.*, **31**, 723–729

Korinek, V., Barker, N., Willert, K., Molenaar, M., Roose, J., Wagenaar, G., Markman, M., Lamers, W., Destree, O. & Clevers, H. (1998) Two members of the Tcf family implicated in Wnt/b-catenin signaling during embryogenesis in the mouse. *Mol. Cell Biol.*, **18**, 1248–1256

Kroymann, J., Textor, S., Tokuhisa, J.G., Falk, K.L., Bartram, S., Gershenzon, J. & Mitchell-Olds, T. (2001) A gene controlling variation in *Arabidopsis* glucosinolate composition is part of the methionine chain elongation pathway. *Plant Physiol.*, **127**, 1077–1088

Kroymann, J., Donnerhacke, S., Schnabelrauch, D. & Mitchell-Olds, T. (2003) Evolutionary dynamics of an *Arabidopsis* insect resistance quantitative trait locus. *Proc. Natl Acad. Sci. USA*, **100** (Suppl. 2), 14587–14592

de Kruif, C.A., Marsman, J.W., Venekamp, J.C., Falke, H.E., Noordhoek, J., Blaauboer, B.J. & Wortelboer, H.M. (1991) Structure elucidation of acid reaction products of indole-3-carbinol: Detection in vivo and enzyme induction in vitro. *Chem.–Biol. Interactions*, **80**, 303–315

Krul, C., Humblot, C., Philippe, C., Vermeulen, M., van Nuenen, M., Havenaar, R. & Rabot, S. (2002) Metabolism of sinigrin (2-propenyl glucosinolate) by the human colonic microflora in a dynamic *in vitro* large-intestinal model. *Carcinogenesis*, **23**, 1009–1016

Kune, S., Kune, G.A. & Watson, L.F. (1987) Case–control study of dietary etiological factors: The Melbourne colorectal cancer study. *Nutr. Cancer*, **9**, 21–42

Kuo, M.L., Lee, K.C. & Lin, J.K. (1992) Genotoxicities of nitropyrenes and their modulation by apigenin, tannic acid, ellagic acid and indole-3-carbinol in the Salmonella and CHO systems. *Mutat. Res.*, **270**, 87–95

Kushad, M.M., Brown, A.F., Kurilich, A.C., Juvik, J.A., Klein, B.P., Wallig, M.A. & Jeffery, E.H. (1999) Variation of glucosinolates in vegetable crops of *Brassica oleracea*. *J. Agric. Food Chem.*, **47**, 1541–1548

Kwak, M.K., Wakabayashi, N., Itoh, K., Motohashi, H., Yamamoto, M. & Kensler, T.W. (2003) Modulation of gene expression by cancer chemopreventive dithiolethiones through the Keap1-Nrf2 pathway. Identification of novel gene clusters for cell survival. *J. Biol. Chem.*, **278**, 8135–8145

Kwon, C.S., Grose, K.R., Riby, J., Chen, Y.H. & Bjeldanes, L.F. (1994) In vivo production and enzyme-inducing activity of indolo(3,2-*b*)carbazole. *J. Agric. Food Chem.*, **42**, 2536–2540

Kyung, K.H. & Fleming, H.P. (1997) Antimicrobial activity of sulfur compounds derived from cabbage. *J. Food Prot.*, **60**, 67–71

Laky, B., Knasmuller, S., Gminiski, R., Mersch-Sundermann, V., Scharf, G., Verkerk, R., Freywald, C., Uhl, M. & Kassie, F. (2002) Protective effects of Brussels sprouts towards benzo(a)pyrene-induced DNA damage. *Food Chem. Toxicol.*, **40**, 1072–1083.

Lambrix, V., Reichelt, M., Mitchell-Olds, T., Kliebenstein, D.J. & Gershenzon, J. (2001) The *Arabidopsis* epithiospecifier protein promotes the hydrolysis of glucosinolates to nitriles and influences *Trichoplusia ni* Herbivory. *Plant Cell*, **13**, 2793–2807

Lampe, J.W., King, I.B., Li, S., Grate, M.T., Barale, K.V., Chen, C., Feng, Z. & Potter, J.D. (2000a) Brassica vegetables increase and apiaceous vegetables decrease cytochrome P450 1A2 activity in humans: Changes in caffeine metabolite ratios in response to controlled vegetable diets. *Carcinogenesis*, **21**, 1157–1162

Lampe, J.W., Chen, C., Li, S., Prunty, J., Grate, M.T., Meehan, D.E., Barale, K.V., Dightman, D.A., Feng, Z. & Potter, J.D. (2000b) Modulation of human glutathione S-transferases by botanically defined vegetable diets. *Cancer Epidemiol. Biomarkers Prev.*, **9**, 787–793

Langer, P. & Stolc, V. (1965) Goitrogenic activity of allylisothiocyanate — A widespread natural mustard oil. *Endocrinology*, **76**, 151–155

Langer, P., Michajlovskij, N., Sedlak, J. & Kutka, M. (1971) Studies on the antithyroid activity of naturally occurring L-5-vinyl-2-thiooxazolidone in man. *Endokrinologie*, **57**, 225–229

Lanza, E., Schatzkin, A., Daston, C., Corle, D., Freedman, L., Ballard-Barbash, R., Caan, B., Lance, P., Marshall, J., Iber, F., Shike, M., Weissfeld, J., Slattery, M., Paskett, E., Mateski, D., Albert, P. & the PPT Study Group (2001) Implementation of a 4-y, high-fiber, high-fruit-and-vegetable, low-fat dietary intervention: Results of dietary changes in the Polyp Prevention Trial. *Am. J. Clin. Nutr.*, **74**, 387–401

Larsen-Su, S. & Williams, D.E. (1996) Dietary indole-3-carbinol inhibits FMO activity and the expression of flavin-containing monooxygenase form 1 in rat liver and intestine. *Drug Metab. Disposition*, **24**, 927–931

Larsen-Su, S.A. & Williams, D.E. (2001) Transplacental exposure to indole-3-carbinol induces sex-specific expression of CYP1A1 and CYP1B1 in the liver of Fischer 344 neonatal rats. *Toxicol. Sci.*, **64**, 162–168

La Vecchia, C., Negri, E., Decarli, A., D'Avanzo, B., Gallotti, L., Gentile, A. & Franceschi, S. (1988) A case–control study of diet and colo-rectal cancer in northern Italy. *Int. J. Cancer*, **41**, 492–498

Le, H.T., Schaldach, C.M., Firestone, G.L. & Bjeldanes, L.F. (2003) Plant derived 3,3′-diindolylmethane is a strong androgen antagonist in human prostate cancer cells. *J. Biol. Chem.*, **278**, 21136–21145

Leclercq, I., Desager, J.P. & Horsmans, Y. (1998) Inhibition of chlorzoxazone metabolism, a clinical probe for CYP2E1, by a single ingestion of watercress. *Clin. Pharmacol. Ther.*, **64**, 144–149

Lee, M.S. (1992) Oxidative conversion by rat liver microsomes of 2-naphthyl isothiocyanate to 2-naphthyl isocyanate, a genotoxicant. *Chem. Res. Toxicol.*, **5**, 791–796

Lee, M.S. (1996) Enzyme induction and comparative oxidative desulfuration of isothiocyanates to isocyanates. *Chem. Res. Toxicol.*, **9**, 1072–1078

Lee, H.P., Gourley, L., Duffy, S.W., Estève, J., Lee, J. & Day, N.E. (1989) Colorectal cancer and diet in an Asian population—A case–control study among Singapore Chinese. *Int. J. Cancer*, **43**, 1007–1016

Lee, J.K., Park, B.J., Yoo, K.Y. & Ahn, Y.O. (1995) Dietary factors and stomach cancer: A case–control study in Korea. *Int. J. Epidemiol.*, **24**, 33–41

Lee, P.J., Alam, J., Wiegand, G.W. & Choi, A.M. (1996) Overexpression of heme oxygenase-1 in human pulmonary epithelial cells results in cell growth arrest and increased resistance to hyperoxia. *Proc. Natl Acad. Sci. USA*, **93**, 10393–10398

Lee, J.M., Calkins, M.J., Chan, K., Kan, Y.W. & Johnson, J.A. (2003) Identification of the NF-E2-related factor-2-dependent genes conferring protection against oxidative stress in primary cortical astrocytes using oligonucleotide microarray analysis. *J. Biol. Chem.*, **278**, 12029–12038

Leibelt, D.A., Hedstrom, O.R., Fischer, K.A., Pereira, C.B. & Williams, D.E. (2003) Evaluation of chronic dietary exposure to indole-3-carbinol and absorption-enhanced 3,3´-diindolylmethane in Sprague-Dawley rats. *Toxicol. Sci.*, **74**, 10–21

Le Marchand, L., Yoshizawa, C.N., Kolonel, L.N., Hankin, J.H. & Goodman, M.T. (1989) Vegetable consumption and lung cancer risk: A population-based case–control study in Hawaii. *J. Natl Cancer Inst.*, **81**, 1158–1164

Le Marchand, L., Hankin, J.H., Kolonel, L.N. & Wilkens, L.R. (1991) Vegetable and fruit consumption in relation to prostate cancer risk in Hawaii: A reevaluation of the effect of dietary beta-carotene. *Am. J. Epidemiol.*, **133**, 215–219

Lenman, M., Rodin, J., Josefsson, L.G. & Rask, L. (1990) Immunological characterization of rapeseed myrosinase. *Eur. J. Biochem.*, **194**, 747–753

Lenman, M., Falk, A., Rödin, J., Höglund, A.S., Ek, B. & Rask, L. (1993) Differential expression of myrosinase gene families. *Plant Physiol.*, **103**, 703–711

Leong, H., Firestone, G.L. & Bjeldanes, L.F. (2001) Cytostatic effects of 3,3´-diindolyl-methane in human endometrial cancer cells result from an estrogen receptor-mediated increase in transforming growth factor-α expression. *Carcinogenesis*, **22**, 1809–1817

Leoni, O., Iori, R., Palmieri, S., Esposito, E., Menegatti, E., Cortesi, R. & Nastruzzi, C. (1997) Myrosinase-generated isothiocyanate from glucosinolates: Isolation, characterization and in vitro antiproliferative studies. *Bioorg. Med. Chem.*, **5**, 1799–1806

Levi, F., La Vecchia, C., Gulie, C. & Negri, E. (1993a) Dietary factors and breast cancer risk in Vaud, Switzerland. *Nutr. Cancer*, **19**, 327–335

Levi, F., Franceschi, S., Negri, E. & La Vecchia, C. (1993b) Dietary factors and the risk of endometrial cancer. *Cancer*, **71**, 3575–3581

Lewerenz, H.J., Plass, R., Bleyl, D.W. & Macholz, R. (1988) Short-term toxicity study of allyl isothiocyanate in rats. *Nahrung*, **32**, 723–728

Lewerenz, H.J., Bleyl, D.W. & Plass, R. (1992) Subacute oral toxicity study of benzyl isothiocyanate in rats. *Nahrung*, **36**, 190–198

Lewis, S., Brennan, P., Nyberg, F., Ahrens, W., Constantinescu, V., Mukeria, A., Benhamou, S., Batura-Gabryel, H., Bruske-Hohlfeld, I., Simonato, L., Menezes, A. & Boffetta, P. (2002) Cruciferous vegetable intake, GSTM1 genotype and lung cancer risk in a non-smoking population. In : Riboli, E. & Lambert, R., eds, *Nutrition and Lifestyle: Opportunities for Cancer Prevention* (IARC Scientific Publications No. 156), Lyon, IARCPress, pp. 507–508

Li, Y., Wang, E.J., Chen, L., Stein, A.P., Reuhl, K.R. & Yang, C.S. (1997) Effects of phenethyl isothiocyanate on acetaminophen metabolism and hepatotoxicity in mice. *Toxicol. Appl. Pharmacol.*, **144**, 306–314

Li, H., Zhu, H., Xu, C.J. & Yuan, J. (1998) Cleavage of BID by caspase 8 mediates the mitochondrial damage in the Fas pathway of apoptosis. *Cell*, **94**, 491–501

Li, Y., Li, X. & Sarkar, F.H. (2003) Gene expression profiles of I3C- and DIM-treated PC3 human prostate cancer cells determined by cDNA microarray analysis. *J. Nutr.*, **133**, 1011–1019

Lichtenstein, E.P., Strong, F.M. & Morgan, D.G. (1962) Identification of 2-phenylethyl isothiocyanate as an insecticide occurring naturally in the edible part of turnips. *J. Agric. Food Chem.*, **10**, 30–33

Liebes, L., Conaway, C.C., Hochster, H., Mendoza, S., Hecht, S.S., Crowell, J. & Chung, F.L. (2001) High-performance liquid chromatography-based determination of total isothiocyanate levels in human plasma: Application to studies with 2-phenethyl isothiocyanate. *Anal. Biochem.*, **291**, 279–289

van Lieshout, E.M., Bedaf, M.M., Pieter, M., Ekkel, C., Nijhoff, W.A. & Peters, W.H. (1998a) Effects of dietary anticarcinogens on rat gastrointestinal glutathione S-transferase theta 1-1 levels. *Carcinogenesis*, **19**, 2055–2057

van Lieshout, E.M., Posner, G.H., Woodard, B.T. & Peters, W.H. (1998b) Effects of the sulforaphane analog compound 30, indole-3-carbinol, D-limonene or relafen on glutathione S-transferases and glutathione peroxidase of the rat digestive tract. *Biochim. Biophys. Acta*, **1379**, 325–336

Lin, J.M., Amin, S., Trushin, N. & Hecht, S.S. (1993) Effects of isothiocyanates on tumorigenesis by benzo[a]pyrene in murine tumour models. *Cancer Lett.*, **74**, 151–159

Lin, H.J., Probst-Hensch, N.M., Louie, A.D., Kau, I.H., Witte, J.S., Ingles, S.A., Frankl, H.D., Lee, E.R. & Haile, R.W. (1998) Glutathione transferase null genotype, broccoli, and lower prevalence of colorectal adenomas. *Cancer Epidemiol. Biomarkers Prev.*, **7**, 647–652

Lin, C.M., Preston, J.F., III & Wei, C.I. (2000a) Antibacterial mechanism of allyl isothiocyanate. *J. Food Prot.*, **63**, 727–734

Lin, C.M., Kim, J., Du, W.X. & Wei, C.I. (2000b) Bactericidal activity of isothiocyanate against pathogens on fresh produce. *J. Food Prot.*, **63**, 25–30

Lin, H.J., Zhou, H., Dai, A., Huang, H.F., Lin, J.H., Frankl, H.D., Lee, E.R. & Haile, R.W. (2002) Glutathione transferase GSTT1, broccoli, and prevalence of colorectal adenomas. *Pharmacogenetics*, **12**, 175–179

Lindblad, P., Wolk, A., Bergström, R. & Adami, H.O. (1997) Diet and risk of renal cell cancer: A population-based case–control study. *Cancer Epidemiol. Biomarkers Prev.*, **6**, 215–223

Lissowska, J., Pilarska, A., Pilarski, P., Samolczyk-Wanyura, D., Piekarczyk, J., Bardin-Mikollajczak, A., Zatonski, W., Herrero, R., Muñoz, N. & Franceschi, S. (2003) Smoking, alcohol, diet, dentition and sexual practices in the epidemiology of oral cancer in Poland. *Eur. J. Cancer Prev.*, **12**, 25–33

Littman, A.J., Beresford, S.A. & White, E. (2001) The association of dietary fat and plant foods with endometrial cancer (United States). *Cancer Causes Control*, **12**, 691–702

Liu, J.Z., Gilbert, K., Parker, H.M., Haschek, W.M. & Milner, J.A. (1991) Inhibition of 7,12-dimethylbenz(a)anthracene-induced mammary tumors and DNA adducts by dietary selenite. *Cancer Res.*, **51**, 4613–4617

Liu, J., Lin, R.I. & Milner, J.A. (1992) Inhibition of 7,12-dimethylbenz[a]anthracene-induced mammary tumors and DNA adducts by garlic powder. *Carcinogenesis*, **13**, 1847–1851

Liu, H., Wormke, M., Safe, S.H. & Bjeldanes, L.F. (1994) Indolo[3,2-b]carbazole: A dietary-derived factor that exhibits both antiestrogenic and estrogenic activity. *J. Natl Cancer Inst.*, **86**, 1758–1765

Loeb, L.A. & Christians, F.C. (1996) Multiple mutations in human cancers. *Mutat. Res.*, **350**, 279–286

Loft, S. & Poulsen, H.E. (2000) Antioxidant intervention studies related to DNA damage, DNA repair and gene expression. *Free Radicals Res.*, **33** (Suppl.), S67–S83

Loft, S., Otte, J., Poulsen, H.E. & Sorensen, H. (1992) Influence of intact and myrosinase-treated indolyl glucosinolates on the metabolism *in vivo* of metronidazole and antipyrine in the rat. *Food Chem. Toxicol.*, **30**, 927–935

London, S.J., Yuan, J.M., Chung, F.L., Gao, Y.T., Coetzee, G.A., Ross, R.K. & Yu, M.C. (2000) Isothiocyanates, glutathione S-transferase M1 and T1 polymorphisms, and lung-cancer risk: A prospective study of men in Shanghai, China. *Lancet*, **356**, 724–729

Lopez, M. & Mazzanti, L. (1955) Experimental investigations on alpha-naphthyl-isothiocyanate as a hyperplastic agent of the biliary ducts in the rat. *J. Pathol. Bacteriol.*, **69**, 243–250

Loub, W.D., Wattenberg, L.W. & Davis, D.W. (1975) Aryl hydrocarbon hydroxylase induction in rat tissues by naturally occurring indoles of cruciferous plants. *J. Natl Cancer Inst.*, **54**, 985–988

Lubet, R.A., Steele, V.E., Eto, I., Juliana, M.M., Kelloff, G.J. & Grubbs, C.J. (1997) Chemopreventive efficacy of anethole trithione, N-acetyl-L-cysteine, miconazole and phenethylisothiocyanate in the DMBA-induced rat mammary cancer model. *Int. J. Cancer*, **72**, 95–101

Lund, E.K., Smith, T.K., Clarke, R.G. & Johnson, I.T. (2001) Cell death in the colorectal cancer cell line HT29 in response to glucosinolate metabolites. *J. Sci. Food Agric.*, **81**, 959–961

Maclure, M. & Willett, W. (1990) A case–control study of diet and risk of renal adenocarcinoma. *Epidemiology*, **1**, 430–440

Maeda, H., Katsuki, T., Akaike, T. & Yasutake, R. (1992) High correlation between lipid peroxide radical and tumor-promoter effect: Suppression of tumor promotion in the Epstein-Barr virus/B-lymphocyte system and scavenging of alkyl peroxide radicals by various vegetable extracts. *Jpn. J. Cancer Res.*, **83**, 923–928

Mahéo, K., Morel, F., Langouët, S., Kramer, H., Le Ferrec, E., Ketterer, B. & Guillouzo, A. (1997) Inhibition of cytochromes P-450 and induction of glutathione S-transferases by sulforaphane in primary human and rat hepatocytes. *Cancer Res.*, **57**, 3649–3652

Malejka-Giganti, D., Niehans, G.A., Reichert, M.A. & Bliss, R.L. (2000) Post-initiation treatment of rats with indole-3-carbinol or β-naphthoflavone does not suppress 7,12-dimethylbenz[a]anthracene-induced mammary gland carcinogenesis. *Cancer Lett.*, **160**, 209–218

Malloy, V.L., Bradlow, H.L. & Orentreich, N. (1997) Interaction between a semisynthetic diet and indole-3-carbinol on mammary tumour incidence in Balb/cfC3H mice. *Anticancer Res.*, **17**, 4333–4337

Manson, M.M., Barrett, M.C., Clark, H.L., Judah, D.J., Williamson, G. & Neal, G.E. (1997) Mechanisms of action of dietary chemoprotective agents in rat liver: Induction of phase I and II drug-metabolising enzymes and aflatoxin B metabolism. *Carcinogenesis*, **18**, 1729–1738

Manson, M.M., Hudson, E.A., Ball, H.W., Barrett, M.C., Clark, H.L., Judah, D.J., Verschoyle, R.D. & Neal, G.E. (1998) Chemoprevention of aflatoxin B_1-induced carcinogenesis by indole-3-carbinol in rat liver—Predicting the outcome using early biomarkers. *Carcinogenesis*, **19**, 1829–1836

Marshall, J.R., Graham, S., Byers, T., Swanson, M. & Brasure, J. (1983) Diet and smoking in the epidemiology of cancer of the cervix. *J. Natl Cancer Inst.*, **70**, 847–851

Martin, C., Connelly, A., Keku, T.O., Mountcastle, S.B., Galanko, J., Woosley, J.T., Schliebe, B., Lund, P.K. & Sandler, R.S. (2002) Nonsteroidal anti-inflammatory drugs, apoptosis, and colorectal adenomas. *Gastroenterology*, **123**, 1770–1777

Mason, J.M., Zeiger, E., Haworth, S., Ivett, J. & Valencia, R. (1987) Genotoxicity studies of methyl isocyanate in Salmonella, Drosophila, and cultured Chinese hamster ovary cells. *Environ. Mutag.*, **9**, 19–28

Masutomi, N., Toyoda, K., Shibutani, M., Niho, N., Uneyama, C., Takahashi, N. & Hirose, M. (2001) Toxic effects of benzyl and allyl isothiocyanates and benzyl-isoform specific metabolites in the urinary bladder after a single intravesical application to rats. *Toxicol. Pathol.*, **29**, 617–622

Matusheski, N.V. & Jeffery, E.H. (2001) Comparison of the bioactivity of two glucoraphanin hydrolysis products found in broccoli, sulforaphane and sulforaphane nitrile. *J. Agric. Food Chem.*, **49**, 5743–5749

Matusheski, N.V., Juvik, J.A. & Jeffery, E.H. (2003) Sulforaphane content and bioactivity of broccoli sprouts are enhanced by heat processing: A role for epithiospecifier protein. *FASEB J.*, **17**, A377–A377

Mawson, R., Heaney, R.K., Zdunczyk, Z. & Kozlowska, H. (1994) Rapeseed meal-glucosinolates and their antinutritional effects. Part 5. Animal reproduction. *Nahrung*, **38**, 588–598

McCullough, M.L., Robertson, A.S., Chao, A., Jacobs, E.J., Stampfer, M.J., Jacobs, D.R., Diver, W.R., Calle, E.E. & Thun, M.J. (2003) A prospective study of whole grains, fruits, vegetables and colon cancer risk. *Cancer Causes Control*, **14**, 959–970

McDanell, R., McLean, A.E., Hanley, A.B., Heaney, R.K. & Fenwick, G.R. (1987) Differential induction of mixed-function oxidase (MFO) activity in rat liver and intestine by diets containing processed cabbage: Correlation with cabbage levels of glucosinolates and glucosinolate hydrolysis products. *Food Chem. Toxicol.*, **25**, 363–368

McDanell, R., McLean, A.E., Hanley, A.B., Heaney, R.K. & Fenwick, G.R. (1989) The effect of feeding Brassica vegetables and intact glucosinolates on mixed-function-oxidase activity in the livers and intestines of rats. *Food Chem. Toxicol.*, **27**, 289–293

McDougal, A., Gupta, M.S., Morrow, D., Ramamoorthy, K., Lee, J.E. & Safe, S.H. (2001) Methyl-substituted diindolylmethanes as inhibitors of estrogen-induced growth of T47D cells and mammary tumours in rats. *Breast Cancer Res. Treat.*, **66**, 147–157

McLaughlin, J.K., Mandel, J.S., Blot, W.J., Schuman, L.M., Mehl, E.S. & Fraumeni, J.F., Jr (1984) A population-based case–control study of renal cell carcinoma. *J. Natl Cancer Inst.*, **72**, 275–284

McLaughlin, J.K., Gridley, G., Block, G., Winn, D.M., Preston-Martin, S., Schoenberg, J.B., Greenberg, R.S., Stemhagen, A., Austin, D.F. & Ershow, A.G. (1988) Dietary factors in oral and pharyngeal cancer. *J. Natl Cancer Inst.*, **80**, 1237–1243

McLaughlin, J.K., Gao, Y.T., Gao, R.N., Zheng, W., Ji, B.T., Blot, W.J. & Fraumeni, J.F., Jr (1992) Risk factors for renal-cell cancer in Shanghai, China. *Int. J. Cancer*, **52**, 562–565

McLean, M.R. & Rees, K.R. (1958) Hyperplasia of bile-ducts induced by alpha-naphthyl-isothiocyanate: Experimental biliary cirrhosis free from biliary obstruction. *J. Pathol. Bacteriol.*, **76**, 175–188

McMahon, M., Itoh, K., Yamamoto, M., Chanas, S.A., Henderson, C.J., McLellan, L.I., Wolf, C.R., Cavin, C. & Hayes, J.D. (2001) The Cap'n'Collar basic leucine zipper transcription factor Nrf2 (NF-E2 p45-related factor 2) controls both constitutive and inducible expression of intestinal detoxification and glutathione biosynthetic enzymes. *Cancer Res.*, **61**, 3299–3307

McMahon, M., Itoh, K., Yamamoto, M. & Hayes, J.D. (2003) Keap1-dependent proteasomal degradation of transcription factor Nrf2 contributes to the negative regulation of antioxidant response element-driven gene expression. *J. Biol. Chem.*, **278**, 21592–21600

McMillan, M., Spinks, E.A. & Fenwick, G.R. (1986) Preliminary observations on the effect of dietary Brussels sprouts on thyroid function. *Hum. Toxicol.*, **5**, 15–19

Meah, M.N., Harrison, N. & Davies, A. (1994) Nitrate and nitrite in foods and the diet. *Food Addit. Contam.*, **11**, 519–532

Mehta, R.G., Liu, J., Constantinou, A., Thomas, C.F., Hawthorne, M., You, M., Gerhuser, C., Pezzuto, J.M., Moon, R.C. & Moriarty, R.M. (1995) Cancer chemopreventive activity of brassinin, a phytoalexin from cabbage. *Carcinogenesis*, **16**, 399–404

Meilahn, E.N., De Stavola, B., Allen, D.S., Fentiman, I., Bradlow, H.L., Sepkovic, D.W. & Kuller, L.H. (1998) Do urinary oestrogen metabolites predict breast cancer? Guernsey III cohort follow-up. *Br. J. Cancer*, **78**, 1250–1255

Mellemgaard, A., McLaughlin, J.K., Overvad, K. & Olsen, J.H. (1996) Dietary risk factors for renal cell carcinoma in Denmark. *Eur. J. Cancer*, **32A**, 673–682

Memon, A., Varghese, A. & Suresh, A. (2002) Benign thyroid disease and dietary factors in thyroid cancer: A case–control study in Kuwait. *Br. J. Cancer*, **86**, 1745–1750

Meng, Q., Qi, M., Chen, D.Z., Yuan, R., Goldberg, I.D., Rosen, E.M., Auborn, K. & Fan, S. (2000a) Suppression of breast cancer invasion and migration by indole-3-carbinol: Associated with up-regulation of BRCA1 and E-cadherin/catenin complexes. *J. Mol. Med.*, **78**, 155–165

Meng, Q., Goldberg, I.D., Rosen, E.M. & Fan, S. (2000b) Inhibitory effects of indole-3-carbinol on invasion and migration in human breast cancer cells. *Breast Cancer Res. Treat.*, **63**, 147–152

Meng, Q., Yuan, F., Goldberg, I.D., Rosen, E.M., Auborn, K. & Fan, S. (2000c) Indole-3-carbinol is a negative regulator of estrogen receptor-alpha signaling in human tumor cells. *J. Nutr.*, **130**, 2927–2931

Mennicke, W.H., Gorler, K. & Krumbiegel, G. (1983) Metabolism of some naturally occurring isothiocyanates in the rat. *Xenobiotica*, **13**, 203–207

Mennicke, W.H., Görler, K., Krumbiegel, G., Lorenz, D. & Rittmann, N. (1988) Studies on the metabolism and excretion of benzyl isothiocyanate in man. *Xenobiotica*, **18**, 441–447

Mettlin, C. & Graham, S. (1979) Dietary risk factors in human bladder cancer. *Am. J. Epidemiol.*, **110**, 255–263

Meyer, D.J., Crease, D.J. & Ketterer, B. (1995) Forward and reverse catalysis and product sequestration by human glutathione S-transferases in the reaction of GSH with dietary aralkyl isothiocyanates. *Biochem. J.*, **306** (Part 2), 565–569

Michaud, D.S., Spiegelman, D., Clinton, S.K., Rimm, E.B., Willett, W.C. & Giovannucci, E.L. (1999) Fruit and vegetable intake and incidence of bladder cancer in a male prospective cohort. *J. Natl Cancer Inst.*, **91**, 605–613

Michaud, D.S., Pietinen, P., Taylor, P.R., Virtanen, M., Virtamo, J. & Albanes, D. (2002) Intakes of fruits and vegetables, carotenoids and vitamins A, E, C in relation to the risk of bladder cancer in the ATBC cohort study. *Br. J. Cancer*, **87**, 960–965

Michels, K.B., Giovannucci, E., Joshipura, K.J., Rosner, B.A., Stampfer, M.J., Fuchs, C.S., Colditz, G.A., Speizer, F.E. & Willett, W.C. (2000) Prospective study of fruit and vegetable consumption and incidence of colon and rectal cancers. *J. Natl Cancer Inst.*, **92**, 1740–1752

Michnovicz, J.J. & Bradlow, H.L. (1990) Induction of estradiol metabolism by dietary indole-3-carbinol in humans. *J. Natl Cancer Inst.*, **82**, 947–949

Michnovicz, J.J. & Bradlow, H.L. (1991) Altered estrogen metabolism and excretion in humans following consumption of indole-3-carbinol. *Nutr. Cancer*, **16**, 59–66

Miller, K.W. & Stoewsand, G.S. (1983) Comparison of the effects of Brussels sprouts, glucosinolates, and glucosinolate metabolite consumption on rat hepatic poly-substrate monooxygenases. *Dev. Toxicol. Environ. Sci.*, **11**, 341–344

Miller, A.B., Howe, G.R., Jain, M., Craib, K.J. & Harrison, L. (1983) Food items and food groups as risk factors in a case–control study of diet and colo-rectal cancer. *Int. J. Cancer*, **32**, 155–161

Miller, A.B., Altenburg, H.P., Bueno de Mesquita, H.B., Boshuizen, H., Agudo, A., Berrino, F., Gram, I. T., Janson, L., Linseisen, J., Overvad, K., Rasmuson, T., Vineis, P., Lukanova, A., Allen, N., Berglund, G., Boeing, H., Clavel-Chapelon, F., Day, N.E., Gonzalez, C.A., Hallmans, G., Lund, E., Martinez, C., Palli, D., Panico, S., Peeters, P.H., Tjonneland, A., Tumino, R., Trichopoulou, A., Trichopoulos, A., Slimani, N. & Riboli, E. (2004) Fruits and vegetables and lung cancer: Findings from the European prospective investigation into cancer and nutrition. *Int. J. Cancer*, **108**, 269–276

Mithen, R. (2001) Glucosinolates and their degradation products. *Adv. Bot. Res.*, **35**, 214–262

Mithen, R., Clarke, J., Lister, C. & Dean, C. (1995) Genetics of aliphatic glucosinolates. III. Side-chain structure of aliphatic glucosinolates in *Arabidopsis thaliana*. *Heredity*, **74**, 210–215

Mithen, R., Faulkner, K., Magrath, R., Rose, P., Williamson, G. & Marquez, J. (2003) Development of isothiocyanate-enriched broccoli, and its enhanced ability to induce phase 2 detoxification enzymes in mammalian cells. *Theor. Appl. Genet.*, **106**, 727–734

Moreno, R.L., Kent, U.M., Hodge, K. & Hollenberg, P.F. (1999) Inactivation of cytochrome P450 2E1 by benzyl isothiocyanate. *Chem. Res. Toxicol.*, **12**, 582–587

Morimitsu, Y., Nakagawa, Y., Hayashi, K., Fujii, H., Kumagai, T., Nakamura, Y., Osawa, T., Horio, F., Itoh, K., Iida, K., Yamamoto, M. & Uchida, K. (2002) A sulforaphane analogue that potently activates the Nrf2-dependent detoxification pathway. *J. Biol. Chem.*, **277**, 3456–3463

Morse, M.A., Wang, C.X., Amin, S.G., Hecht, S.S. & Chung, F.L. (1988) Effects of dietary sinigrin or indole-3-carbinol on O^6-methylguanine–DNA transmethylase activity and 4-(methylnitrosamino)-1-(3-pyridyl)-1-butanone-induced DNA methylation and tumorigenicity in Fischer 344 rats. *Carcinogenesis*, **9**, 1891–1895

Morse, M.A., Wang, C.X., Stoner, G.D., Mandal, S., Conran, P.B., Amin, S.G., Hecht, S.S. & Chung, F.L. (1989a) Inhibition of 4-(methylnitrosamino)-1-(3-pyridyl)-1-butanone-induced DNA adduct formation and tumorigenicity in the lung of Fischer 344 rats by dietary phenethyl isothiocyanate. *Cancer Res.*, **49**, 549–553

Morse, M.A., Amin, S.G., Hecht, S.S. & Chung, F.L. (1989b) Effects of aromatic isothiocyanates on tumorigenicity, O^6-methylguanine formation, and metabolism of the tobacco-specific nitrosamine 4-(methylnitrosamino)-1-(3-pyridyl)-1-butanone in A/J mouse lung. *Cancer Res.*, **49**, 2894–2897

Morse, M.A., Eklind, K.I., Amin, S.G., Hecht, S.S. & Chung, F.L. (1989c) Effects of alkyl chain length on the inhibition of NNK-induced lung neoplasia in A/J mice by arylalkyl isothiocyanates. *Carcinogenesis*, **10**, 1757–1759

Morse, M.A., Reinhardt, J.C., Amin, S.G., Hecht, S.S., Stoner, G.D. & Chung, F.L. (1990a) Effect of dietary aromatic isothiocyanates fed subsequent to the administration of 4-(methylnitrosamino)-1-(3-pyridyl)-1-butanone on lung tumorigenicity in mice. *Cancer Lett.*, **49**, 225–230

Morse, M.A., LaGreca, S.D., Amin, S.G. & Chung, F.L. (1990b) Effects of indole-3-carbinol on lung tumorigenesis and DNA methylation induced by 4-(methylnitrosamino)-1-(3-pyridyl)-1-butanone (NNK) and on the metabolism and disposition of NNK in A/J mice. *Cancer Res.*, **50**, 2613–2617

Morse, M.A., Eklind, K.I., Hecht, S.S., Jordan, K.G., Choi, C.I., Desai, D.H., Amin, S.G. & Chung, F.L. (1991) Structure–activity relationships for inhibition of 4-(methylnitrosamino)-1-(3-pyridyl)-1-butanone lung tumorigenesis by arylalkyl isothiocyanates in A/J mice. *Cancer Res.*, **51**, 1846–1850

Morse, M.A., Eklind, K.I., Amin, S.G. & Chung, F.L. (1992) Effect of frequency of isothiocyanate administration on inhibition of 4-(methylnitrosamino)-1-(3-pyridyl)-1-butanone-induced pulmonary adenoma formation in A/J mice. *Cancer Lett.*, **62**, 77–81

Morse, M.A., Zu, H., Galati, A.J., Schmidt, C.J. & Stoner, G.D. (1993) Dose-related inhibition by dietary phenethyl isothiocyanate of esophageal tumorigenesis and DNA methylation induced by *N*-nitrosomethylbenzylamine in rats. *Cancer Lett.*, **72**, 103–110

Muda, M., Theodosiou, A., Rodrigues, N., Boschert, U., Camps, M., Gillieron, C., Davies, K., Ashworth, A. & Arkinstall, S. (1996) The dual specificity phosphatases M3/6 and MKP-3 are highly selective for inactivation of distinct mitogen-activated protein kinases. *J. Biol. Chem.*, **271**, 27205–27208

Murata, M., Yamashita, N., Inoue, S. & Kawanishi, S. (2000) Mechanism of oxidative DNA damage induced by carcinogenic allyl isothiocyanate. *Free Radicals Biol. Med.*, **28**, 797–805

Murillo, G. & Mehta, R.G. (2001) Cruciferous vegetables and cancer prevention. *Nutr. Cancer*, **41**, 17–28

Murray, S., Lake, B.G., Gray, S., Edwards, A.J., Springall, C., Bowey, E.A., Williamson, G., Boobis, A.R. & Gooderham, N.J. (2001) Effect of cruciferous vegetable consumption on heterocyclic aromatic amine metabolism in man. *Carcinogenesis*, **22**, 1413–1420

Musk, S.R. & Johnson, I.T. (1993) The clastogenic effects of isothiocyanates. *Mutat. Res.*, **300**, 111–117

Musk, S.R., Smith, T.K. & Johnson, I.T. (1995a) On the cytotoxicity and genotoxicity of allyl and phenethyl isothiocyanates and their parent glucosinolates sinigrin and gluconasturtiin. *Mutat. Res.*, **348**, 19–23

Musk, S.R., Astley, S.B., Edwards, S.M., Stephenson, P., Hubert, R.B. & Johnson, I.T. (1995b) Cytotoxic and clastogenic effects of benzyl isothiocyanate towards cultured mammalian cells. *Food Chem. Toxicol.*, **33**, 31–37

Muti, P., Bradlow, H.L., Micheli, A., Krogh, V., Freudenheim, J.L., Schunemann, H.J., Stanulla, M., Yang, J., Sepkovic, D.W., Trevisan, M. & Berrino, F. (2000) Estrogen metabolism and risk of breast cancer: A prospective study of the 2:16alpha-hydroxy-estrone ratio in premenopausal and postmenopausal women. *Epidemiology*, **11**, 635–640

Nachshon-Kedmi, M., Yannai, S., Haj, A. & Fares, F.A. (2003) Indole-3-carbinol and 3,3′-diindolylmethane induce apoptosis in human prostate cancer cells. *Food Chem. Toxicol.*, **41**, 745–752

Nagle, C.M., Purdie, D.M., Webb, P.M., Green, A., Harvey, P.W. & Bain, C.J. (2003) Dietary influences on survival after ovarian cancer. *Int. J. Cancer*, **106**, 264–269

Nakajima, M., Yoshida, R., Shimada, N., Yamazaki, H. & Yokoi, T. (2001) Inhibition and inactivation of human cytochrome P450 isoforms by phenethyl isothiocyanate. *Drug Metab. Dispos.*, **29**, 1110–1113

Nakamura, Y., Morimitsu, Y., Uzu, T., Ohigashi, H., Murakami, A., Naito, Y., Nakagawa, Y., Osawa, T. & Uchida, K. (2000a) A glutathione S-transferase inducer from papaya: Rapid screening, identification and structure–activity relationship of isothiocyanates. *Cancer Lett.*, **157**, 193–200

Nakamura, Y., Ohigashi, H., Masuda, S., Murakami, A., Morimitsu, Y., Kawamoto, Y., Osawa, T., Imagawa, M. & Uchida, K. (2000b) Redox regulation of glutathione S-transferase induction by benzyl isothiocyanate: Correlation of enzyme induction with the formation of reactive oxygen intermediates. *Cancer Res.*, **60**, 219–225

Nakamura, Y., Kawakami, M., Yoshihiro, A., Miyoshi, N., Ohigashi, H., Kawai, K., Osawa, T. & Uchida, K. (2002) Involvement of the mitochondrial death pathway in chemopreventive benzyl isothiocyanate-induced apoptosis. *J. Biol. Chem.*, **277**, 8492–8499

Nastruzzi, C., Cortesi, R., Esposito, E., Menegatti, E., Leoni, O., Iori, R. & Palmieri, S. (2000) *In vitro* antiproliferative activity of isothiocyanates and nitriles generated by myrosinase-mediated hydrolysis of glucosinolates from seeds of cruciferous vegetables. *J. Agric. Food Chem.*, **48**, 3572–3575

National Institute of Health & Nutrition (2002) *National Nutrition Survey Search for Household Food Intake*, available at http://www.nihn-jst.nih.go.jp:8888/nns/-owa/nns_main_e.hm01, Tokyo

National Toxicology Program (1982) *NTP Technical Report on the Carcinogenicity of Allyl Isothiocyanate (CAS No. 57-06-7) in F344/n Rats and B6C3F1 Mice (Gavage Study)*, Bethesda, Maryland, Department of Health and Human Services

Natural Resources Conservation Services (2003) *Plants Database*, Department of Agriculture, available at http://plants.usda.-gov/index.html, Washington DC

Negrusz, A., Moore, C.M., McDonagh, N.S., Woods, E.F., Crowell, J.A. & Levine, B.S. (1998) Determination of phenethylamine, a phenethyl isothiocyanate marker, in dog plasma using solid-phase extraction and gas chromatography–mass spectrometry with chemical ionization. *J. Chromatogr. B. Biomed. Sci. Appl.*, **718**, 193–198

Nesnow, S., Ross, J.A., Mass, M.J. & Stoner, G.D. (1998) Mechanistic relationships between DNA adducts, oncogene mutations, and lung tumorigenesis in strain A mice. *Exp. Lung Res.*, **24**, 395–405

Neudecker, T. & Henschler, D. (1985) Allyl isothiocyanate is mutagenic in *Salmonella typhimurium*. *Mutat. Res.*, **156**, 33–37

Neuhouser, M.L., Patterson, R.E., Thornquist, M.D., Omenn, G.S., King, I.B. & Goodman, G.E. (2003) Fruits and vegetables are associated with lower lung cancer

risk only in the placebo arm of the β–carotene and retinol efficacy trial (CARET). *Cancer Epidemiol. Biomarkers Prev.*, **12**, 350–358

Newfield, L., Bradlow, H.L., Sepkovic, D.W. & Auborn, K. (1998) Estrogen metabolism and the malignant potential of human papillomavirus immortalized keratinocytes. *Proc. Soc. Exp. Biol. Med.*, **217**, 322–326

Nguyen, T., Sherratt, P.J., Huang, H.C., Yang, C.S. & Pickett, C.B. (2003) Increased protein stability as a mechanism that enhances Nrf2-mediated transcriptional activation of the antioxidant response element. Degradation of Nrf2 by the 26 S proteasome. *J. Biol. Chem.*, **278**, 4536–4541

Nho, C.W. & Jeffery, E. (2001) The synergistic upregulation of phase II detoxification enzymes by glucosinolate breakdown products in cruciferous vegetables. *Toxicol. Appl. Pharmacol.*, **174**, 146–152

Nijhoff, W.A., Grubben, M.J., Nagengast, F.M., Jansen, J.B., Verhagen, H., van Poppel, G. & Peters, W.H. (1995a) Effects of consumption of Brussels sprouts on intestinal and lymphocytic glutathione S-transferases in humans. *Carcinogenesis*, **16**, 2125–2128

Nijhoff, W.A., Mulder, T.P., Verhagen, H., van Poppel, G. & Peters, W.H. (1995b) Effects of consumption of Brussels sprouts on plasma and urinary glutathione S-transferase class -α and -π in humans. *Carcinogenesis*, **16**, 955–957

Nioi, P., McMahon, M., Itoh, K., Yamamoto, M. & Hayes, J.D. (2003) Identification of a novel Nrf2-regulated antioxidant response element (ARE) in the mouse NAD(P)H:quinone oxidoreductase 1 gene: Reassessment of the ARE consensus sequence. *Biochem. J.*, **374**, 337–348

Nishie, K. & Daxenbichler, M.E. (1980) Toxicology of glucosinolates, related compounds (nitriles, *R*-goitrin, isothiocyanates) and vitamin U found in Cruciferae. *Food Cosmet. Toxicol.*, **18**, 159–172

Nishikawa, A., Furukawa, F., Ikezaki, S., Tanakamaru, Z.Y., Chung, F.L., Takahashi, M. & Hayashi, Y. (1996a) Chemopreventive effects of 3-phenylpropyl isothiocyanate on hamster lung tumorigenesis initiated with *N*-nitrosobis(2-oxopropyl)amine. *Jpn. J. Cancer Res.*, **87**, 122–126

Nishikawa, A., Furukawa, F., Uneyama, C., Ikezaki, S., Tanakamaru, Z., Chung, F.L., Takahashi, M. & Hayashi, Y. (1996b) Chemopreventive effects of phenethyl isothiocyanate on lung and pancreatic tumorigenesis in *N*-nitrosobis(2-oxopropyl)amine-treated hamsters. *Carcino-genesis*, **17**, 1381–1384

Nishikawa, A., Lee, I.S., Uneyama, C., Furukawa, F., Kim, H.C., Kasahara, K., Huh, N. & Takahashi, M. (1997) Mechanistic insights into chemopreventive effects of phenethyl isothiocyanate in *N*-nitrosobis(2-oxopropyl)amine-treated hamsters. *Jpn. J. Cancer Res.*, **88**, 1137–1142

Nishikawa, A., Furukawa, F., Kasahara, K., Tanakamaru, Z., Miyauchi, M., Nakamura, H., Ikeda, T., Imazawa, T. & Hirose, M. (1999) Failure of phenethyl isothiocyanate to inhibit hamster tumorigenesis induced by *N*-nitrosobis(2-oxopropyl)amine when given during the post-initiation phase. *Cancer Lett.*, **141**, 109–115

Nishikawa, A., Morse, M.A. & Chung, F.L. (2003) Inhibitory effects of 2-mercaptoethane sulfonate and 6-phenylhexyl isothiocyanate on urinary bladder tumorigenesis in rats induced by *N*-butyl-*N*-(4-hydroxy-butyl)nitrosamine. *Cancer Lett.*, **193**, 11–16

Niwa, T., Swaneck, G. & Bradlow, H.L. (1994) Alterations in estradiol metabolism in MCF-7 cells induced by treatment with indole-3-carbinol and related compounds. *Steroids*, **59**, 523–527

Nixon, J.E., Hendricks, J.D., Pawlowski, N.E., Pereira, C.B., Sinnhuber, R.O. & Bailey, G.S. (1984) Inhibition of aflatoxin B_1 carcinogenesis in rainbow trout by flavone and indole compounds. *Carcinogenesis*, **5**, 615–619

Nordfeldt, S., Gellerstedt, N. & Falkmer, S. (1954) Studies on rape-seed meal and its goitrogenic effect on pig. *Acta Pathol. Microbiol. Scand.*, **35**, 217–236

Nugon-Baudon, L., Rabot, S., Flinois, J.P., Lory, S. & Beaune, P. (1998) Effects of the bacterial status of rats on the changes in some liver cytochrome P450 (EC 1.14.14.1) apoproteins consequent to a glucosinolate-rich diet. *Br. J. Nutr.*, **80**, 231–234

Nyberg, F., Agrenius, V., Svartengren, K., Svensson, C. & Pershagen, G. (1998)

Dietary factors and risk of lung cancer in never-smokers. *Int. J. Cancer*, **78**, 430–436

Ocké, M.C. & Kaaks, R.J. (1997) Biochemical markers as additional measurements in dietary validity studies: Application of the method of triads with examples from the European Prospective Investigation into Cancer and Nutrition. *Am. J. Clin. Nutr.*, **65**, 1240S–1245S

Oganesian, A., Hendricks, J.D. & Williams, D.E. (1997) Long term dietary indole-3-carbinol inhibits diethylnitrosamine-initiated hepatocarcinogenesis in the infant mouse model. *Cancer Lett.*, **118**, 87–94

Oganesian, A., Hendricks, J.D., Pereira, C.B., Orner, G.A., Bailey, G.S. & Williams, D.E. (1999) Potency of dietary indole-3-carbinol as a promoter of aflatoxin B_1-initiated hepatocarcinogenesis: Results from a 9000 animal tumor study. *Carcinogenesis*, **20**, 453–458

Ogawa, K., Futakuchi, M., Hirose, M., Boonyaphiphat, P., Mizoguchi, Y., Miki, T. & Shirai, T. (1998) Stage and organ dependent effects of 1-*O*-hexyl-2,3,5-trimethylhydroquinone, ascorbic acid derivatives, n-heptadecane-8-10-dione and phenylethyl isothiocyanate in a rat multiorgan carcinogenesis model. *Int. J. Cancer*, **76**, 851–856

Ogawa, K., Hirose, M., Sugiura, S., Cui, L., Imaida, K., Ogiso, T. & Shirai, T. (2001) Dose-dependent promotion by phenylethyl isothiocyanate, a known chemopreventer, of two-stage rat urinary bladder and liver carcinogenesis. *Nutr. Cancer*, **40**, 134–139

Okazaki, K., Yamagishi, M., Son, H.Y., Imazawa, T., Furukawa, F., Nakamura, H., Nishikawa, A., Masegi, T. & Hirose, M. (2002) Simultaneous treatment with benzyl isothiocyanate, a strong bladder promoter, inhibits rat urinary bladder carcinogenesis by *N*-butyl-*N*-(4-hydroxybutyl)nitrosamine. *Nutr. Cancer*, **42**, 211–216

Olsen, G.W., Mandel, J.S., Gibson, R.W., Wattenberg, L.W. & Schuman, L.M. (1989) A case–control study of pancreatic cancer and cigarettes, alcohol, coffee and diet. *Am. J. Public Health*, **79**, 1016–1019

Ono, H., Tesaki, S., Tanabe, S. & Watanabe, M. (1998) 6-Methylsulfinylhexyl isothiocyanate and its homologues as food-originated compounds with antibacterial activity against *Escherichia coli* and *Staphylococcus aureus*. *Biosci. Biotechnol. Biochem.*, **62**, 363–365

Ovesen, L., Lyduch, S. & Idorn, M.L. (1988) The effect of a diet rich in Brussels sprouts on warfarin pharmacokinetics. *Eur. J. Clin. Pharmacol.*, **34**, 521–523

Pacin, A., Martínez, E., Martín de Portela, M.L. & Neira, M.S. (1999) [Food consumption and ingestion of various nutrients in the population of the National University of Luján, Argentina.] *Arch. Latinoam. Nutr.*, **49**, 31–39 (in Spanish)

Pantuck, E.J., Pantuck, C.B., Garland, W.A., Min, B.H., Wattenberg, L.W., Anderson, K.E., Kappas, A. & Conney, A.H. (1979) Stimulatory effect of Brussels sprouts and cabbage on human drug metabolism. *Clin. Pharmacol. Ther.*, **25**, 88–95

Pantuck, E.J., Pantuck, C.B., Anderson, K.E., Wattenberg, L.W., Conney, A.H. & Kappas, A. (1984) Effect of Brussels sprouts and cabbage on drug conjugation. *Clin. Pharmacol. Ther.*, **35**, 161–169

Park, J.Y. & Bjeldanes, L.F. (1992) Organ-selective induction of cytochrome P-450-dependent activities by indole-3-carbinol-derived products: Influence on covalent binding of benzo[a]pyrene to hepatic and pulmonary DNA in the rat. *Chem.–Biol. Interactions*, **83**, 235–247

Payen, L., Courtois, A., Loewert, M., Guillouzo, A. & Fardel, O. (2001) Reactive oxygen species-related induction of multidrug resistance-associated protein 2 expression in primary hepatocytes exposed to sulforaphane. *Biochem. Biophys. Res. Commun.*, **282**, 257–263

Pence, B.C., Buddingh, F. & Yang, S.P. (1986) Multiple dietary factors in the enhancement of dimethylhydrazine carcinogenesis: Main effect of indole-3-carbinol. *J. Natl Cancer Inst.*, **77**, 269–276

Pereira, M.A. (1995) Chemoprevention of diethylnitrosamine-induced liver foci and hepatocellular adenomas in C3H mice. *Anticancer Res.*, **15**, 1953–1956

Pereira, M.A. & Khoury, M.D. (1991) Prevention by chemopreventive agents of azoxymethane-induced foci of aberrant crypts in rat colon. *Cancer Lett.*, **61**, 27–33

Pereira, F.M., Rosa, E., Fahey, J.W., Stephenson, K.K., Carvalho, R. & Aires, A. (2002) Influence of temperature and ontogeny on the levels of glucosinolates in broccoli (*Brassica oleracea* var. *italica*) sprouts and their effect on the induction of mammalian phase 2 enzymes. *J. Agric. Food Chem.*, **50**, 6239–6244

Perocco, P., Iori, R., Barillari, J., Broccoli, M., Sapone, A., Affatato, A. & Paolini, M. (2002) In vitro induction of benzo(a)pyrene cell-transforming activity by the glucosinolate gluconasturtiin found in cruciferous vegetables. *Cancer Lett.*, **184**, 65–71

Peters, R.K., Pike, M.C., Garabrant, D. & Mack, T.M. (1992) Diet and colon cancer in Los Angeles County, California. *Cancer Causes Control*, **3**, 457–473

Pietinen, P., Malila, N., Virtanen, M., Hartman, T.J., Tangrea, J.A., Albanes, D. & Virtamo, J. (1999) Diet and risk of colorectal cancer in a cohort of Finnish men. *Cancer Causes Control*, **10**, 387–396

Piironen, E. & Virtanen, A.I. (1962) The synthesis of ascorbigen from ascorbic acid and 3-hydroxymethylindoles. *Acta Chem. Scand.*, **16**, 1286–1287

Platz, E.A., Giovannucci, E., Rimm, E.B., Rockett, H.R., Stampfer, M.J., Colditz, G.A. & Willett, W.C. (1997) Dietary fiber and distal colorectal adenoma in men. *Cancer Epidemiol. Biomarkers Prev.*, **6**, 661–670

Plumb, G.W., Lambert, N., Chambers, S.J., Wanigatunga, S., Heaney, R.K., Plumb, J.A., Aruoma, O.I., Halliwell, B., Miller, N.J. & Williamson, G. (1996) Are whole extracts and purified glucosinolates from cruciferous vegetables antioxidants? *Free Radicals Res.*, **25**, 75–86

Pohjanvirta, R., Korkalainen, M., McGuire, J., Simanainen, U., Juvonen, R., Tuomisto, J.T., Unkila, M., Viluksela, M., Bergman, J., Poellinger, L. & Tuomisto, J. (2002) Comparison of acute toxicities of indolo[3,2-b]carbazole (ICZ) and 2,3,7,8-tetrachloro-dibenzo-*p*-dioxin (TCDD) in TCDD-sensitive rats. *Food Chem. Toxicol.*, **40**, 1023–1032

van Poppel, G., Verhoeven, D.T., Verhagen, H. & Goldbohm, R.A. (1999) *Brassica* vegetables and cancer prevention. Epidemiology and mechanisms. *Adv. Exp. Med. Biol.*, **472**, 159–168

Posner, G.H., Cho, C.G., Green, J.V., Zhang, Y. & Talalay, P. (1994) Design and synthesis of biofunctional isothiocyanate analogies of sulforaphane: Correlation between structure and potency as inducers of anticarcinogenic detoxification enzymes. *J. Med. Chem.*, **37**, 170–176

Potischman, N., Swanson, C.A., Brinton, L.A., McAdams, M., Barrett, R.J., Berman, M.L., Mortel, R., Twiggs, L.B., Wilbanks, G.D. & Hoover, R.N. (1993) Dietary associations in a case–control study of endometrial cancer. *Cancer Causes Control*, **4**, 239–250

Potischman, N., Swanson, C.A., Coates, R.J., Gammon, M.D., Brogan, D.R., Curtin, J. & Brinton, L.A. (1999) Intake of food groups and associated micronutrients in relation to risk of early-stage breast cancer. *Int. J. Cancer*, **82**, 315–321

Preobrazhenskaya, M.N., Bukhman, V.M., Korolev, A.M. & Efimov, S.A. (1993a) Ascorbigen and other indole-derived compounds from *Brassica* vegetables and their analogs as anticarcinogenic and immuno-modulating agents. *Pharmacol. Ther.*, **60**, 301–313

Preobrazhenskaya, M.N., Korolev, A.M., Lazhko, E.I., Aleksandrova, L.G., Bergman, J. & Lindström, J.O. (1993b) Ascorbigen as a precursor of 5,11-dihydroindolo[3,2-b]car-bazole. *Food Chem.*, **48**, 57–62

Prestera, T., Holtzclaw, W.D., Zhang, Y. & Talalay, P. (1993) Chemical and molecular regulation of enzymes that detoxify carcinogens. *Proc. Natl Acad. Sci. USA*, **90**, 2965–2969

Prestera, T., Talalay, P., Alam, J., Ahn, Y.I., Lee, P.J. & Choi, A.M. (1995) Parallel induction of heme oxygenase-1 and chemoprotective phase 2 enzymes by electrophiles and antioxidants: Regulation by upstream antioxidant-responsive elements (ARE). *Mol. Med.*, **1**, 827–837

Probst-Hensch, N.M., Tannenbaum, S.R., Chan, K.K., Coetzee, G.A., Ross, R.K. & Yu, M.C. (1998) Absence of the glutathione S-transferase *M1* gene increases cytochrome P4501A2 activity among frequent consumers of cruciferous vegetables in a Caucasian population. *Cancer Epidemiol. Biomarkers Prev.*, **7**, 635–638

Prochaska, H.J. & Santamaria, A.B. (1988) Direct measurement of NAD(P)H:quinone reductase from cells cultured in microtiter wells: A screening assay for anticarcinogenic enzyme inducers. *Anal. Biochem.*, **169**, 328–336

Prochaska, H.J., Santamaria, A.B. & Talalay, P. (1992) Rapid detection of inducers of enzymes that protect against carcinogens. *Proc. Natl Acad. Sci. USA*, **89**, 2394–2398

Qiblawi, S. & Kumar, A. (1999) Chemopreventive action by an extract from *Brassica compestris* (var *Sarason*) on 7,12-dimethyl-benz(a)anthracene induced skin papillomagenesis in mice. *Phytother. Res.*, **13**, 261–263

Rahman, K.M. & Sarkar, F.H. (2002) Steroid hormone mimics molecular mechanisms of cell growth and apoptosis in normal and malignant mammary epithelial cells. *J. Steroid Biochem. Mol. Biol.*, **80**, 191–201

Rahman, K.M., Aranha, O., Glazyrin, A., Chinni, S.R. & Sarkar, F.H. (2000) Translocation of Bax to mitochondria induces apoptotic cell death in indole-3-carbinol (I3C) treated breast cancer cells. *Oncogene*, **19**, 5764–5771

Rahman, K.M., Aranha, O. & Sarkar, F.H. (2003) Indole-3-carbinol (I3C) induces apoptosis in tumorigenic but not in non-tumorigenic breast epithelial cells. *Nutr. Cancer*, **45**, 101–112

Rajkumar, T., Sridhar, H., Balaram, P., Vaccarella, S., Gajalakshmi, V., Nandakumar, A., Ramdas, K., Jayshree, R., Muñoz, N., Herrero, R., Franceschi, S. & Weiderpass, E. (2003) Oral cancer in southern India: The influence of body size, diet, infections and sexual practices. *Eur. J. Cancer Prev.*, **12**, 135–143

Rannug, U., Sjogren, M., Rannug, A., Gillner, M., Toftgard, R., Gustafsson, J.A., Rosenkranz, H. & Klopman, G. (1991) Use of artificial intelligence in structure–affinity correlations of 2,3,7,8-tetrachlorodibenzo-p-dioxin (TCDD) receptor ligands. *Carcinogenesis*, **12**, 2007–2015

Rao, C.V., Rivenson, A., Simi, B., Zang, E., Hamid, R., Kelloff, G.J., Steele, V. & Reddy, B.S. (1995) Enhancement of experimental colon carcinogenesis by dietary 6-phenylhexyl isothiocyanate. *Cancer Res.*, **55**, 4311–4318

Rask, L., Andreasson, E., Ekbom, B., Eriksson, S., Pontoppidan, B. & Meijer, J. (2000) Myrosinase: Gene family evolution and herbivore defense in Brassicaceae. *Plant Mol. Biol.*, **42**, 93–113

Reed, D.W., Davin, L., Jain, J.C., Deluca, V., Nelson, L. & Underhill, E.W. (1993) Purification and properties of UDP-glucose:thiohydroximate glucosyltransferase from *Brassica napus* L. seedlings. *Arch. Biochem. Biophys.*, **305**, 526–532

Renwick, A.B., Mistry, H., Barton, P.T., Mallet, F., Price, R.J., Beamand, J.A. & Lake, B.G. (1999) Effect of some indole derivatives on xenobiotic metabolism and xenobiotic-induced toxicity in cultured rat liver slices. *Food Chem. Toxicol.*, **37**, 609–618

Reznikova, M.I., Korolev, A.M., Bodyagin, D.A. & Preobrazhenskaya, M.N. (2000) Transformations of ascorbigen *in vivo* into ascorbigen acid and 1-deoxy-1-(indol-3-yl)keoses. *Food Chem.*, **71**, 469–474

Riboli, E., Hunt, K.J., Slimani, N., Ferrari, P., Norat, T., Fahey, M., Charrondiere, U.R., Hemon, B., Casagrande, C., Vignat, J., Overvad, K., Tjonneland, A., Clavel-Chapelon, F., Thiebaut, A., Wahrendorf, J., Boeing, H., Trichopoulos, D., Trichopoulou, A., Vineis, P., Palli, D., Bueno de Mesquita, H.B., Peeters, P.H., Lund, E., Engeset, D., Gonzalez, C.A., Barricarte, A., Berglund, G., Hallmans, G., Day, N.E., Key, T.J., Kaaks, R. & Saracci, R. (2002) European Prospective Investigation into Cancer and Nutrition (EPIC): Study populations and data collection. *Public Health Nutr.*, **5**, 1113–1124

Riby, J.E., Feng, C., Chang, Y.C., Schaldach, C.M., Firestone, G.L. & Bjeldanes, L.F. (2000a) The major cyclic trimeric product of indole-3-carbinol is a strong agonist of the estrogen receptor signaling pathway. *Biochemistry*, **39**, 910–918

Riby, J.E., Chang, G.H., Firestone, G.L. & Bjeldanes, L.F. (2000b) Ligand-independent activation of estrogen receptor function by 3,3′-diindolylmethane in human breast cancer cells. *Biochem. Pharmacol.*, **60**, 167–177

Rijken, P.J., Timmer, W.G., van de Kooij, A.J., van Benschop, I.M., Wiseman, S.A., Meijers, M. & Tijburg, L.B. (1999) Effect of vegetable and carotenoid consumption on aberrant crypt multiplicity, a surrogate end-point marker for colorectal cancer in azoxymethane-induced rats. *Carcinogenesis*, **20**, 2267–2272

Risch, H.A., Jain, M., Choi, N.W., Fodor, J.G., Pfeiffer, C.J., Howe, G.R., Harrison, L.W., Craib, K.J. & Miller, A.B. (1985) Dietary factors and the incidence of cancer of the stomach. *Am. J. Epidemiol.*, **122**, 947–959

Ritter, C.L., Prigge, W.F., Reichert, M.A. & Malejka-Giganti, D. (2001) Oxidations of 17beta-estradiol and estrone and their interconversions catalyzed by liver, mammary gland and mammary tumour after acute and chronic treatment of rats with indole-3-carbinol or beta-naphthoflavone. *Can. J. Physiol. Pharmacol.*, **79**, 519–532

Ron, E., Kleinerman, R.A., Boice, J.D., Jr, LiVolsi, V.A., Flannery, J.T. & Fraumeni, J.F., Jr (1987) A population-based case–control study of thyroid cancer. *J. Natl Cancer Inst.*, **79**, 1–12

Ronco, A., De Stefani, E., Boffetta, P., Deneo-Pellegrini, H., Mendilaharsu, M. & Leborgne, F. (1999) Vegetables, fruits, and related nutrients and risk of breast cancer: A case–control study in Uruguay. *Nutr. Cancer*, **35**, 111–119

Rosa, E.A., Heaney, R.K., Fenwick, G.R. & Portas, C.A. (1997) Glucosinolates in crop plants. *Hortic. Rev.*, **19**, 99–215

Rose, P., Faulkner, K., Williamson, G. & Mithen, R. (2000) 7-Methylsulfinylheptyl and 8-methylsulfinyloctyl isothiocyanates from watercress are potent inducers of phase II enzymes. *Carcinogenesis*, **21**, 1983–1988

Rosen, C.A., Woodson, G.E., Thompson, J.W., Hengesteg, A.P. & Bradlow, H.L. (1998) Preliminary results of the use of indole-3-carbinol for recurrent respiratory papillomatosis. *Otolaryngol. Head Neck Surg.*, **118**, 810–815

Rosenblatt, K.A., Thomas, D.B., Jimenez, L.M., Fish, B., McTiernan, A., Stalsberg, H., Stemhagen, A., Thompson, W.D., Curnen, M.G., Satariano, W., Austin, D.F., Greenberg, R.S., Key, C., Kolonel, L.N. & West, D.W. (1999) The relationship between diet and breast cancer in men (United States). *Cancer Causes Control*, **10**, 107–113

Ross, R.K., Shimizu, H., Paganini-Hill, A., Honda, G. & Henderson, B.E. (1987) Case–control studies of prostate cancer in blacks and whites in Southern California. *J. Natl Cancer Inst.*, **78**, 869–874

Rouimi, P., Tulliez, J. & Gamet-Payrastre, L. (2001) Sulforaphane induces glutathione S-transferase a in subconfluent CaCo-2 colon cancer cells. *Chem.–Biol. Interactions*, **133**, 312–314

Rouzaud, G., Rabot, S., Ratcliffe, B. & Duncan, A.J. (2003) Influence of plant and bacterial myrosinase activity on the metabolic fate of glucosinolates in gnotobiotic rats. *Br. J. Nutr.*, **90**, 395–404

Ruddick, J.A., Newsome, W.H. & Nash, L. (1976) Correlation of teratogenicity and molecular structure: Ethylenethiourea and related compounds. *Teratology*, **13**, 263–266

Rushmore, T.H., Morton, M.R. & Pickett, C.B. (1991) The antioxidant responsive element. Activation by oxidative stress and identification of the DNA consensus sequence required for functional activity. *J. Biol. Chem.*, **266**, 11632–11639

Sadek, I., Abdel-Salam, F. & al Qattan, K. (1995) Chemopreventive effects of cabbage on 7,12-dimethylbenz(a)-anthracene-induced hepatocarcinogenesis in toads (*Bufo viridis*). *J. Nutr. Sci. Vitaminol. (Tokyo)*, **41**, 163–168

Safe, S.H. (1998) Development validation and problems with the toxic equivalency factor approach for risk assessment of dioxins and related compounds. *J. Anim. Sci.*, **76**, 134–141

Salbe, A.D. & Bjeldanes, L.F. (1986) Dietary influences on rat hepatic and intestinal DT-diaphorase activity. *Food Chem. Toxicol.*, **24**, 851–856

Samaha, H.S., Kelloff, G.J., Steele, V., Rao, C.V. & Reddy, B.S. (1997) Modulation of apoptosis by sulindac, curcumin, phenylethyl-3-methylcaffeate, and 6-phenylhexyl isothiocyanate: Apoptotic index as a biomarker in colon cancer chemoprevention and promotion. *Cancer Res.*, **57**, 1301–1305

Sánchez, M.J., Martínez, C., Nieto, A., Castellsagué, X., Quintana, M.J., Bosch, F.X., Muñoz, N., Herrero, R. & Franceschi, S. (2003) Oral and oropharyngeal cancer in Spain: Influence of dietary patterns. *Eur. J. Cancer Prev.*, **12**, 49–56

Sanderson, J.T., Slobbe, L., Lansbergen, G.W., Safe, S. & van den Berg, M. (2001) 2,3,7,8-Tetrachlorodibenzo-p-dioxin and diindolylmethanes differentially induce cytochrome P450 1A1, 1B1, and 19 in H295R human adrenocortical carcinoma cells. *Toxicol. Sci.*, **61**, 40–48

Sarkar, F.H., Rahman, K.M. & Li, Y. (2003) Bax translocation to mitochondria is an important event in inducing apoptotic cell death by indole-3-carbinol (I3C) treatment of breast cancer cells. *J. Nutr.*, **133**, 2434S–2439S

Sasagawa, C. & Matsushima, T. (1991) Mutagen formation on nitrite treatment of indole compounds derived from indole-glucosinolate. *Mutat. Res.*, **250**, 169–174

Sasaki, S. (1963) Inhibitory effects by α-naphthyl-isothiocyanate on liver tumorigenesis in rats treated with 3′-methyl-4-dimethyl-aminoazobenzene. *J. Nara Med. Assoc.*, **14**, 101–115

Scharf, G., Prustomersky, S., Knasmuller, S., Schulte-Hermann, R. & Huber, W.W. (2003) Enhancement of glutathione and γ-glutamylcysteine synthetase, the rate limiting enzyme of glutathione synthesis, by chemoprotective plant-derived food and beverage components in the human hepatoma cell line HepG2. *Nutr. Cancer*, **45**, 74–83

Schneider, J., Kinne, D., Fracchia, A., Pierce, V., Anderson, K.E., Bradlow, H.L. & Fishman, J. (1982) Abnormal oxidative metabolism of estradiol in women with breast cancer. *Proc. Natl Acad. Sci. USA*, **79**, 3047–3051

Scholar, E.M., Wolterman, K., Birt, D.F. & Bresnick, E. (1989) The effect of diets enriched in cabbage and collards on murine pulmonary metastasis. *Nutr. Cancer*, **12**, 121–126

Schuman, L.M., Radke, A. & Halberg, F. (1982) Some selected features of the epidemiology of prostatic cancer: Minneapolis–St Paul, Minnesota case–control study, 1976–1979. In: *Trends in Cancer Incidence: Causes and Practical Implications*, Washington DC, Hemisphere, pp. 345–354

Schut, H.A. & Dashwood, R.H. (1995) Inhibition of DNA adduct formation of 2-amino-1-methyl-6-phenylimidazo[4,5-*b*]-pyridine (PhIP) by dietary indole-3-carbinol (I3C) in the mammary gland, colon, and liver of the female F-344 rat. *Ann. N.Y. Acad. Sci.*, **768**, 210–214

Schut, H.A. & Snyderwine, E.G. (1999) DNA adducts of heterocyclic amine food mutagens: Implications for mutagenesis and carcinogenesis. *Carcinogenesis*, **20**, 353–368

Schuurman, A.G., Goldbohm, R.A., Dorant, E. & van den Brandt, P.A. (1998) Vegetable and fruit consumption and prostate cancer risk: A cohort study in The Netherlands. *Cancer Epidemiol. Biomarkers Prev.*, **7**, 673–680

Scorrano, L. & Korsmeyer, S.J. (2003) Mechanisms of cytochrome c release by proapoptotic BCL-2 family members. *Biochem. Biophys. Res. Commun.*, **304**, 437–444

Seo, K.W., Kim, J.G., Park, M., Kim, T.W. & Kim, H.J. (2000) Effects of phenethylisothiocyanate on the expression of glutathione S-transferases and hepatotoxicity induced by acetaminophen. *Xenobiotica*, **30**, 535–545

Seow, A., Shi, C.Y., Chung, F.L., Jiao, D., Hankin, J.H., Lee, H.P., Coetzee, G.A. & Yu, M.C. (1998) Urinary total isothiocyanate (ITC) in a population-based sample of middle-aged and older Chinese in Singapore: Relationship with dietary total ITC and glutathione S-transferase *M1/T1/P1* genotypes. *Cancer Epidemiol. Biomarkers Prev.*, **7**, 775–781

Seow, A., Yuan, J.M., Sun, C.L., Van Den Berg, D., Lee, H.P. & Yu, M.C. (2002a) Dietary isothiocyanates, glutathione S-transferase polymorphisms and colorectal cancer risk in the Singapore Chinese Health Study. *Carcinogenesis*, **23**, 2055–2061

Seow, A., Poh, W.T., Teh, M., Eng, P., Wang, Y.T., Tan, W.C., Chia, K.S., Yu, M.C. & Lee, H.P. (2002b) Diet, reproductive factors and lung cancer risk among Chinese women in Singapore: Evidence for a protective effect of soy in nonsmokers. *Int. J. Cancer*, **97**, 365–371

Sepkovic, D.W., Bradlow, H.L., Ho, G., Hankinson, S.E., Gong, L., Osborne, M.P. & Fishman, J. (1995) Estrogen metabolite ratios and risk assessment of hormone-related cancers. Assay validation and prediction of cervical cancer risk. *Ann. N.Y. Acad. Sci.*, **768**, 312–316

Sepkovic, D.W., Bradlow, H.L. & Bell, M. (2001) Quantitative determination of 3,3′-diindolylmethane in urine of individuals receiving indole-3-carbinol. *Nutr. Cancer*, **41**, 57–63

Shannon, J., Thomas, D.B., Ray, R.M., Kestin, M., Koetsawang, A., Koetsawang, S., Chitnarong, K., Kiviat, N. & Kuypers, J. (2002) Dietary risk factors for invasive and in-situ cervical carcinomas in Bangkok, Thailand. *Cancer Causes Control*, **13**, 691–699

Shapiro, T.A., Fahey, J.W., Wade, K.L., Stephenson, K.K. & Talalay, P. (1998) Human metabolism and excretion of cancer chemoprotective glucosinolates and isothiocyanates of cruciferous vegetables. *Cancer Epidemiol. Biomarkers Prev.*, **7**, 1091–1100

Shapiro, T.A., Fahey, J.W., Wade, K.L., Stephenson, K.K. & Talalay, P. (2001) Chemoprotective glucosinolates and isothiocyanates of broccoli sprouts: Metabolism and excretion in humans. *Cancer Epidemiol. Biomarkers Prev.*, **10**, 501–508

Sharma, S., Stutzman, J.D., Kelloff, G.J. & Steele, V.E. (1994) Screening of potential chemopreventive agents using biochemical markers of carcinogenesis. *Cancer Res.*, **54**, 5848–5855

Shattuck, V.I. & Wang, W. (1994) Growth stress induces glucosinolate changes in pakchoy (*Brassica campestris* ssp. *chinensis*). *Can. J. Plant Sci.*, **74**, 595–601

Sherratt, P.J., McLellan, L.I. & Hayes, J.D. (2003) Positive and negative regulation of prostaglandin E2 biosynthesis in human colorectal carcinoma cells by cancer chemopreventive agents. *Biochem. Pharmacol.*, **66**, 51–61

Shertzer, H.G. (1982) Indole-3-carbinol and indole-3-acetonitrile influence on hepatic microsomal metabolism. *Toxicol. Appl. Pharmacol.*, **64**, 353–361

Shertzer, H.G. (1983) Protection by indole-3-carbinol against covalent binding of benzo[*a*]pyrene metabolites to mouse liver DNA and protein. *Food Chem. Toxicol.*, **21**, 31–35

Shertzer, H.G. (1984) Indole-3-carbinol protects against covalent binding of benzo[a]pyrene and *N*-nitrosodimethylamine metabolites to mouse liver macromolecules. *Chem.–Biol. Interactions*, **48**, 81–90

Shertzer, H.G. & Sainsbury, M. (1991a) Intrinsic acute toxicity and hepatic enzyme inducing properties of the chemoprotectants indole-3-carbinol and 5,10-dihydroindeno[1,2-b]indole in mice. *Food Chem. Toxicol.*, **29**, 237–242

Shertzer, H.G. & Sainsbury, M. (1991b) Chemoprotective and hepatic enzyme induction properties of indole and indenoindole antioxidants in rats. *Food Chem. Toxicol.*, **29**, 391–400

Shertzer, H.G., Niemi, M.P. & Tabor, M.W. (1986) Indole-3-carbinol inhibits lipid peroxidation in cell-free systems. *Adv. Exp. Med. Biol.*, **197**, 347–356

Shertzer, H.G., Berger, M.L. & Tabor, M.W. (1988) Intervention in free radical mediated hepatotoxicity and lipid peroxidation by indole-3-carbinol. *Biochem. Pharmacol.*, **37**, 333–338

Shertzer, H.G., Sainsbury, M., Graupner, P.R. & Berger, M.L. (1991) Mechanisms of chemical mediated cytotoxicity and chemoprotection in isolated rat hepatocytes. *Chem.–Biol. Interactions*, **78**, 123–141

Shilling, A.D., Carlson, D.B., Katchamart, S. & Williams, D.E. (2001) 3,3′-Diindolylmethane, a major condensation product of indole-3-carbinol, is a potent estrogen in the rainbow trout. *Toxicol. Appl. Pharmacol.*, **170**, 191–200

Shimkin, M.B. & Stoner, G.D. (1975) Lung tumors in mice: Application to carcinogenesis bioassay. *Adv. Cancer Res.*, **21**, 1–58

Shofran, B.G., Purrington, S.T., Breidt, F. & Fleming, H.P. (1998) Antimicrobial properties of sinigrin and its hydrolysis products. *J. Food Sci.*, **63**, 621–624

Shu, X.O., Gao, Y.T., Yuan, J.M., Ziegler, R.G. & Brinton, L.A. (1989) Dietary factors and epithelial ovarian cancer. *Br. J. Cancer*, **59**, 92–96

Shu, X.O., Zheng, W., Potischman, N., Brinton, L.A., Hatch, M.C., Gao, Y.T. & Fraumeni, J.F., Jr (1993) A population-based case–control study of dietary factors and endometrial cancer in Shanghai,

People's Republic of China. *Am. J. Epidemiol.*, **137**, 155–165

Shukla, Y., Arora, A. & Taneja, P. (2003) Antigenotoxic potential of certain dietary constituents. *Teratog. Carcinog. Mutag.*, **23** (Suppl. 1), 323–335

Sidransky, H., Ito, N. & Verney, E. (1966) Influence of alpha-naphthyl-isothiocyanate on liver tumorigenesis in rats ingesting ethionine and *N*-2-fluorenylacetamide. *J. Natl Cancer Inst.*, **37**, 677–686

Siglin, J.C., Barch, D.H. & Stoner, G.D. (1995) Effects of dietary phenethyl isothiocyanate, ellagic acid, sulindac and calcium on the induction and progression of *N*-nitrosomethylbenzylamine-induced esophageal carcinogenesis in rats. *Carcinogenesis*, **16**, 1101–1106

Silverman, D.T., Swanson, C.A., Gridley, G., Wacholder, S., Greenberg, R.S., Brown, L.M., Hayes, R.B., Swanson, G.M., Schoenberg, J.B., Pottern, L.M., Schwartz, A.G., Fraumeni, J.F., Jr & Hoover, R.N. (1998) Dietary and nutritional factors and pancreatic cancer: A case–control study based on direct interviews. *J. Natl Cancer Inst.*, **90**, 1710–1719

Singletary, K. & MacDonald, C. (2000) Inhibition of benzo[a]pyrene- and 1,6-dinitropyrene-DNA adduct formation in human mammary epithelial cells by dibenzoylmethane and sulforaphane. *Cancer Lett.*, **155**, 47–54

Singletary, K.W. & Nelshoppen, J.M. (1991) Inhibition of 7,12-dimethylbenz[a]anthracene (DMBA)-induced mammary tumorigenesis and of in vivo formation of mammary DMBA–DNA adducts by rosemary extract. *Cancer Lett.*, **60**, 169–17

Slattery, M.L., Kampman, E., Samowitz, W., Caan, B.J. & Potter, J.D. (2000) Interplay between dietary inducers of GST and the *GSTM-1* genotype in colon cancer. *Int. J. Cancer*, **87**, 728–733

Slimani, N., Kaaks, R., Ferrari, P., Casagrande, C., Clavel-Chapelon, F., Lotze, G., Kroke, A., Trichopoulos, D., Trichopoulou, A., Lauria, C., Bellegotti, M., Ocké, M.C., Peeters, P.H., Engeset, D., Lund, E., Agudo, A., Larranaga, N., Mattisson, I., Andren, C., Johansson, I., Davey, G., Welch, A.A., Overvad, K., Tjonneland, A., van Staveren, W.A., Saracci, R. & Riboli, E. (2002) European Prospective Investigation into Cancer and Nutrition (EPIC) calibration study: Rationale, design and population characteristics. *Public Health Nutr.*, **5**, 1125–1145

Smith, R.H. (1980) Kale poisoning: The Brassica anaemia factor. *Vet. Rec.*, **107**, 12–15

Smith, T.J. & Yang, C.S. (2000) Effect of organosulfur compounds from garlic and cruciferous vegetables on drug metabolism enzymes. *Drug Metab. Drug Interactions*, **17**, 23–49

Smith, T., Guo, Z., Thomas, P., Chung, F., Morse, M., Elkind, K. & Yang, C. (1990) Metabolism of 4-(methylnitrosamino)-1-(3-pyridyl)-1-butanone in mouse lung microsomes and its inhibition by isothiocyanates. *Cancer Res*, **50**, 6817–4333

Smith, T.J., Guo, Z., Li, C., Ning, S.M., Thomas, P.E. & Yang, C.S. (1993) Mechanisms of inhibition of 4-(methylnitrosamino)-1-(3-pyridyl)-1-butanone bioactivation in mouse by dietary phenethyl isothiocyanate. *Cancer Res.*, **53**, 3276–3282

Smith, T.J., Guo, Z., Guengerich, F.P. & Yang, C.S. (1996) Metabolism of 4-(methylnitrosamino)-1-(3-pyridyl)-1-butanone (NNK) by human cytochrome P450 1A2 and its inhibition by phenethyl isothiocyanate. *Carcinogenesis*, **17**, 809–813

Smith, T.K., Lund, E.K. & Johnson, I.T. (1998) Inhibition of dimethylhydrazine-induced aberrant crypt foci and induction of apoptosis in rat colon following oral administration of the glucosinolate sinigrin. *Carcinogenesis*, **19**, 267–273

Smith, T.K., Mithen, R. & Johnson, I.T. (2003) Effects of Brassica vegetable juice on the induction of apoptosis and aberrant crypt foci in rat colonic mucosal crypts in vivo. *Carcinogenesis*, **24**, 491–495

Smith-Warner, S.A., Elmer, P.J., Tharp, T.M., Fosdick, L., Randall, B., Gross, M., Wood, J. & Potter, J.D. (2000) Increasing vegetable and fruit intake: Randomized intervention and monitoring in an at-risk population. *Cancer Epidemiol. Biomarkers Prev.*, **9**, 307–317

Smith-Warner, S.A., Spiegelman, D., Yaun, S.S., Adami, H.O., Beeson, W.L., van den Brandt, P.A., Folsom, A.R., Fraser, G.E., Freudenheim, J.L., Goldbohm, R.A., Graham, S., Miller, A.B., Potter, J.D., Rohan, T.E., Speizer, F.E., Toniolo, P., Willett, W.C., Wolk, A., Zeleniuch-Jacquotte, A. & Hunter, D.J. (2001) Intake of fruits and vegetables and risk of breast cancer: A pooled analysis of cohort studies. *JAMA*, **285**, 769–776

Smith-Warner, S.A., Elmer, P.J., Fosdick, L., Randall, B., Bostick, R.M., Grandits, G., Grambsch, P., Louis, T.A., Wood, J.R. & Potter, J.D. (2002) Fruits, vegetables, and adenomatous polyps: The Minnesota Cancer Prevention Research Unit case–control study. *Am. J. Epidemiol.*, **155**, 1104–1113

Smith-Warner, S.A., Spiegelman, D., Yaun, S.S., Albanes, D., Beeson, W.L., van den Brandt, P.A., Feskanich, D., Folsom, A.R., Fraser, G.E., Freudenheim, J.L., Giovannucci, E., Goldbohm, R.A., Graham, S., Kushi, L.H., Miller, A.B., Pietinen, P., Rohan, T.E., Speizer, F.E., Willett, W.C. & Hunter, D.J. (2003) Fruits, vegetables and lung cancer: A pooled analysis of cohort studies. *Int. J. Cancer*, **107**, 1001–1011

Son, H.Y., Nishikawa, A., Furukawa, F., Lee, I.S., Ikeda, T., Miyauchi, M., Nakamura, H. & Hirose, M. (2000) Modi-fying effects of 4-phenylbutyl isothiocyanate on *N*-nitrosobis(2-oxopropyl)-amine-induced tumorigenesis in hamsters. *Cancer Lett.*, **160**, 141–147

Sones, K., Heaney, R.K. & Fenwick, G.R. (1984) An estimate of the mean daily intake of glucosinolates from cruciferous vegetables in the UK. *J. Sci. Food Agric.*, **35**, 712–720

Sorensen, M., Jensen, B.R., Poulsen, H.E., Deng, X., Tygstrup, N., Dalhoff, K. & Loft, S. (2001) Effects of a Brussels sprouts extract on oxidative DNA damage and metabolising enzymes in rat liver. *Food Chem. Toxicol.*, **39**, 533–540

Sparnins, V.L., Venegas, P.L. & Wattenberg, L.W. (1982a) Glutathione S-transferase activity: Enhancement by compounds inhibiting chemical carcinogenesis and by dietary constituents. *J. Natl Cancer Inst.*, **68**, 493–496

Sparnins, V.L., Chuan, J. & Wattenberg, L.W. (1982b) Enhancement of glutathione S-transferase activity of the esophagus by phenols, lactones, and benzyl isothiocyanate. *Cancer Res.*, **42**, 1205–1207

Spitz, M.R., Duphorne, C.M., Detry, M.A., Pillow, P.C., Amos, C.I., Lei, L., de Andrade, M., Gu, X., Hong, W.K. & Wu, X. (2000) Dietary intake of isothiocyanates: Evidence of a joint effect with glutathione S-transferase polymorphisms in lung cancer risk. *Cancer Epidemiol. Biomarkers Prev.*, **9**,1017–1020

Srisangnam, C., Hendricks, D.G., Sharma, R.P., Salunkhe, D.K. & Mahoney, A.W. (1980) Effects of cabbage *(Brassica oleracea* L.) on the tumorigenicity of 1,2-dimethylhydrazine in mice. *J. Food Saf.*, **4**, 235–245

Srivastava, B. & Shukla, Y. (1998) Antitumour promoting activity of indole-3-carbinol in mouse skin carcinogenesis. *Cancer Lett.*, **134**, 91–95

Srivastava, S.K., Xiao, D. , Lew, K.L., Hershberger, P., Kokkinakis, D.M., Johnson, C.S., Trump, D.L. & Singh, S.V. (2003) Allyl isothiocyanate, a constituent of cruciferous vegetables, inhibits growth of PC-3 human prostate cancer xenografts *in vivo*. *Carcinogenesis,* **24**, 1665-1670

Staack, R., Kingston, S., Wallig, M.A. & Jeffery, E.H. (1998) A comparison of the individual and collective effects of four glucosinolate breakdown products from Brussels sprouts on induction of detoxication enzymes. *Toxicol. Appl. Pharmacol.*, **149**, 17–23

Staretz, M.E. & Hecht, S.S. (1995) Effects of phenethyl isothiocyanate on the tissue distribution of 4-(methylnitrosamino)-1-(3-pyridyl)-1-butanone and metabolites in F344 rats. *Cancer Res.*, **55**, 5580-5588

Staretz, M.E., Foiles, P.G., Miglietta, L.M. & Hecht, S.S. (1997a) Evidence for an important role of DNA pyridyloxobutylation in rat lung carcinogenesis by 4-(methylnitrosamino)-1-(3-pyridyl)-1-butanone: Effects of dose and phenethyl isothiocyanate. *Cancer Res.*, **57**, 259–266

Staretz, M.E., Koenig, L.A. & Hecht, S.S. (1997b) Effects of long term dietary phenethyl isothiocyanate on the microsomal metabolism of 4-(methylnitrosamino)-1-(3-pyridyl)-1-butanone and 4-(methylnitrosamino)-1-(3-pyridyl)-1-butanol in F344 rats. *Carcinogenesis,* **18**, 1715-1722

Staub, R.E., Feng, C., Onisko, B., Bailey, G.S., Firestone, G.L. & Bjeldanes, L.F. (2002) Fate of indole-3-carbinol in cultured human breast tumor cells. *Chem. Res. Toxicol.*, **15**, 101–109

Steinmetz, K.A. & Potter, J.D. (1993) Food-group consumption and colon cancer in the Adelaide case–control study. I. Vegetables and fruit. *Int. J. Cancer*, **53**, 711–719

Steinmetz, K.A., Kushi, L.H., Bostick, R.M., Folsom, A.R. & Potter, J.D. (1994) Vegetables, fruit, and colon cancer in the Iowa Women's Health Study. *Am. J. Epidemiol.*, **139**, 1–15

Stephensen, P.U., Bonnesen, C., Bjeldanes, L.F. & Vang, O. (1999) Modulation of cytochrome P4501A1 activity by ascorbigen in murine hepatoma cells. *Biochem. Pharmacol.*, **58**, 1145–1153

Stephensen, P.U., Bonnesen, C., Schaldach, C., Andersen, O., Bjeldanes, L.F. & Vang, O. (2000) N-Methoxyindole-3-carbinol is a more efficient inducer of cytochrome P-450 1A1 in cultured cells than indol-3-carbinol. *Nutr. Cancer*, **36**, 112–121

Steyn, N.P., Nel, J.H. & Casey, A. (2003) Secondary data analyses of dietary surveys undertaken in South Africa to determine usual food consumption of the population. *Public Health Nutr.*, **6,** 631-644

Sticha, K.R., Staretz, M.E., Wang, M., Liang, H., Kenney, P.M. & Hecht, S.S. (2000) Effects of benzyl isothiocyanate and phenethyl isothiocyanate on benzo-[a]pyrene metabolism and DNA adduct formation in the A/J mouse. *Carcinogenesis*, **21**, 1711–1719

Sticha, K.R., Kenney, P.M., Boysen, G., Liang, H., Su, X., Wang, M., Upadhyaya, P. & Hecht, S.S. (2002) Effects of benzyl isothiocyanate and phenethyl isothiocyanate on DNA adduct formation by a mixture of benzo[a]pyrene and 4-(methylnitrosamino)-1-(3-pyridyl)-1-butanone in A/J mouse lung. *Carcinogenesis*, **23**, 1433–1439

Stoewsand, G.S. (1995) Bioactive organosulfur phytochemicals in *Brassica oleracea* vegetables—A review. *Food Chem. Toxicol.*, **33**, 537–543

Stoewsand, G.S., Babish, J.B. & Wimberly, H.C. (1978) Inhibition of hepatic toxicities from polybrominated biphenyls and aflatoxin B in rats fed cauliflower. *J. Environ. Pathol. Toxicol.*, **2**, 399–406

Stoewsand, G.S., Anderson, J.L. & Munson, L. (1988) Protective effect of dietary Brussels sprouts against mammary carcinogenesis in Sprague-Dawley rats. *Cancer Lett.*, **39**, 199–207

Stoewsand, G.S., Anderson, J.L., Munson, L. & Lisk, D.J. (1989) Effect of dietary Brussels sprouts with increased selenium content on mammary carcinogenesis in the rat. *Cancer Lett.*, **45**, 43–48

Stolzenberg-Solomon, R.Z., Pietinen, P., Taylor, P.R., Virtamo, J. & Albanes, D. (2002) Prospective study of diet and pancreatic cancer in male smokers. *Am. J. Epidemiol.*, **155**, 783–792

Stoner, G.D. & Morse, M.A. (1997) Isothiocyanates and plant polyphenols as inhibitors of lung and esophageal cancer. *Cancer Lett.*, **114**, 113–119

Stoner, G.D., Morrissey, D.T., Heur, Y.H., Daniel, E.M., Galati, A.J. & Wagner, S.A. (1991) Inhibitory effects of phenethyl isothiocyanate on N-nitrosobenzylmethylamine carcinogenesis in the rat esophagus. *Cancer Res.*, **51**, 2063–2068

Stoner, G.D., Siglin, J.C. , Morse, M.A., Desai, D.H., Amin, S.G., Kresty, L.A., Toburen, A.L., Heffner, E.M. & Francis, D.J. (1995) Enhancement of esophageal carcinogenesis in male F344 rats by dietary phenylhexyl isothiocyanate. *Carcinogenesis*, **16,** 2473-2476

Stoner, G., Casto, B., Ralston, S., Roebuck, B., Pereira, C. & Bailey, G. (2002) Development of a multi-organ rat model for evaluating chemopreventive agents: Efficacy of indole-3-carbinol. *Carcinogenesis*, **23**, 265–272

Strassman, M. & Ceci, L.N. (1963) Enzymic formation of α-isopropylmalic acid, an intermediate in leucine biosynthesis. *J. Biol. Chem.*, **238**, 2445–2452

Stresser, D.M., Bailey, G.S. & Williams, D.E. (1994a) Indole-3-carbinol and β-naphthoflavone induction of aflatoxin B$_1$ metabolism and cytochromes P-450 associated with bioactivation and detoxication of aflatoxin B1 in the rat. *Drug Metab. Disposition*, **22**, 383–391

Stresser, D.M., Williams, D.E., McLellan, L.I., Harris, T.M. & Bailey, G.S. (1994b) Indole-3-carbinol induces a rat liver glutathione transferase subunit (Yc2) with high activity toward aflatoxin B_1 exo-epoxide. Association with reduced levels of hepatic aflatoxin–DNA adducts *in vivo*. *Drug Metab. Disposition*, **22**, 392–399

Stresser, D.M., Bjeldanes, L.F., Bailey, G.S. & Williams, D.E. (1995a) The anticarcinogen 3,3´-diindolylmethane is an inhibitor of cytochrome P-450. *J. Biochem. Toxicol.*, **10**, 191–201

Stresser, D.M., Williams, D.E., Griffin, D.A. & Bailey, G.S. (1995b) Mechanisms of tumor modulation by indole-3-carbinol. Disposition and excretion in male Fischer 344 rats. *Drug Metab. Disposition*, **23**, 965–975

Sugie, S., Okumura, A., Yoshimi, N., Ohono, T., Tanaka, T. & Mori, H. (1991) Inhibitory effects of benzyl thiocyanate (BTC) and benzyl isothiocyanate (BIT) on methylazoxymethanol (MAM) acetate-induced intestinal carcinogenesis in rats. *Proc. Am. Assoc. Cancer Res.*, **32**, 128

Sugie, S., Okamoto, K., Okumura, A., Tanaka, T. & Mori, H. (1994) Inhibitory effects of benzyl thiocyanate and benzyl isothiocyanate on methylazoxymethanol acetate-induced intestinal carcinogenesis in rats. *Carcinogenesis*, **15**, 1555–1560

Sugiura, S., Ogawa, K., Hirose, M., Takeshita, F., Asamoto, M. & Shirai, T. (2003) Reversibility of proliferative lesions and induction of non-papillary tumors in rat urinary bladder treated with phenylethyl isothiocyanate. *Carcinogenesis*, **24**, 547–553

Suto, A., Bradlow, H.L., Wong, G.Y., Osborne, M.P. & Telang, N.T. (1993) Experimental down-regulation of intermediate biomarkers of carcinogenesis in mouse mammary epithelial cells. *Breast Cancer Res. Treat.*, **27**, 193–202

Swanson, H.I. & Bradfield, C.A. (1993) The Ah-receptor: Genetics, structure and function. *Pharmacogenetics*, **3**, 213–230

Tabor, M.W., Coats, E., Sainsbury, M. & Shertzer, H.G. (1991) Antioxidation potential of indole compounds—Structure activity studies. *Adv. Exp. Med. Biol.*, **283**, 833–836

Taioli, E., Garte, S.J., Trachman, J., Garbers, S., Sepkovic, D.W., Osborne, M.P., Mehl, S. & Bradlow, H.L. (1996) Ethnic differences in estrogen metabolism in healthy women. *J. Natl Cancer Inst.*, **88**, 617

Taioli, E., Garbers, S., Bradlow, H.L., Carmella, S.G., Akerkar, S. & Hecht, S.S. (1997) Effects of indole-3-carbinol on the metabolism of 4-(methylnitrosamino)-1-(3-pyridyl)-1-butanone in smokers. *Cancer Epidemiol. Biomarkers Prev.*, **6**, 517–522

Takahashi, H. & Echizen, H. (2001) Pharmacogenetics of warfarin elimination and its clinical implications. *Clin. Pharmacokinet.*, **40**, 587-603

Takahashi, N., Dashwood, R.H., Bjeldanes, L.F., Bailey, G.S. & Williams, D.E. (1995a) Regulation of hepatic cytochrome *P4501A* by indole-3-carbinol: Transient induction with continuous feeding in rainbow trout. *Food Chem. Toxicol.*, **33**, 111–120

Takahashi, N., Stresser, D.M., Williams, D.E. & Bailey, G.S. (1995b) Induction of hepatic CYP1A by indole-3-carbinol in protection against aflatoxin B_1 hepatocarcinogenesis in rainbow trout. *Food Chem. Toxicol.*, **33**, 841–850

Takahashi, N., Dashwood, R.H., Bjeldanes, L.F., Williams, D.E. & Bailey, G.S. (1995c) Mechanisms of indole-3-carbinol (I3C) anticarcinogenesis: Inhibition of aflatoxin B_1-DNA adduction and mutagenesis by I3C acid condensation products. *Food Chem. Toxicol.*, **33**, 851–857

Talalay, P. & Fahey, J.W. (2001) Phytochemicals from cruciferous plants protect against cancer by modulating carcinogen metabolism. *J. Nutr.*, **131**, 3027S–3033S

Tan, W., Lin, D.X., Xiao, Y., Kadlubar, F. & Chen, J.S. (1999) Chemoprevention of 2-amino-1-methyl-6-phenyli-midazo 4,5-b pyridine-induced carcinogen–DNA adducts by Chinese cabbage in rats. *World J. Gastroenterol.*, **5**, 138–142

Tanaka, T., Mori, Y., Morishita, Y., Hara, A., Ohno, T. & Kojima, T. (1990) Inhibitory effect of sinigrin and indole-3-carbinol on diethylnitrosamine-induced hepatocarcinogenesis in male ACI/N rats. *Carcinogene-sis*, **11**, 1403–1406

Tanaka, T., Kojima, T., Morishita, Y. & Mori, H. (1992) Inhibitory effects of the natural products indole-3-carbinol and sinigrin during initiation and promotion phases of 4-nitroquinoline 1-oxide-induced rat tongue carcinogenesis. *Jpn. J. Cancer Res.*, **83**, 835–842

Tanida, N., Kawaura, A., Takahashi, A., Sawada, K. & Shimoyama, T. (1991) Suppressive effect of wasabi (pungent Japanese spice) on gastric carcinogenesis induced by MNNG in rats. *Nutr. Cancer*, **16**, 53–58

Tawfiq, N., Wanigatunga, S., Heaney, R.K., Musk, S.R., Williamson, G. & Fenwick, G.R. (1994) Induction of the anti-carcinogenic enzyme quinone reductase by food extracts using murine hepatoma cells. *Eur. J. Cancer Prev.*, **3**, 285–292

Tawfiq, N., Heaney, R.K., Plumb, J.A., Fenwick, G.R., Musk, S.R. & Williamson, G. (1995) Dietary glucosinolates as blocking agents against carcinogenesis: Glucosinolate breakdown products assessed by induction of quinone reductase activity in murine hepa1c1c7 cells. *Carcinogenesis*, **16**, 1191–1194

Telang, N.T., Suto, A., Wong, G.Y., Osborne, M.P. & Bradlow, H.L. (1992) Induction by estrogen metabolite 16 alpha-hydroxyestrone of genotoxic damage and aberrant proliferation in mouse mammary epithelial cells. *J. Natl Cancer Inst.*, **84**, 634–638

Telang, N.T., Katdare, M., Bradlow, H.L. & Osborne, M.P. (1997a) Estradiol metabolism: An endocrine biomarker for modulation of human mammary carcinogenesis. *Environ. Health Perspectives*, **105** (Suppl. 3), 559–564

Telang, N.T., Inoue, S., Bradlow, H.L. & Osborne, M.P. (1997b) Negative growth regulation of oncogene-transformed mammary epithelial cells by tumor inhibitors. *Adv. Exp. Med. Biol.*, **400A**, 409–418

Telang, N.T., Katdare, M., Bradlow, H.L., Osborne, M.P. & Fishman, J. (1997c) Inhibition of proliferation and modulation of estradiol metabolism: Novel mechanisms for breast cancer prevention by the phytochemical indole-3-carbinol. *Proc. Soc. Exp. Biol. Med.*, **216**, 246–252

Temmink, J.H., Bruggeman, I.M. & van Bladeren, P.J. (1986) Cytomorphological changes in liver cells exposed to allyl and benzyl isothiocyanate and their cysteine and glutathione conjugates. *Arch. Toxicol.*, **59**, 103–110

Temple, N.J. & Basu, T.K. (1987) Selenium and cabbage and colon carcinogenesis in mice. *J. Natl Cancer Inst.*, **79**, 1131–1134

Temple, N.J. & El–Khatib, S.M. (1987) Cabbage and vitamin E: Their effect on colon tumor formation in mice. *Cancer Lett.*, **35**, 71–77

Terry, P., Wolk, A., Persson, I. & Magnusson, C. (2001) Brassica vegetables and breast cancer risk. *JAMA*, **285**, 2975–2977

Terry, P., Vainio, H., Wolk, A. & Weiderpass, E. (2002) Dietary factors in relation to endometrial cancer: A nationwide case–control study in Sweden. *Nutr. Cancer*, **42**, 25–32

Thimmulappa, R.K., Mai, K.H., Srisuma, S., Kensler, T.W., Yamamoto, M. & Biswal, S. (2002) Identification of Nrf2-regulated genes induced by the chemopreventive agent sulforaphane by oligonucleotide microarray. *Cancer Res.*, **62**, 5196–5203

Thornalley, P.J. (2002) Isothiocyanates: Mechanism of cancer chemopreventive action. *Anticancer Drugs*, **13**, 331–338

Thummel, K.E., Lee, C.A., Kunze, K.L., Nelson, S.D. & Slattery, J.T. (1993) Oxidation of acetaminophen to *N*-acetyl-*p*-aminobenzoquinone imine by human CYP3A4. *Biochem. Pharmacol.*, **45**, 1563–1569

Tiedink, H.G., Davies, J.A., van Broekhoven, L.W., van der Kamp, H.J. & Jongen, W.M. (1988) Formation of mutagenic *N*-nitroso compounds in vegetable extracts upon nitrite treatment: A comparison with the glucosinolate content. *Food Chem. Toxicol.*, **26**, 947–954

Tiedink, H.G., Hissink, A.M., Lodema, S.M., van Broekhoven, L.W. & Jongen, W.M. (1990) Several known indole compounds are not important precursors of direct mutagenic *N*-nitroso compounds in green cabbage. *Mutat. Res.*, **232**, 199–207

Tiedink, H.G., Malingre, C.E., van Broekhoven, L.W., Jongen, W.M., Lewis, J. & Fenwick, G.R. (1991) Role of glucosinolates in the formation of *N*-nitroso compounds. *J. Agric. Food Chem.*, **39**, 922–926

Tiwari, R.K., Guo, L., Bradlow, H.L., Telang, N.T. & Osborne, M.P. (1994) Selective responsiveness of human breast cancer cells to indole-3-carbinol, a chemopreventive agent. *J. Natl Cancer Inst.*, **86**, 126–131

Tookey, H.L. (1973) Crambe thioglucoside glucohydrolase (EC 3.2.3.1): Separation of a protein required for epithiobutane formation. *Can. J. Biochem.*, **51**, 1654–1660

Toroser, D., Thormann, C.E., Osborn, T.C. & Mithen, R. (1995) RFLP mapping of quantitative trait loci controlling seed aliphatic-glucosinolate content in oilseed rape (*Brassica napus* L.). *Theor. Appl. Genet.*, **91**, 802–808

Tseng, E., Kamath, A. & Morris, M.E. (2002) Effect of organic isothiocyanates on the P-glycoprotein- and MRP1-mediated transport of daunomycin and vinblastine. *Pharm. Res.*, **19**, 1509–1515

Uhl, M., Laky, B., Lhoste, E., Kassie, F., Kundi, M. & Knasmüller, S. (2003) Effects of mustard sprouts and allylisothiocyanate on benzo(a)pyrene-induced DNA damage in human-derived cells: A model study with the single cell gel electrophoresis/Hep G2 assay. *Teratog. Carcinog. Mutag.*, **23** (Suppl. 1), 273–282

United Nations (2002) *World Population Prospects: The 2002 Revision,* New York, Department of Economic and Social Affairs, Population Division

Ursin, G., London, S., Stanczyk, F.Z., Gentzschein, E., Paganini-Hill, A., Ross, R.K. & Pike, M.C. (1999) Urinary 2-hydroxyestrone/16α-hydroxyestrone ratio and risk of breast cancer in postmenopausal women. *J. Natl Cancer Inst.*, **91**, 1067–1072

Vallejo, F., Tomas-Barberan, F.A., Benavente-Garcia, A.G. & Garcia-Viguera, C. (2003a) Total and individual glucosinolate contents in inflorescences of eight broccoli cultivars grown under various climatic and fertilisation conditions. *J. Sci. Food Agric.*, **83**, 307–313

Vallejo, F., Garcia-Viguera, C. & Tomas-Barberan, F.A. (2003b) Changes in broccoli (*Brassica oleracea* L. var. *italica*) health-promoting compounds with inflorescence development. *J. Agric. Food Chem.*, **51**, 3776–3782

Vallejo, F., Tomas-Barberan, F.A. & Garcia-Viguera, C. (2003c) Health-promoting compounds in broccoli as influenced by refrigerated transport and retail sale period. *J. Agric. Food Chem.*, **51**, 3029–3034

Vang, O. & Dragsted, L. (1996) *Naturally Occurring Antitumorigens. III. Indoles.* Copenhagen, Nordic Council of Ministers

Vang, O., Jensen, M.B. & Autrup, H. (1990) Induction of cytochrome P450IA1 in rat colon and liver by indole-3-carbinol and 5,6-benzoflavone. *Carcinogenesis*, **11**, 1259–1263

Vang, O., Jensen, H. & Autrup, H. (1991) Induction of cytochrome *P*-450IA1, IA2, IIB1, IIB2 and IIE1 by broccoli in rat liver and colon. *Chem.–Biol. Interactions*, **78**, 85–96

Vang, O., Frandsen, H., Hansen, K.T., Nielsen, J.B. & Andersen, O. (1999) Modulation of drug-metabolising enzyme expression by condensation products of indole-3-ylcarinol, an inducer in cruciferous vegetables. *Pharmacol. Toxicol.*, **84**, 59–65

Vang, O., Frandsen, H., Hansen, K.T., Sorensen, J.N., Sørensen, H. & Andersen, O. (2001) Biochemical effects of dietary intake of different broccoli samples. I. Differential modulation of cytochrome P-450 activities in rat liver, kidney, and colon. *Metabolism*, **50**, 1123–1129

Verhagen, H., Poulsen, H.E., Loft, S., van Poppel, G., Willems, M.I. & van Bladeren, P.J. (1995) Reduction of oxidative DNA-damage in humans by Brussels sprouts. *Carcinogenesis*, **16**, 969–970

Verhagen, H., de Vries, A., Nijhoff, W.A., Schouten, A., van Poppel, G., Peters, W.H. & van den Berg, H. (1997) Effect of Brussels sprouts on oxidative DNA-damage in man. *Cancer Lett.*, **114**, 127–130

Verhoeven, D.T., Verhagen, H., Goldbohm, R.A., van den Brandt, P.A. & van Poppel, G. (1997) A review of mechanisms underlying anticarcinogenicity by Brassica vegetables. *Chem.–Biol. Interactions*, **103**, 79–129

Verkerk, R., Dekker, M. & Jongen, W.M. (2001) Post-harvest increase of indolyl glucosinolates in response to chopping and storage of *Brassica* vegetables. *J. Sci. Food Agric.*, **81**, 953–958

Vermeulen, M., Van Rooijen, H.J. & Vaes, W.H. (2003) Analysis of isothiocyanate mercapturic acids in urine: A biomarker for cruciferous vegetable intake. *J. Agric. Food Chem.*, **51**, 3554–3559

Vermorel, M., Heaney, R.K. & Fenwick, G.R. (1986) Nutritive value of rapeseed meal: Effects of individual glucosinolates. *J. Sci. Food Agric.*, **37**, 1197–1202

Vilkki, P., Kreula, M. & Piironen, E. (1962) Studies on the goitrogenic influence of cow's milk on man. In: *Annales Academiae Scientiarum Fennicae*, Series A, Helsinki, Suomalainen Tiedeakatemia

Villeneuve, P.J., Johnson, K.C., Kreiger, N. & Mao, Y. (1999) Risk factors for prostate cancer: Results from the Canadian National Enhanced Cancer Surveillance System. The Canadian Cancer Registries Epidemiology Research Group. *Cancer Causes Control*, **10**, 355–367

Vistisen, K., Poulsen, H.E. & Loft, S. (1992) Foreign compound metabolism capacity in man measured from metabolites of dietary caffeine. *Carcinogenesis*, **13**, 1561–1568

Voorrips, L.E., Goldbohm, R.A., van Poppel, G., Sturmans, F., Hermus, R.J. & van den Brandt, P.A. (2000a) Vegetable and fruit consumption and risks of colon and rectal cancer in a prospective cohort study: The Netherlands cohort study on diet and cancer. *Am. J. Epidemiol.*, **152**, 1081–1092

Voorrips, L.E., Goldbohm, R.A., Verhoeven, D.T., van Poppel, G.A., Sturmans, F., Hermus, R.J. & van den Brandt, P.A. (2000b) Vegetable and fruit consumption and lung cancer risk in the Netherlands cohort study on diet and cancer. *Cancer Causes Control*, **11**, 101–115

Wakabayashi, K., Nagao, M., Ochiai, M., Tahira, T., Yamaizumi, Z. & Sugimura, T. (1985) A mutagen precursor in Chinese cabbage, indole-3-acetonitrile, which becomes mutagenic on nitrite treatment. *Mutat. Res.*, **143**, 17–21

Wakabayashi, K., Nagao, M., Tahira, T., Yamaizumi, Z., Katayama, M., Marumo, S. & Sugimura, T. (1986) 4-Methoxyindole derivatives as nitrosable precursors of mutagens in Chinese cabbage. *Mutagenesis*, **1**, 423–426

Wakabayashi, N., Itoh, K., Wakabayashi, J., Motohashi, H., Noda, S., Takahashi, S., Imakado, S., Kotsuji, T., Otsuka, F., Roop, D.R., Harada, T., Engel, J.D. & Yamamoto, M. (2003) *Keap1*-null mutation leads to postnatal lethality due to constitutive Nrf2 activation. *Nat. Genet.*, **35**, 238–245

Wallig, M.A., Kingston, S., Staack, R. & Jefferey, E.H. (1998) Induction of rat pancreatic glutathione S-transferase and quinone reductase activities by a mixture of glucosinolate breakdown derivatives found in Brussels sprouts. *Food Chem. Toxicol.*, **36**, 365–373

Ward, S.M., Delaquis, P.J., Holley, R.A. & Mazza, G. (1998) Inhibition of spoilage and pathogenic bacteria on agar and pre-cooked roast beef by volatile horseradish distillates. *Food Res. Int.*, **31**, 19–26

Wargovich, M.J., Chen, C.D., Jimenez, A., Steele, V.E., Velasco, M., Stephens, L.C., Price, R., Gray, K. & Kelloff, G.J. (1996) Aberrant crypts as a biomarker for colon cancer: Evaluation of potential chemopreventive agents in the rat. *Cancer Epidemiol. Biomarkers Prev.*, **5**, 355–360

Wasserman, W.W. & Fahl, W.E. (1997) Functional antioxidant responsive elements. *Proc. Natl Acad. Sci. USA*, **94**, 5361–5366

Wattenberg, L.W. (1977) Inhibition of carcinogenic effects of polycyclic hydrocarbons by benzyl isothiocyanate and related compounds. *J. Natl Cancer Inst.*, **58**, 395–398

Wattenberg, L.W. (1981) Inhibition of carcinogen-induced neoplasia by sodium cyanate, tert-butyl isocyanate, and benzyl isothiocyanate administered subsequent to carcinogen exposure. *Cancer Res.*, **41**, 2991–2994

Wattenberg, L.W. (1983) Inhibition of neoplasia by minor dietary constituents. *Cancer Res.*, **43**, 2448s–2453s

Wattenberg, L.W. (1987) Inhibitory effects of benzyl isothiocyanate administration shortly before diethyl-nitrosamine or benzo(a)pyrene on pulmonary and forestomach neoplasia in A/J mice. *Carcinogenesis*, **8**, 1971–1973

Wattenberg, L. (1990) Inhibition of carcinogenesis by minor nutrient constituents of the diet. *Proc. Nutr. Soc.*, **49**, 173–183

Wattenberg, L.W. & Loub, W.D. (1978) Inhibition of polycyclic aromatic hydrocarbon-induced neoplasia by naturally occurring indoles. *Cancer Res.*, **38**, 1410–1413

Wattenberg, L.W., Hanley, A.B., Barany, G., Sparnins, V.L., Lam, L.K.T. & Fenwick, G.R. (1986) Inhibition of carcinogenesis by some minor dietary constituents. In: Hayashi, Y., Nagao, M., Sugimura, T., Takayama, S., Tomatis, L., Wattenberg, L.W. & Wogan, G.N., eds, *Diet, Nutrition and Cancer*,

Tokyo, Japan Scientific Societies Press, pp. 193–203

Wei, Y.D., Helleberg, H., Rannug, U. & Rannug, A. (1998) Rapid and transient induction of CYP1A1 gene expression in human cells by the tryptophan photoproduct 6-formylindolo[3,2-b]carbazole. *Chem.–Biol. Interactions*, **110**, 39–55

Wellejus, A. & Loft, S. (2002) Receptor-mediated ethinylestradiol-induced oxidative DNA damage in rat testicular cells. *FASEB J.*, **16**, 195–201

Whalen, R. & Boyer, T.D. (1998) Human glutathione S-transferases. *Semin. Liver Dis.*, **18**, 345–358

Whitty, J.P. & Bjeldanes, L.F. (1987) The effects of dietary cabbage on xenobiotic-metabolizing enzymes and the binding of aflatoxin B1 to hepatic DNA in rats. *Food Chem. Toxicol.*, **25**, 581–587

Wilker, C., Johnson, L. & Safe, S. (1996) Effects of developmental exposure to indole-3-carbinol or 2,3,7,8-tetrachloro-dibenzo-p-dioxin on reproductive potential of male rat offspring. *Toxicol. Appl. Pharmacol.*, **141,** 68-75

Wilkinson, J.T., Morse, M.A., Kresty, L.A. & Stoner, G.D. (1995) Effect of alkyl chain length on inhibition of N-nitrosomethylbenzylamine-induced esophageal tumorigenesis and DNA methylation by isothiocyanates. *Carcinogenesis*, **16**, 1011–1015

Williams, C. (1995) Healthy eating: Clarifying advice about fruit and vegetables. *Br. Med. J*, **310**, 1453–1455

Wingren, G., Hatschek, T. & Axelson, O. (1993) Determinants of papillary cancer of the thyroid. *Am. J. Epidemiol.*, **138**, 482–491

Witschi, H., Espiritu, I., Yu, M. & Willits, N.H. (1998) The effects of phenethyl isothiocyanate, N-acetylcysteine and green tea on tobacco smoke-induced lung tumours in strain A/J mice. *Carcinogenesis*, **19**, 1789–1794

Witte, J.S., Longnecker, M.P., Bird, C.L., Lee, E.R., Frankl, H.D. & Haile, R.W. (1996) Relation of vegetable, fruit, and grain consumption to colorectal adenomatous polyps. *Am. J. Epidemiol.*, **144**, 1015–1025

Wolk, A., Gridley, G., Niwa, S., Lindblad, P., McCredie, M., Mellemgaard, A., Mandel, J.S., Wahrendorf, J., McLaughlin, J.K. & Adami, H.O. (1996) International renal cell cancer study. VII. Role of diet. *Int. J. Cancer*, **65**, 67–73

Wong, B.K., Fei, P. & Kong, A.N. (1995) Differential induction of UDP-glucuronosyl-transferase activity and gene expression in rat liver. *Pharm. Res.*, **12**, 1105–1108

Wong, G.Y., Bradlow, L., Sepkovic, D., Mehl, S., Mailman, J. & Osborne, M.P. (1997) Dose-ranging study of indole-3-carbinol for breast cancer prevention. *J. Cell Biochem.*, **28–29** (Suppl.), 111–116

Wortelboer, H.M., de Kruif, C.A., van Iersel, A.A., Noordhoek, J., Blaauboer, B.J., van Bladeren, P.J. & Falke, H.E. (1992a) Effects of cooked Brussels sprouts on cytochrome P-450 profile and phase II enzymes in liver and small intestinal mucosa of the rat. *Food Chem. Toxicol.*, **30**, 17–27

Wortelboer, H.M., van der Linden, E.C., de Kruif, C.A., Noordhoek, J., Blaauboer, B.J., van Bladeren, P.J. & Falke, H.E. (1992b) Effects of indole-3-carbinol on biotransformation enzymes in the rat: *In vivo* changes in liver and small intestinal mucosa in comparison with primary hepatocyte cultures. *Food Chem. Toxicol.*, **30**, 589–599

Wortelboer, H.M., de Kruif, C.A., van Iersel, A.A., Falke, H.E., Noordhoek, J. & Blaauboer, B.J. (1992c) Acid reaction products of indole-3-carbinol and their effects on cytochrome P450 and phase II enzymes in rat and monkey hepatocytes. *Biochem. Pharmacol.*, **43**, 1439–1447

Xiao, D. & Singh, S.V. (2002) Phenethyl isothiocyanate-induced apoptosis in p53-deficient PC-3 human prostate cancer cell line is mediated by extracellular signal-regulated kinases. *Cancer Res.*, **62**, 3615–3619

Xu, K. & Thornalley, P.J. (2000a) Studies on the mechanism of the inhibition of human leukaemia cell growth by dietary isothiocyanates and their cysteine adducts *in vitro*. *Biochem. Pharmacol.*, **60**, 221–231

Xu, K. & Thornalley, P.J. (2000b) Antitumour activity of sphingoid base adducts of phenethyl isothiocyanate. *Bioorg. Med. Chem. Lett.*, **10**, 53–54

Xu, K. & Thornalley, P.J. (2001a) Involvement of glutathione metabolism in the cytotoxicity of the phenethyl isothiocyanate and its cysteine conjugate to human leukaemia cells *in vitro*. *Biochem. Pharmacol.*, **61**, 165–177

Xu, K. & Thornalley, P.J. (2001b) Signal transduction activated by the cancer chemopreventive isothiocyanates: Cleavage of BID protein, tyrosine phosphorylation and activation of JNK. *Br. J. Cancer*, **84**, 670–673

Xu, M., Bailey, A.C., Hernaez, J.F., Taoka, C.R., Schut, H.A. & Dashwood, R.H. (1996) Protection by green tea, black tea, and indole-3-carbinol against 2-amino-3-methylimidazo[4,5-*f*]quinoline-induced DNA adducts and colonic aberrant crypts in the F344 rat. *Carcinogenesis*, **17**, 1429–1434

Xu, M., Schut, H.A., Bjeldanes, L.F., Williams, D.E., Bailey, G.S. & Dashwood, R.H. (1997) Inhibition of 2-amino-3-methylimidazo[4,5-*f*]quinoline–DNA adducts by indole-3-carbinol: Dose–response studies in the rat colon. *Carcinogenesis*, **18**, 2149–2153

Xu, M., Orner, G.A., Bailey, G.S., Stoner, G.D., Horio, D.T. & Dashwood, R.H. (2001) Post-initiation effects of chlorophyllin and indole-3-carbinol in rats given 1,2-dimethylhydrazine or 2-amino-3-methylimidazo[4,5-*f*]quinoline. *Carcinogenesis*, **22**, 309–314

Xue, J.P., Lenman, M., Falk, A. & Rask, L. (1992) The glucosinolate-degrading enzyme myrosinase in Brassicaceae is encoded by a gene family. *Plant Mol. Biol.*, **27**, 911–922

Xue, J.P., Jorgensen, M., Pihlgren, U. & Rask, L. (1995) The myrosinase gene family in *Arabidopsis thaliana* gene organization, expression and evolution. *Plant Mol. Biol.*, **27**, 911-922

Yamaguchi, T. (1980) Mutagenicity of isothiocyanates, isocyanates and thioureas on *Salmonella typhimurium*. *Agric. Biol. Chem.*, **44**, 3017–3018

Yamashita, K., Wakabayashi, K., Kitagawa, Y., Nagao, M. & Sugimura, T. (1988) ^{32}P-Postlabeling analysis of DNA adducts in rat stomach with 1-nitrosoindole-3-acetonitrile, a direct-acting mutagenic indole compound formed by nitrosation. *Carcinogenesis*, **9**, 1905–1907

Yang, Y.M., Conaway, C.C., Chiao, J.W., Wang, C.X., Amin, S., Whysner, J., Dai, W.,

Reinhardt, J. & Chung, F.L. (2002) Inhibition of benzo(*a*)pyrene-induced lung tumorigenesis in A/J mice by dietary *N*-acetylcysteine conjugates of benzyl and phenethyl isothiocyanates during the postinitiation phase is associated with activation of mitogen-activated protein kinases and p53 activity and induction of apoptosis. *Cancer Res.*, **62**, 2–7

Yano, T., Yajima, S., Virgona, N., Yano, Y., Otani, S., Kumagai, H., Sakurai, H., Kishimoto, M. & Ichikawa, T. (2000) The effect of 6-methylthiohexyl isothiocyanate isolated from *Wasabia japonica* (wasabi) on 4-(methylnitrosamino)-1-(3-pyridyl)-1-butanone-induced lung tumorigenesis in mice. *Cancer Lett.*, **155**, 115–120

Ye, L. & Zhang, Y. (2001) Total intracellular accumulation levels of dietary isothiocyanates determine their activity in elevation of cellular glutathione and induction of Phase 2 detoxification enzymes. *Carcinogenesis*, **22**, 1987–1992

Ye, L., Dinkova-Kostova, A.T., Wade, K.L., Zhang, Y., Shapiro, T.A. & Talalay, P. (2002) Quantitative determination of dithiocarbamates in human plasma, serum, erythrocytes and urine: Pharmacokinetics of broccoli sprout isothiocyanates in humans. *Clin. Chim. Acta*, **316**, 43–53

Young, T.B. (1989) A case–control study of breast cancer and alcohol consumption habits. *Cancer*, **64**, 552–558

Young, T.B. & Wolf, D.A. (1988) Case–control study of proximal and distal colon cancer and diet in Wisconsin. *Int. J. Cancer*, **42**, 167–175

Yu, R., Jiao, J.J., Duh, J.L., Tan, T.H. & Kong, A.N. (1996) Phenethyl isothiocyanate, a natural chemopreventive agent, activates c-Jun N-terminal kinase 1. *Cancer Res.*, **56**, 2954–2959

Yu, R., Mandlekar, S., Harvey, K.J., Ucker, D.S. & Kong, A.N. (1998) Chemopreventive isothiocyanates induce apoptosis and caspase-3-like protease activity. *Cancer Res.*, **58**, 402–408

Yu, R., Lei, W., Mandlekar, S., Weber, M.J., Der, C.J., Wu, J. & Kong, A.T. (1999) Role of a mitogen-activated protein kinase pathway in the induction of phase II detoxifying enzymes by chemicals. *J. Biol. Chem.*, **274**, 27545–27552

Yu, R., Mandlekar, S., Lei, W., Fahl, W.E., Tan, T.H. & Kong, A.T. (2000) p38 mitogen-activated protein kinase negatively regulates the induction of phase II drug-metabolizing enzymes that detoxify carcinogens. *J. Biol. Chem.*, **275**, 2322–2327

Yuan, J.M., Gago-Dominguez, M., Castelao, J.E., Hankin, J.H., Ross, R.K. & Yu, M.C. (1998) Cruciferous vegetables in relation to renal cell carcinoma. *Int. J. Cancer*, **77**, 211–216

Yuan, F., Chen, D.Z., Liu, K., Sepkovic, D.W., Bradlow, H.L. & Auborn, K. (1999) Anti-estrogenic activities of indole-3-carbinol in cervical cells: Implication for prevention of cervical cancer. *Anticancer Res.*, **19**, 1673–1680

Zeligs, M.A., Fulfs, J.C., Peterson, R., Wilson, S.M., McIntyre, L., Sepkovic, D.W. & Bradlow, H.L. (2003) In vivo, uterine-protective activity of absorption-enhanced diindolylmethane: Animal and preliminary human use in combination with Tamoxifen. *Proc. Am. Assoc. Cancer Res.*, **44**, 1268

Zhang, Y. (2000) Role of glutathione in the accumulation of anticarcinogenic isothiocyanates and their glutathione conjugates by murine hepatoma cells. *Carcinogenesis*, **21**, 1175–1182

Zhang, Y. (2001) Molecular mechanism of rapid cellular accumulation of anticarcinogenic isothiocyanates. *Carcinogenesis*, **22**, 425–431

Zhang, Y. & Callaway, E.C. (2002) High cellular accumulation of sulphoraphane, a dietary anticarcinogen, is followed by rapid transporter-mediated export as a glutathione conjugate. *Biochem. J.*, **364**, 301–307

Zhang, X. & Malejka-Giganti, D. (2003) Effects of treatment of rats with indole-3-carbinol on apoptosis in the mammary gland and mammary adenocarcinomas. *Anticancer Res.*, **23**, 2473–2479

Zhang, Y. & Talalay, P. (1994) Anti-carcinogenic activities of organic isothiocyanates: Chemistry and mechanisms. *Cancer Res.*, **54**, 1976S–1981S

Zhang, Y. & Talalay, P. (1998) Mechanism of differential potencies of isothiocyanates as inducers of anticarcinogenic Phase 2 enzymes. *Cancer Res.*, **58**, 4632–4639

Zhang, Y., Cho, C.G., Posner, G.H. & Talalay, P. (1992a) Spectroscopic quantitation of organic isothiocyanates by cyclocondensation with vicinal dithiols. *Anal. Biochem.*, **205**, 100–107

Zhang, Y., Talalay, P., Cho, C.G. & Posner, G.H. (1992b) A major inducer of anticarcinogenic protective enzymes from broccoli: Isolation and elucidation of structure. *Proc. Natl Acad. Sci. USA*, **89**, 2399–2403

Zhang, Y., Kensler, T.W., Cho, C.G., Posner, G.H. & Talalay, P. (1994) Anticar-cinogenic activities of sulforaphane and structurally related synthetic norbornyl isothiocyanates. *Proc. Natl Acad. Sci. USA*, **91**, 3147–3150

Zhang, Y., Kolm, R.H., Mannervik, B. & Talalay, P. (1995) Reversible conjugation of isothiocyanates with glutathione catalyzed by human glutathione transferases. *Biochem. Biophys. Res. Commun*, **206**, 748–755

Zhang, Y., Wade, K.L., Prestera, T. & Talalay, P. (1996) Quantitative determination of isothiocyanates, dithiocarbamates, carbon disulfide, and related thiocarbonyl compounds by cyclocondensation with 1,2-benzenedithiol. *Anal. Biochem.*, **239**, 160–167

Zhang, S., Hunter, D.J., Forman, M.R., Rosner, B.A., Speizer, F.E., Colditz, G.A., Manson, J.E., Hankinson, S.E. & Willett, W.C. (1999) Dietary carotenoids and vitamins A, C, and E and risk of breast cancer. *J. Natl Cancer Inst.*, **91**, 547–556

Zhang, S.M., Hunter, D.J., Rosner, B.A., Giovannucci, E.L., Colditz, G.A., Speizer, F.E. & Willett, W.C. (2000) Intakes of fruits, vegetables, and related nutrients and the risk of non-Hodgkin's lymphoma among women. *Cancer Epidemiol. Biomarkers Prev.*, **9**, 477–485

Zhang, M., Yang, Z.Y., Binns, C.W. & Lee, A.H. (2002) Diet and ovarian cancer risk: A case–control study in China. *Br. J. Cancer*, **86**, 712–717

Zhang, J., Svehlikova, V., Bao, Y., Howie, A.F., Beckett, G.J. & Williamson, G. (2003) Synergy between sulforaphane and selenium in the induction of thioredoxin reductase 1 requires both transcriptional and translational modulation. *Carcinogenesis*, **24**, 497–503

Zhao, F.J., Evans, E.J., Bilsborrow, P.E. & Syers, J.K. (1994) Influence of nitrogen and sulfur on the glucosinolate profile of rapeseed (*Brassica napus* L.). *J. Sci. Food Agric.*, **64**, 295–304

Zhao, B., Seow, A., Lee, E.J., Poh, W.T., Teh, M., Eng, P., Wang, Y.T., Tan, W.C., Yu, M.C. & Lee, H.P. (2001) Dietary isothiocyanates, glutathione S-transferase-M1, -T1 polymorphisms and lung cancer risk among Chinese women in Singapore. *Cancer Epidemiol. Biomarkers Prev.*, **10**, 1063–1067

Zheng, G.Q., Kenney, P.M. & Lam, L.K. (1992) Phenylalkyl isothiocyanate–cysteine conjugates as glutathione S-transferase stimulating agents. *J. Med. Chem.*, **35**, 185–188

Zheng, W., Blot, W.J., Shu, X.O., Diamond, E.L., Gao, Y.T., Ji, B.T. & Fraumeni, J.F., Jr (1992a) Risk factors for oral and pharyngeal cancer in Shanghai, with emphasis on diet. *Cancer Epidemiol. Biomarkers Prev.*, **1**, 441–448

Zheng, W., Blot, W.J., Shu, X.O., Gao, Y.T., Ji, B.T., Ziegler, R.G. & Fraumeni, J.F., Jr (1992b) Diet and other risk factors for laryngeal cancer in Shanghai, China. *Am. J. Epidemiol.*, **136**, 178–191

Zheng, W., Shu, X.O., Ji, B.T. & Gao, Y.T. (1996) Diet and other risk factors for cancer of the salivary glands: A population-based case–control study. *Int. J. Cancer*, **67**, 194–198

Zhu, B.T. & Conney, A.H. (1998) Functional role of estrogen metabolism in target cells: Review and perspectives. *Carcinogenesis*, **19**, 1–27

Zhu, C.Y. & Loft, S. (2001) Effects of Brussels sprouts extracts on hydrogen peroxide-induced DNA strand breaks in human lymphocytes. *Food Chem. Toxicol.*, **39**, 1191–1197

Zhu, C.Y. & Loft, S. (2003) Effect of chemopreventive compounds from *Brassica* vegetables on NAD(P)H:quinone reductase and induction of DNA strand breaks in murine hepa1c1c7 cells. *Food Chem. Toxicol.*, **41**, 455–462

Zhu, C., Poulsen, H.E. & Loft, S. (2000) Inhibition of oxidative DNA damage in vitro by extracts of Brussels sprouts. *Free Radicals Res.*, **33**, 187–196

Appendix: Chemical and physical properties

Isothiocyanates

2-Propenyl (allyl) isothiocyanate

Chemical name: 3-isothiocyanato-1-propene

CAS: 57-06-7

Structure:

$$CH_2{=}CH{-}CH_2{-}CH_2{-}N{=}C{=}S$$

Composition: C_4H_5NS

Relative molecular mass: 99.2

Boiling-point: 148–154 °C

Partition coefficient: 2.3 (Jiao *et al.,* 1994; Zhang, 2001)

Comments: Lipophillic, highly volatile and very pungent

3-Methylsulfinylpropyl isothiocyanate (iberin)

Chemical name: 1-isothiocyanato-3 (methylsulfinyl)propane

CAS: 505-44-2

Structure:

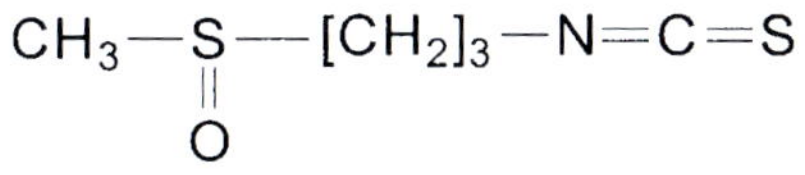

$$CH_3{-}\overset{\displaystyle}{\underset{\overset{\|}{O}}{S}}{-}[CH_2]_3{-}N{=}C{=}S$$

Composition: $C_5H_9NOS_2$

Relative molecular mass: 163.3

Comments: Water-soluble, non-volatile

4-Methylthiobutyl isothiocyanate (erucin)

Chemical name: 1-isothiocyanato-4-(methylthio)butane

CAS: 4430-36-8

Structure:

$$CH_3{-}S{-}[CH_2]_4{-}N{=}C{=}S$$

Composition: $C_6H_{11}NS_2$

Relative molecular mass: 161.3

Boiling-point: 136 °C

Comments: Volatile

4-Methylsulfinylbutyl isothiocyanate (sulforaphane)

Chemical name: 1-isothiocyanato-4-(methylsulfinyl)butane

CAS: 4478-93-7

Structure:

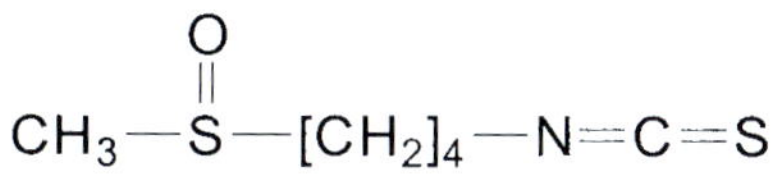

$$CH_3{-}\overset{\overset{\displaystyle O}{\|}}{S}{-}[CH_2]_4{-}N{=}C{=}S$$

Composition: $C_6H_{11}NOS_2$

Relative molecular mass: 177.3

Boiling-point: 125–135 °C

Partition coefficient: 0.45 (Zhang, 2001)

Comments: Water-soluble, non-volatile

Benzyl isothiocyanate

Chemical name: benzyl isothiocyanate

CAS: 622-78-6

Structure:

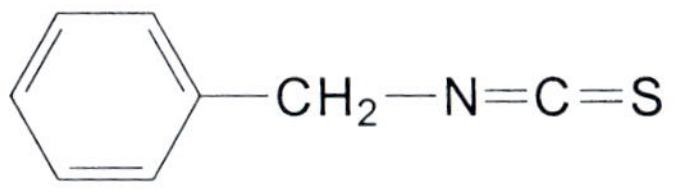

Composition: C_8H_7NS

Relative molecular mass: 149.2

Boiling-point: 242 °C

Partition coefficient: 3.0 (Jiao *et al.*, 1994; Zhang, 2001)

Comments: Lipophillic, partially volatile

2-Phenethyl isothiocyanate

Chemical name: 2-isothiocyanato-ethylbenzene

CAS: 2257-09-2

Structure:

Composition: C_9H_9NS

Relative molecular mass: 163.2

Boiling-point: 140 °C

Partition coefficient: 3.1 (Jiao *et al.*, 1994; Zhang, 2001)

Comments: Lipophillic, highly volatile

Indoles

Glucobrassicin

Chemical names: Indole-3-ylcarbinol glucosinolate; 3-indolylacet-thio-(*S*-β-glucopyranosido)hydroximyl-*O*-sulfate

CAS: 4356-52-9

Structure:

Composition: $C_{16}H_{20}N_2O_9S_2$

Relative molecular mass: 448.5

Melting-point: 148–150 °C (Gmelin & Virtanen, 1961; Hanley *et al.*, 1990)

Ultraviolet absorption spectra: (Gmelin & Virtanen, 1961; Agerbirk *et al.*, 1998)

Nuclear magnetic resonance spectra: (Hanley *et al.*, 1990; Agerbirk *et al.*, 1998)

Infrared absorption spectra: (Gmelin & Virtanen, 1961; Hanley *et al.*, 1990)

Mass spectrometry (m/z): (Hanley *et al.*, 1990)

Neoglucobrassicin

Chemical names: 1-methoxyindole-3-ylcarbinol glucosinolate; β-D-glucopyranose, 1-thio-,1-[1-methoxy-*N*-(sulfoxy)-1*H*-indole-3-ethanimidate]

CAS: 5187-84-8

Structure:

Composition: $C_{17}H_{22}N_2O_{10}S_2$

Relative molecular mass: 478.5

Melting-point: 158–162 °C (Hanley *et al.*, 1990)

Ultravioletabsorption spectra: (Agerbirk *et al.*, 1998)

Nuclear magnetic resonance spectra: (Hanley *et al.*, 1990; Agerbirk *et al.*, 1998)

Infrared absorption spectra: (Hanley *et al.*, 1990)

Mass spectrometry (m/z): (Hanley *et al.*, 1990)

Indole-3-carbinol

Chemical names: 1*H*-indole-3-methanol; 3-hydroxymethyl-indole; indol-3-ylmethanol

CAS: 700-06-1

Structure:

Composition: C_9H_9NO

Relative molecular mass: 147.2

Description: White crystals (Leete & Marion, 1953), colourless crystals (Styngach *et al.*, 1973)

Melting-point: 99–100 °C (Leete & Marion, 1953; Thesing, 1954; Silverstein *et al.*, 1954; Ames *et al.*, 1956; Henry & Leete, 1957; Styngach *et al.*, 1973; Le Borgne *et al.*, 1997)

Ultraviolet absorption spectra: (Leete & Marion, 1953; (Mendez, 1970; Goyal *et al.*, 2001)

Nuclear magnetic resonance spectra: (Hinman & Lang, 1965; Burton *et al.*, 1986; Hwu *et al.*, 1996; Le Borgne *et al.*, 1997)

Infrared absorption spectra: (Leete & Marion, 1953; Styngach *et al.*, 1973; Hwu *et al.*, 1996; Le Borgne *et al.*, 1997)

Mass spectrometry: (m/z): (Hwu *et al.*, 1996; Prinsen *et al.*, 1997; Delonga *et al.*, 2001)

Stability: Unstable in hot alkali and sensitive to acids (Leete & Marion, 1953)

N-Methoxyindole-3-carbinol

Chemical names: 1-methoxyindole-3-methanol; 1*H*-indole-3-methanol

CAS: 110139-35-0

Structure:

Composition: $C_{10}H_{11}NO_2$

Relative molecular mass: 177.2

Melting-point: 92–94 °C (0.1 Torr) (Hanley *et al.*, 1990)

Solubility: Sparingly soluble

Nuclear magnetic resonance spectra: (Hanley *et al.*, 1990; Stephensen *et al.*, 2000)

Infrared absorption spectra: (Hanley *et al.*, 1990)

Mass spectrometry (m/z): (Hanley *et al.*, 1990)

Ascorbigen

Chemical name: 2-*C*-(1*H*-indol-3-ylmethyl)-β-L-lyxo-3-hexulofuranosonic acid g-lactone

CAS: 8075-98-7

Structure:

Composition: $C_{15}H_{15}NO_6$

Relative molecular mass: 305.3

Nuclear magnetic resonance spectra: (Agerbirk *et al.*, 1998)

Infrared absorption spectra: (Gmelin & Virtanen, 1961)

Mass spectrometry (m/z): (Agerbirk *et al.*, 1998)

Stability: 90% present in acidic medium (pH < 1, 37 °C) after 3 h, whereas only 15% present after 3 days (Yudina *et al.*, 2000a)

3,3´-Diindolylmethane

Chemical name: 3,3´-diindolylmethane

CAS: 1968-05-4

Structure:

Composition: $C_{17}H_{14}N_2$

Relative molecular mass: 246.3

Description: White to off-white crystal

Melting-point: 164–165 °C (Leete & Marion, 1953; Thesing, 1954)

Ultraviolet absorption spectra: (Leete & Marion, 1953)

Nuclear magnetic resonance spectra: (Grose & Bjeldanes, 1992)

Infrared absorption spectra: (Leete & Marion, 1953)

Mass spectrometry (m/z): (Grose & Bjeldanes, 1992)

Indolo[3,2-*b*]carbazole

Chemical name: 6,12-diaza-indeno[1,2-*b*]fluorene

CAS: 241-55-4

Structure:

Composition: $C_{18}H_{10}N_2$

Relative molecular mass: 254.3

Ultraviolet absorption spectra: (Robinson, 1963; Hünig & Steinmetzer, 1976)

Nuclear magnetic resonance spectra: (Hünig & Steinmetzer, 1976; Yudina *et al.*, 2000b)

Mass spectrometry (m/z): (Gardner *et al.*, 1957; Hünig & Steinmetzer, 1976)

References

Agerbirk, N., Olsen, C. E. & Sørensen, H. (1998) Initial and final products, nitriles, and ascorbigens produced in myrosinase-catalyzed hydrolysis of indole glucosinolates. *J. Agric. Food Chem.*, **46**, 1563–1571

Ames, D.E., Bowman, R.E., Evans, D.D. & Jones, W.A. (1956) The synthesis of some indolylalkylamines. *J. Chem. Soc.*, 1984–1989

Burton, G., Ghini, A.A. & Gros, E.G. (1986) Carbon-13 NMR spectra of substituted indoles. *Magn. Reson. Chem.* **24**, 829–831

Delonga, K., Smit, Z., Dragovic-Uzelac, V., Mrkic, V. & Vorkapic-Furac, J. (2001) Hydrolysis products of glucosinolates from white cabbage (*Brassica oleracea* L. var capitata) and cauliflower (*Brassica oleracea* L. var. botrytis) analyzed by HPLC and GC/MS. In: Pfannhauser, W., Fenwick, G.R. & Khokhar S., eds, *Biologically Active Phytochemicals in Food*, London, Royal Society of Chemistry, pp. 213–216

Gardner, P.D., Haynes, G.R. & Brandon, R.L. (1957) Formation of Dieckmann reaction products under acyloin conditions. Competition of the two reactions. *J. Org. Chem.*, **22**, 1206–1210

Gmelin, R. & Virtanen, A.I. (1961) Glucobrassicin, the precursor of the thiocyanate ion, 3-acetonitrile, and ascorbigen in *Brassica oleracea* (and related) species. *Ann. Acad. Sci. Fenn.* A II, 1–25

Goyal, R.N., Kumar, A. & Gupta, P. (2001) Oxidation chemistry of indole-3-methanol. *J. Chem. Soc. Perkin Trans.*, 2, 618–623

Grose, K.R. & Bjeldanes, L.F. (1992) Oligomerization of indole-3-carbinol in aqueous acid. *Chem. Res. Toxicol.*, **5**, 188–193

Hanley, A. B., Parsley, K. R., Lewis, J. A. & Fenwick, G. R. (1990) Chemistry of indole glucosinolates: Intermediacy of indole-3-ylmethyl isothiocyanates in the enzymatic hydrolysis of indole glucosinolates. J. *Chem. Soc. Perkin Trans.* 1, 2273–2276

Henry, D.W. & Leete, E. (1957) Amine oxides. 1. Gramine oxide. *J. Am. Chem. Soc.*, **79**, 5254–5256

Hinman, R.L. & Lang, J. (1965) Peroxidase-catalyzed oxidation of indole-3-acetic acid. *Biochemistry*, **4**, 144–158

Hünig, S. Steinmetzer, H.C. (1976) [Two step redox systems. XXIII. Fused nitrogen heterocycles]. *Justus Liebigs Ann. Chem.*, 1090–1102 (in German)

Hwu, J.R., Wein, Y.S. & Leu, Y.J. (1996) Calcium metal in liquid ammonia for selective reduction of organic compounds. *J. Org. Chem.*, **61**, 1493–1499

Jiao, D., Ho, C.T., Foiles, P. & Chung, F.L. (1994) Identification and quantification of the N-acetylcysteine conjugate of allyl isothiocyanate in human urine after ingestion of mustard. *Cancer Epidemiol. Biomarkers Prev.*, **3**, 487–492

Le Borgne, M., Marchand, P., Duflos, M., Delevoye-Seiller, B., Piessard-Robert, S., Le Baut, G., Hartmann, R.W. & Palzer, M. (1997) Synthesis and in vitro evaluation of 3-(1-azolylmethyl)-1H-indoles and 3-(1-azolyl-1-phenylmethyl)-1H-indoles as inhibitors of P450 arom. *Arch. Pharm.*, **330**, 141–145

Leete, E. & Marion, L. (1953) The hydrogenolysis of 3-hydroxymethylindole and other indole derivatives with lithium aluminium hydride. *Can. J. Chem.*, **31**, 775–784

Mendez, J. (1970) Ultraviolet spectral study of indoles. *Microchem. J.*, **15**, 1–5

Prinsen, E., Van Dongen, W., Esmans, E.L. & Van Onckelen, H.A. (1997) HPLC linked electrospray tandem mass spectrometry: A rapid and reliable method to analyse indole-3-acetic acid metabolism in bacteria. *J. Mass Spectrom.*, **32**, 12–22

Robinson, B. (1963) The Fischer indolisation of cyclohexane-1,4-dione bis-phenyl-hydrazone. *J. Chem. Soc.*, 3097–3099

Silverstein, R.M., Ryskiewicz, E.E. & Chaikin, S.W. (1954) 2-Pyrrolealdehyde, 3-hydroxymethylindole and 2-hydroxymethylpyrrole. *J. Am. Chem. Soc.*, **76**, 4485–4486

Stephensen, P.U., Bonnesen, C., Schaldach, C., Andersen, O., Bjeldanes, L. F. & Vang, O. (2000) *N*-Methoxyindole-3-carbinol is a more efficient inducer of cytochrome P-450 1A1 in cultured cells than indol-3-carbinol. *Nutr. Cancer*, **36**, 112–121

Styngach, E.P., Kuchkova, K.I., Efremova, T.M. & Semenov, A.A. (1973) Carbolines. 6. Study of synthesis of 4-hetaryl-beta-carbolines. *Khim. Geterotsikl. Soedin.*, 1523–1527

Thesing, J. (1954) [Chemistry of indoles. 3. Action of alkali on quaternary salts in gramine]. *Chem. Ber./Rec.*, **87**, 692–699 (in German)

Yudina, L.N., Korolev, A.M., Reznikova, M.I. & Preobrazhenskaya, M.N. (2000a) Investigation of neoascorbigen. *Khim. Geterotsikl. Soedin.*, **36**, 144–151

Yudina, L.N., Preobrazhenskaya, M.N. & Korolev, A.M. (2000b) Transformation of 5H,11H-indolo[3,2-b]carbazole via 5,11-didehydroindolo[3,2-b]carbazole. *Khim. Geterotsikl. Soedin.*, **36**, 1275–1277

Zhang, Y. (2001) Molecular mechanism of rapid cellular accumulation of anticarcinogenic isothiocyanates. *Carcinogenesis*, **22**, 425–431

Abbreviations

AC	aberrant crypts	EPIC	European Prospective Investigation into Cancer and Nutrition
ACF	aberrant crypt foci	ER	estrogen receptor
Akt	serine–threonine protein kinase	ERE	estrogen response element
AFAR	aflatoxin B_1 aldehyde reductase	ETS	environmental tobacco smoke
AFB_1	aflatoxin B_1		
Ah	aryl hydrocarbon	F	female
AKR	aldo–keto reductase	F_1	first filial generation
AOM	azoxymethane	FAA	N-2-fluorenylacetamide
ARE	antioxidant response element	FFQ	food frequency questionnaire
AT	N-acetyltransferase	FMO	flavin-related monooxygenase
ATF	activating transcription factor		
AUC	area under the time–plasma concentration curve	GADD	growth arrest in response to DNA damage
		GCL	glutamate cysteine ligase
B[a]P	benzo[a]pyrene	GCLC	glutamate cysteine ligase catalytic
BBN	N-butyl-N-(4-hydroxybutyl)nitrosamine	GCS	γ-glutamylcysteine synthetase
BOP	N-nitrosobis(2-oxopropyl)amine	GGT	γ-glutamyl transferase
BPDE	7,8-dihydroxy-9,10-epoxy-7,8,9,10-tetrahydrobenzo[a]pyrene	GSH	glutathione
		GSSG	reduced glutathione
BROD	benzyloxyresorufin-O-dealkylase	GST	glutathione S-transferase
bw	body weight	GST-P	glutathione S-transferase placental form
bZIP	cap 'n' collar basic region leucine zipper [transcription factor]		
		HPLC	high-performance liquid chromatography
		HPV	human papillomavirus
CARET	β-carotene and retinol efficacy trial		
CAT	chloramphenicol acetyltransferase	I3C	indole-3-carbinol
CC	case–control study	i.p.	intraperitoneally
CDK	cyclin-dependent kinase	IQ	2-amino-3-methylimidazo[4,5-f]quinoline
CG	cysteinylglycinase	ITC	isothiocyanate
CI	confidence interval	i.v.	intravenously
COX	cyclo-oxygenase		
CT	5,6,11,12,17,18-hexahydrocyclononal-[1,2-b:4,5-b':7,8-b'']triindole	LD_{50}	median lethal dose
		LTr1	2-(indol-3-ylmethyl)-3,3′-diindolyl methane
CYP	cytochrome P450		
		M	men or male
DHPN	dihydroxydi-N-propylnitrosamine	MAM	methylalkylthiomalate
DIM	3,3′-diindolylmethane	MAP	M-associated protein
DMABP	3′,2′-dimethyl-4-aminobiphenyl	MeIQx	2-amino-3,8-dimethylimidazo[4,5-f]quinoxaline
DMBA	7,12-dimethylbenz[a]anthracene		
DMH	1,2-dimethylhydrazine	Min	multiple intestinal neoplasia
		MNNG	N-methyl-N′-nitro-N-nitrosoguanidine
EROD	ethoxyresorufin O-dealkylase	MNU	N-methyl-N-nitrosourea
EGF	epithelial growth factor	MROD	methoxyresorufin-O-dealkylase
EGFR	epithelial growth factor receptor		
EMSA	electrophoretic mobility-shift analysis		

MRP	multidrug-resistance-associated protein
NAC	*N*-acetylcysteine
NDEA	*N*-nitrosodiethylamine
NDMA	*N*-nitrosodimethylamine
NF-IL6	nuclear factor–interleukin 6
NIFOX	nifedipine oxidation
NMBA	*N*-nitrosomethylbenzylamine
NNAL	4-(methylnitrosamino)-1-(3-pyridyl)-1-butanol
NNK	4-(methylnitrosamino)-1-(3-pyridyl)-1-butanone
NQO1	NAD(P)H:quinone oxidoreductase
NR	not reported
Nrf2	nuclear factor–erythroid 2 p45-related factor 2
NSAID	non-steroidal anti-inflammatory drug
ODC	ornithine decarboxylase
OR	odds ratio
8-oxodG	8-oxo-7,8-dihydro-2´-deoxyguanosine
PCNA	proliferating cell nuclear antigen
PhIP	2-amino-1-methyl-6-phenylimidazo[4,5-*b*]pyridine
PI3K	phosphatidyl inositol 3-kinase
PROD	pentoxyresorufin *O*-dealkylase

PSA	prostate-specific antigen
PTEN	phosphatase and tensin homologue deleted on chromosome 10
Rb	retinoblastoma
RR	relative risk
S9 mix	$9000 \times g$ supernatant of rodent liver
s.c.	subcutaneously
TBRM	total binding of radioactive material
TCDD	2,3,7,8-tetrachloro-*para*-dibenzodioxin
TGF	transforming growth factor
TPA	12-*O*-tetradecanoylphorbol 13-acetate
TRAIL	tumour necrosis factor-related apoptosis-inducing ligand
UGT	UDP-glucuronosyl transferase
v/v	volume per volume
W	women
w/w	weight per weight
XRE	xenobiotic response element

Working Procedures for the *IARC Handbooks of Cancer Prevention*

The prevention of cancer is one of the key objectives of the International Agency for Research on Cancer (IARC). This may be achieved by avoiding exposures to known cancer-causing agents, by increasing host defences through immunization or chemoprevention or by modifying lifestyle. The aim of the series of *IARC Handbooks of Cancer Prevention* is to evaluate scientific information on agents and interventions that may reduce the incidence of or mortality from cancer.

Scope

Cancer-preventive strategies embrace chemical, immunological, dietary and behavioural interventions that may retard, block or reverse carcinogenic processes or reduce underlying risk factors. The term 'chemoprevention' is used to refer to interventions with pharmaceuticals, vitamins, minerals and other chemicals to reduce cancer incidence. The *IARC Handbooks* address the efficacy, safety and mechanisms of cancer-preventive strategies and the adequacy of the available data, including those on timing, dose, duration and indications for use.

Preventive strategies can be applied across a continuum of: (1) the general population; (2) subgroups with particular predisposing host or environmental risk factors, including genetic susceptibility to cancer; (3) persons with precancerous lesions; and (4) cancer patients at risk for second primary tumours. Use of the same strategies or agents in the treatment of cancer patients to control the growth, metastasis and recurrence of tumours is considered to be patient management, not prevention, although data from clinical trials may be relevant when making a *Handbook* evaluation.

Objective

The objective of the *Handbooks* programme is the preparation of critical reviews and evaluations of evidence for cancer-prevention and other relevant properties of a wide range of potential cancer-preventive agents and strategies by international working groups of experts. The resulting Handbooks may also indicate when additional research is needed.

The *Handbooks* may assist national and international authorities in devising programmes of health promotion and cancer prevention and in making benefit–risk assessments. The evaluations of IARC working groups are scientific judgements about the available evidence for cancer-preventive efficacy and safety. No recommendation is given with regard to national and international regulation or legislation, which are the responsibility of individual governments and/or other international authorities.

Working Groups

Reviews and evaluations are formulated by international working groups of experts convened by the IARC. The tasks of each group are: (1) to ascertain that all appropriate data have been collected; (2) to select the data relevant for the evaluation on the basis of scientific merit; (3) to prepare accurate summaries of the data to enable the reader to follow the reasoning of the Working Group; (4) to evaluate the significance of the available data from human studies and experimental models on cancer-preventive activity, and other beneficial effects and also on adverse effects; and (5) to evaluate data relevant to the understanding of the mechanisms of preventive activity.

Approximately 13 months before a working group meets, the topics of the *Handbook* are announced, and participants are selected by IARC staff in consultation with other experts. Subsequently, relevant clinical, experimental and human data are collected by the IARC from all available sources of published information. Representatives of producer or consumer associations may assist in the preparation of sections on production and use, as appropriate.

Working Group participants who contributed to the considerations and evaluations within a particular *Handbook* are listed, with their addresses, at the beginning of each publication. Each participant serves as an individual scientist and not as a representative of any organization, government or industry. In addition, scientists nominated by national and international agencies, industrial associations and consumer and/or environmental organizations may be invited as observers. IARC staff involved in the preparation of the *Handbooks* are listed.

About eight months before the meeting, the material collected is sent to meeting participants to prepare sections for the first drafts of the *Handbooks*. These are then compiled by IARC staff and sent, before the meeting, to all participants of the Working Group for review. There is an opportunity to return the compiled specialized sections of the draft to the experts, inviting preliminary comments, before the complete first-draft document is distributed to all members of the Working Group.

Data for Handbooks

The *Handbooks* do not necessarily cite all of the literature on the agent or strategy being evaluated. Only those data considered by the Working Group to be relevant to making the evaluation are included. In principle, meeting abstracts and other reports that do not provide sufficient detail upon which to base an assessment of their quality are not considered.

With regard to data from toxicological, epidemiological and experimental studies and from clinical trials, only reports that have been published or accepted for publication in the openly available scientific literature are reviewed by the Working Group. In certain instances, government agency reports that have undergone peer review and are widely available are considered. Exceptions may be made on an ad-hoc basis to include unpublished reports that are in their final form and publicly available, if their inclusion is considered pertinent to making a final evaluation. In the sections on chemical and physical properties, on production, on use, on analysis and on human exposure, unpublished sources of information may be used.

The available studies are summarized by the Working Group. In general, numerical findings are indicated as they appear in the original report; units are converted when necessary for easier comparison. The Working Goup may conduct additional analyses of the published data and use them in their assessment of the evidence. Important aspects of a study, directly impinging on its interpretation, are brought to the attention of the reader.

Criteria for selection of topics for evaluation

Agents, classes of agents and interventions to be evaluated in the *Handbooks* are selected on the basis of one or more of the following criteria.

- The available evidence suggests potential for significantly reducing the incidence of cancers.
- There is a substantial body of human, experimental, clinical and/or mechanistic data suitable for evaluation.
- The agent is in widespread use and of putative protective value, but of uncertain efficacy and safety.
- The agent shows exceptional promise in experimental studies but has not been used in humans.
- The agent is available for further studies of human use.

Evaluation of cancer-preventive agents

A wide range of findings must be taken into account before a particular agent can be recognized as preventing cancer and a systematized approach to data presentation has been adopted for *Handbook* evaluations.

Characteristics of the agent or intervention

Chemical identity and other definitive information (such as genus and species of plants) are given as appropriate. Data relevant to identification, occurrence and biological activity are included. Technical products of chemicals, including trade names, relevant specifications and information on composition and impurities are mentioned. Preventive interventions can be broad, community based interventions, or interventions targeted to individuals (counselling, behavioural, chemopreventive).

Occurrence, trends, analysis
Occurrence
Information on the occurrence of an agent in the environment is obtained from monitoring and surveillance in occupational environments, air, water, soil, foods and animal and human tissues. When available, data on the generation, persistence and bioaccumulation of the agent are included. For interventions, data on prevalence are supplied. The data on the prevalence of a factor (e.g., overweight) in different populations are collected as widely as possible.

Production and use
The dates of first synthesis and of first commercial production of a chemical or mixture are provided, the dates of first reported occurrence. In addition, methods of synthesis used in past and present commercial production and methods of production that may give rise to various impurities are described. For interventions, the dates of first mention of their use are given.

Data on the production, international trade and uses and applications of agents are obtained for representative regions. In the case of drugs, mention of their therapeutic applications does not necessarily represent current practice, nor does it imply judgement as to their therapeutic efficacy.

If an agent is used as a prescribed or over-the-counter pharmaceutical product, then the type of person receiving the product in terms of health status, age, sex and medical condition being treated are described. For non-pharmaceutical agents, particularly those taken because of cultural traditions, the characteristics of use or exposure and the relevant populations are described. In all cases, quantitative data, such as dose–response relationships, are considered to be of special importance.

Metabolism of and metabolic responses to the agent or metabolic consequences of an intervention

In evaluating the potential utility of a suspected cancer-preventive agent or strategy, a number of different properties, in addition to direct effects upon cancer incidence, are described and weighed. Furthermore, as many of the data leading to an evaluation are expected to come from studies in experimental animals, information that facilitates interspecies extrapolation is particularly important; this includes metabolic, kinetic and genetic data. Whenever possible, quantitative data, including information on dose, duration and potency, are considered.

Information is given on absorption, distribution (including placental transfer), metabolism and excretion in humans and experimental animals. Kinetic properties within the target species may affect the interpretation and extrapolation of dose–response relationships, such as blood concentrations, protein binding, tissue concentrations, plasma half-lives and elimination rates. Comparative information on the relationship between use or exposure and the dose that reaches the target site may be of particular importance for extrapolation between species. Studies that indicate the metabolic pathways and fate of an agent in humans and experimental animals are summarized, and data on humans and experimental animals are compared when possible. Observations are made on inter-individual vari-

ations and relevant metabolic polymorphisms. Data indicating long-term accumulation in human tissues are included. Physiologically based pharmacokinetic models and their parameter values are relevant and are included whenever they are available. Information on the fate of the compound within tissues and cells (transport, role of cellular receptors, compartmentalization, binding to macromolecules) is given.

The metabolic consequences of interventions are described.

Genotyping will be used increasingly, not only to identify subpopulations at increased or decreased risk for cancers but also to characterize variation in the biotransformation of and responses to cancer-preventive agents. This subsection can include effects of the compound on gene expression, enzyme induction or inhibition, or prooxidant status, when such data are not described elsewhere. It covers data obtained in humans and experimental animals, with particular attention to effects of long-term use and exposure.

Cancer-preventive effects
Human studies
Types of study considered

Human data are derived from experimental and non-experimental study designs and are focused on cancer, precancer or intermediate biological end-points. The experimental designs include randomized controlled trials and short-term experimental studies; non-experimental designs include cohort, case–control and cross-sectional studies.

Cohort and case–control studies relate individual use of, or exposure to, the agent or invervention under study to the occurrence of cancer in individuals and provide an estimate of relative risk (ratio of incidence or mortality in those exposed to incidence or mortality in those not exposed) as the main measure of association. Cohort

and case–control studies follow an observational approach, in which the use of, or exposure to, the agent is not controlled by the investigator.

Intervention studies are experimental in design — that is, the use of, or exposure to, the agent or intervention is assigned by the investigator. The intervention study or clinical trial is the design that can provide the strongest and most direct evidence of a protective or preventive effect; however, for practical and ethical reasons, such studies are limited to observation of the effects among specifically defined study subjects of interventions of 10 years or fewer, which is relatively short when compared with the overall lifespan.

Intervention studies may be undertaken in individuals or communities and may or may not involve randomization to use or exposure. The differences between these designs is important in relation to analytical methods and interpretation of findings.

In addition, information can be obtained from reports of correlation (ecological) studies and case series; however, limitations inherent in these approaches usually mean that such studies carry limited weight in the evaluation of a preventive effect.

Quality of studies considered

The *Handbooks* are not intended to summarize all published studies. The Working Group consider the following aspects: (1) the relevance of the study; (2) the appropriateness of the design and analysis to the question being asked; (3) the adequacy and completeness of the presentation of the data; and (4) the degree to which chance, bias and confounding may have affected the results.

Studies that are judged to be inadequate or irrelevant to the evaluation are generally omitted. They may be mentioned briefly, particularly when the information is considered to be a useful supplement to that in other reports or when it provides the only data available. Their inclusion does not imply acceptance of the adequacy of the study design, nor of the analysis and interpretation of the results, and their limitations are outlined.

Assessment of the cancer-preventive effect at different doses and durations
The Working Group gives special attention to quantitative assessment of the preventive effect of the agent under study, by assessing data from studies at different doses. The Working Group also addresses issues of timing and duration of use or exposure. Such quantitative assessment is important to clarify the circumstances under which a preventive effect can be achieved, as well as the dose at which a toxic effect has been shown.

Criteria for a cancer-preventive effect
After summarizing and assessing the individual studies, the Working Group makes a judgement concerning the evidence that the agent or intervention in question prevents cancer in humans. In making their judgement, the Working Group considers several criteria for each relevant cancer site.

Evidence of protection derived from intervention studies of good quality is particularly informative. Evidence of a substantial and significant reduction in risk, including a 'dose'–response relationship, is more likely to indicate a real effect. Nevertheless, a small effect, or an effect without a dose–response relationship, does not imply lack of real benefit and may be important for public health if the cancer is common.

Evidence is frequently available from different types of study and is evaluated as a whole. Findings that are replicated in several studies of the same design or using different approaches are more likely to provide evidence of a true protective effect than isolated observations from single studies.

The Working Group evaluates possible explanations for inconsistencies across studies, including differences in use of, or exposure to, the agent, differences in the underlying risk of cancer and metabolism and genetic differences in the population.

The results of studies judged to be of high quality are given more weight. Note is taken of both the applicability of preventive action to several cancers and of possible differences in activity, including contradictory findings, across cancer sites.

Data from human studies (as well as from experimental models) that suggest plausible mechanisms for a cancer-preventive effect are important in assessing the overall evidence.

The Working Group may also determine whether, on aggregate, the evidence from human studies is consistent with a lack of preventive effect.

Experimental models

Experimental animals
Animal models are an important component of research into cancer prevention. They provide a means of identifying effective compounds, of carrying out fundamental investigations into their mechanisms of action, of determining how they can be used optimally, of evaluating toxicity and, ultimately, of providing an information base for developing intervention trials in humans. Models that permit evaluation of the effects of cancer-preventive agents on the occurrence of cancer in most major organ sites are available. Major groups of animal models include: those in which cancer is produced by the administration of chemical or physical carcinogens; those involving genetically engineered animals; and those in which tumours develop spontaneously. Most cancer-preventive agents investigated in such studies can be placed into one of three categories: compounds that prevent molecules from reaching or reacting with critical target sites (blocking agents); compounds that decrease the sensitivity of target tissues to carcinogenic stimuli; and compounds that prevent evolution of the neoplastic process (suppressing agents). There is increasing interest in the use of combinations of agents as a means of improving efficacy and minimizing toxicity. Animal models are useful in evaluating such combinations. The development of optimal strategies for human intervention trials can be facilitated by the use of animal models that mimic the neoplastic process in humans.

Specific factors to be considered in such experiments are: (1) the temporal requirements of administration of the cancer-preventive agents; (2) dose–response effects; (3) the site-specificity of cancer-preventive activity; and (4) the number and structural diversity of carcinogens whose activity can be reduced by the agent being evaluated.

An important variable in the evaluation of the cancer-preventive response is the time and the duration of administration of the agent or intervention in relation to any carcinogenic treatment, or in transgenic or other experimental models in which no carcinogen is administered. Furthermore, concurrent administration of a cancer-preventive agent may result in a decreased incidence of tumours in a given organ and an increase in another organ of the same animal. Thus, in these experiments it is important that multiple organs be examined.

For all these studies, the nature and extent of impurities or contaminants present in the cancer-preventive agent or agents being evaluated are given when available. For experimental studies of mixtures, consideration is given to the possibility of changes in the physicochemical properties of the test substance during collection, storage, extraction, concentration and delivery. Chemical and toxicological interactions of the components of mixtures may result in nonlinear dose–response relationships.

As certain components of commonly used diets of experimental animals are themselves known to have cancer-preventive activity, particular consideration should be given to the interaction between the diet and the apparent effect of the agent or intervention being studied. Likewise, restriction of diet may be important. The appropriateness of the diet given relative to the composition of human diets may be commented on by the Working Group.

Qualitative aspects. An assessment of the experimental prevention of cancer involves several considerations of qualitative importance, including: (1) the experimental conditions under which the test was performed (route and schedule of exposure, species, strain, sex and age of animals studied, duration of the exposure, and duration of the study); (2) the consistency of the results, for example across species and target organ(s); (3) the stage or stages of the neoplastic process, from preneoplastic lesions and benign tumours to malignant neoplasms, studied and (4) the possible role of modifying factors.

Considerations of importance to the Working Group in the interpretation and evaluation of a particular study include: (1) how clearly the agent was defined and, in the case of mixtures, how adequately the sample composition was reported; (2) the composition of the diet and the stability of the agent in the diet; (3) whether the source, strain and quality of the animals was reported; (4) whether the dose and schedule of treatment with the known carcinogen were appropriate in assays of combined treatment; (5) whether

the doses of the cancer-preventive agent were adequately monitored; (6) whether the agent(s) was absorbed, as shown by blood concentrations; (7) whether the survival of treated animals was similar to that of controls; (8) whether the body and organ weights of treated animals were similar to those of controls; (9) whether there were adequate numbers of animals, of appropriate age, per group; (10) whether animals of each sex were used, if appropriate; (11) whether animals were allocated randomly to groups; (12) whether appropriate respective controls were used; (13) whether the duration of the experiment was adequate; (14) whether there was adequate statistical analysis; and (15) whether the data were adequately reported. If available, recent data on the incidence of specific tumours in historical controls, as well as in concurrent controls, are taken into account in the evaluation of tumour response.

Quantitative aspects. The probability that tumours will occur may depend on the species, sex, strain and age of the animals, the dose of carcinogen (if any), the dose of the agent and the route and duration of exposure. A decreased incidence and/or decreased multiplicity of neoplasms in adequately designed studies provides evidence of a cancer-preventive effect. A dose-related decrease in incidence and/or multiplicity further strengthens this association.

Statistical analysis. Major factors considered in the statistical analysis by the Working Group include the adequacy of the data for each treatment group: (1) the initial and final effective numbers of animals studied and the survival rate; (2) body weights; and (3) tumour incidence and multiplicity. The statistical methods used should be clearly stated and should be the generally accepted techniques refined for

this purpose. In particular, the statistical methods should be appropriate for the characteristics of the expected data distribution and should account for interactions in multifactorial studies. Consideration is given as to whether the appropriate adjustment was made for differences in survival.

In-vitro models
Cell systems *in vitro* contribute to the early identification of potential cancer-preventive agents and to elucidation of mechanisms of cancer prevention. A number of assays in prokaryotic and eukaryotic systems are used for this purpose. Evaluation of the results of such assays includes consideration of: (1) the nature of the cell type used; (2) whether primary cell cultures or cell lines (tumorigenic or nontumorigenic) were studied; (3) the appropriateness of controls; (4) whether toxic effects were considered in the outcome; (5) whether the data were appropriately summated and analysed; (6) whether appropriate quality controls were used; (7) whether appropriate concentration ranges were used; (8) whether adequate numbers of independent measurements were made per group; and (9) the relevance of the end-points, including inhibition of mutagenesis, morphological transformation, anchorage-independent growth, cell– cell communication, calcium tolerance and differentiation.

Intermediate biomarkers
Other types of study include experiments in which the end-point is not cancer but a defined preneoplastic lesion or tumour-related, intermediate biomarker.

The observation of effects on the occurrence of lesions presumed to be preneoplastic or the emergence of benign or malignant tumours may aid in assessing the mode of action of the presumed cancer-preventive agent or intervention. Particular attention is given to assessing the reversibility of these lesions and their predictive value in relation to cancer development.

Mechanisms of cancer prevention

Data on mechanisms can be derived from both human studies and experimental models. For a rational implementation of cancer-preventive measures, it is essential not only to assess protective end-points but also to understand the mechanisms by which the agents or interventions exert their anticarcinogenic action. Information on the mechanisms of cancer-preventive activity can be inferred from relationships between chemical structure and biological activity, from analysis of interactions between agents and specific molecular targets, from studies of specific end-points in vitro, from studies of the inhibition of tumorigenesis in vivo, from the effects of modulating intermediate biomarkers, and from human studies. Therefore, the Working Group takes account of data on mechanisms in making the final evaluation of cancer prevention.

Several classifications of mechanisms have been proposed, as have several systems for evaluating them. Cancer-preventive agents may act at several distinct levels. Their action may be: (1) extracellular, for example, inhibiting the uptake or endogenous formation of carcinogens, or forming complexes with, diluting and/or deactivating carcinogens; (2) intracellular, for example, trapping carcinogens in non-target cells, modifying transmembrane transport, modulating metabolism, blocking reactive molecules, inhibiting cell replication or modulating gene expression or DNA metabolism; or (3) at the level of the cell, tissue or organism, for example, affecting cell differentiation, intercellular communication, proteases, signal trans-duction, growth factors, cell adhesion molecules, angiogenesis, interactions with the extracellular matrix, hormonal status and the immune system.

Many cancer-preventive agents are known or suspected to act by several mechanisms, which may operate in a coordinated manner and allow them a broader spectrum of anticarcinogenic activity. Therefore, multiple mechanisms of action are taken into account in the evaluation of cancer-prevention.

Beneficial interactions, generally resulting from exposure to inhibitors that work through complementary mechanisms, are exploited in combined cancer-prevention. Because organisms are naturally exposed not only to mixtures of carcinogenic agents but also to mixtures of protective agents, it is also important to understand the mechanisms of interactions between inhibitors.

Other beneficial effects

An expanded description is given, when appropriate, of the efficacy of the agent in the maintenance of a normal healthy state and the treatment of particular diseases. Information on the mechanisms involved in these activities is described. Reviews, rather than individual studies, may be cited as references.

The physiological functions of agents such as vitamins and micronutrients can be described briefly, with reference to reviews. Data on the therapeutic effects of drugs approved for clinical use are summarized.

Toxic effects

Toxic effects are of particular importance in the case of agents or interventions that may be used widely over long periods in healthy populations. Data are given on acute and chronic toxic effects, such as organ toxicity, increased cell proliferation, immunotoxicity and adverse endocrine effects. Some agents or interventions may have both carcinogenic and anticarcinogenic activities. If the agent has been evaluated within the *IARC Monographs on the Evaluation of Carcinogenic Risks to Humans*, that evaluation is accepted, unless significant new data have appeared that may lead the Working Group to reconsider the evidence. If the agent occurs naturally or has been in clinical use previously, the doses and durations used in cancer-prevention trials are compared with intakes from the diet, in the case of vitamins, and previous clinical exposure, in the case of drugs already approved for human use. When extensive data are available, only summaries are presented; if adequate reviews are available, reference may be made to these. If there are no relevant reviews, the evaluation is made on the basis of the same criteria as are applied to epidemiological studies of cancer. Differences in response as a consequence of species, sex, age and genetic variability are presented when the information is available.

Data demonstrating the presence or absence of adverse effects in humans are included; equally, lack of data on specific adverse effects is stated clearly.

Information is given on carcinogenicity, immunotoxicity, neurotoxicity, cardiotoxicity, haematological effects and toxicity to other target organs. Specific case reports in humans and any previous clinical data are noted. Other biochemical effects thought to be relevant to adverse effects are mentioned.

The results of studies of genetic and related effects in mammalian and nonmammalian systems in vivo and in vitro are summarized. Information on whether DNA damage occurs via direct interaction with the agent or via indirect mechanisms (e.g. generation of free radicals) is included, as is information on other genetic effects such as mutation, recombination, chromosomal damage, aneuploidy, cell immortalization and transformation, and effects on cell–cell communication. The presence and toxicological significance of cellular receptors for the cancer-preventive agent are described.

Structure–activity relationships that may be relevant to the evaluation of the toxicity of an agent are described.

Summary of data

In this section, the relevant human and experimental data are summarized. Inadequate studies are generally not included but are identified in the preceding text.

Evaluation

Evaluations of the strength of the evidence for cancer-preventive activity and carcinogenic effects from studies in humans and experimental models are made, using standard terms. These terms may also be applied to other beneficial and adverse effects, when indicated. When appropriate, reference is made to specific organs and populations.

It is recognized that the criteria for these evaluation categories, described below, cannot encompass all factors that may be relevant to an evaluation of cancer-preventive activity. In considering all the relevant scientific data, the Working Group may assign the agent or intervention to a higher or lower category than a strict interpretation of these criteria would indicate.

Cancer-preventive activity

The evaluation categories refer to the strength of the evidence that an agent or intervention prevents cancer. The evaluations may change as new information becomes available.

Evaluations are inevitably limited to the cancer sites, conditions and levels of exposure and length of observation covered by the available studies. An evaluation of degree of evidence, whether for an agent or inter-

vention, is limited to the materials tested, as defined physically, chemically or biologically, or to the intensity of frequency of an intervention. When agents are considered by the Working Group to be sufficiently closely related, they may be grouped for the purpose of a single evaluation of degree of evidence.

Information on mechanisms of action is taken into account when evaluating the strength of evidence in humans and in experimental animals, as well as in assessing the consistency of results between studies in humans and experimental models.

Cancer-preventive activity in humans

The evidence relevant to cancer prevention in humans is classified into one of the following categories.

- *Sufficient evidence of cancer-preventive activity*

The Working Group considers that a causal relationship has been established between use of the agent or intervention and the prevention of human cancer in studies in which chance, bias and confounding could be ruled out with reasonable confidence.

- *Limited evidence of cancer-preventive activity*

The data suggest a reduced risk for cancer with use of the agent or intervention but are limited for making a definitive evaluation either because chance, bias or confounding could not be ruled out with reasonable confidence or because the data are restricted to intermediary biomarkers of uncertain validity in the putative pathway to cancer.

- *Inadequate evidence of cancer-preventive activity*

The available studies are of insufficient quality, consistency or statistical

power to permit a conclusion regarding a cancer-preventive effect of the agent or intervention, or no data on the prevention of cancer in humans are available.

- *Evidence suggesting lack of cancer-preventive activity*

Several adequate studies of use pr or exposure to the agent or intervention are mutually consistent in not showing a preventive effect.

The strength of the evidence for any carcinogenic effect is assessed in parallel.

Both cancer-preventive activity and carcinogenic effects are identified and, when appropriate, tabulated by organ site. The evaluation also cites the population subgroups concerned, specifying age, sex, genetic or environmental predisposing risk factors and the relevance of precancerous lesions.

Cancer-preventive activity in experimental animals

Evidence for cancer prevention in experimental animals is classified into one of the following categories.

- *Sufficient evidence of cancer-preventive activity*

The Working Group considers that a causal relationship has been established between the agent and a decreased incidence and/or multiplicity of neoplasms.

- *Limited evidence of cancer-preventive activity*

The data suggest a cancer-preventive effect but are limited for making a definitive evaluation because, for example, the evidence of cancer prevention is restricted to a single experiment, the agent decreases the incidence and/or multiplicity only of benign neoplasms or lesions of uncertain neoplastic potential or there is conflicting evidence.

- *Inadequate evidence of cancer-preventive activity*

The studies cannot be interpreted as showing either the presence or absence of a preventive effect because of major or quantitative limitations (unresolved questions regarding the adequacy of the design, conduct or interpretation of the study), or no data on cancer prevention in experimental animals are available.

- *Evidence suggesting lack of cancer-preventive activity*

Adequate evidence from conclusive studies in several models shows that, within the limits of the tests used, the agent does not prevent cancer.

Overall evaluation

Finally, the body of evidence is considered as a whole, and summary statements are made that encompass the effects of the agents in humans with regard to cancer-preventive activity, carcinogenic effects and other beneficial and adverse effects, as appropriate.

Recommendations

During the evaluation process, it is likely that opportunities for further research will be identified. These are clearly stated, with the understanding that the areas are recommended for future investigation. It is made clear that these research opportunities are identified in general terms on the basis of the data currently available.

Recommendations for public health action are listed, based on the analysis of the existing scientific data.